Immune Restoration Handbook

2nd Edition

December, 2004

ISBN: 1-887831-08-8

Copyright, 2004
Keep Hope Alive, Ltd
Library of Congress
All Rights Reserved

(First Edition printed March, 2003)

Published in the United States by:
Keep Hope Alive
PO Box 270041
West Allis, WI 53227
Voice mail – 414-545-6539
Internet: www.keephopealive.org

All profits from the sale of this book are donated or used for non-profit (charitable, educational or scientific) purposes

TABLE OF CONTENTS

Foreword i
Chapter 1 The Immune System 1
Chapter 2 Selenium in the prevention & treatment of chronic illness 15
Chapter 3 The Immune System Cure for Candidiasis 31
Chapter 4 The Role of HHV-6 in AIDS, CFIDS and Candidiasis 37
Chapter 5 Immune Response in AIDS and CFIDS 44
Chapter 6 Diagnostics – Monitoring Immune Health 48
Chapter 7 Balance your pH 53
Chapter 8 Adrenal Cortisol helps restore and balance immunity 60
Chapter 9 Thyroid function, body temperature and immunity 85
Chapter 10 Free Radicals and Anti-oxidants 98
Chapter 11 Detoxification of the Liver and Colon 105
Chapter 12 Good and Bad Immune profiles 119
Chapter 13 How to heal a leaky gut and implant friendly flora 122
Chapter 14 Complementary therapies from Africa & America 129
Chapter 15 Immune-based therapies 151
Chapter 16 Chronic Fatigue Syndrome, CFIDS and FM 174
Chapter 17 Pharmaceutical drugs to treat HIV 185
Chapter 18 Osteoporosis and bone mineral density 193
Chapter 19 Bio-Oxidative Therapies 197
Chapter 20 Nutrition for immunity and weight gain 209
Chapter 21 Immune Enhancement Diet 221
Chapter 22 Symptoms and Remedies 235
Chapter 23 Cancer – Complementary and Alternative therapies 261
Chapter 24 Prayers, Promises and Miracles 274
Appendix 281
Index 284

Foreword

It was a very fortunate day in 2001 when someone lead me to the Keep Hope Alive website. Consequently I struck up an email friendship with Mark and began to delve deep into the vast amount of material he has gathered together over the years. In Kenya, where AIDS is rampant, some of the biggest obstacles we face - as over all of Africa - is the tremendous poverty, ignorance and stigma connected to AIDS. People do not know how to treat themselves and they lack courage and the money to get help.

In my work in Kenya, we have used the information of the IRH to its best advantage for the poor. Through the Kenyan publication of IRH information (Great Health, Naturally!), now thousands of Kenyans and Africans have learned how to restore their immune system and keep it up at the lowest possible cost. Korogocho is one of the poorest squatter slums of Nairobi. Here people have no water, no sewage system, no electricity. Whole families live in one-room huts made of mud, sticks, iron sheets and cardboard. Yet it is here that the IRH book having a tremendous impact.

Sixty PLWHA clients of the Medical Mission Sisters home-based care project, in third and fourth stages of HIV, were put on a simple regimen added to their usual medications. This humble regimen is what the project could afford to give their clients. Within the first month, 75% of those clients gained weight and within the next 3 months virtually ALL experienced better appetite, better sleep, recovered energy, weight gain and a reduction of various symptoms including diarrhea, coughs, vomiting, skin rashes, etc. The information in IRH is invaluable in the global fight against AIDS. As you read this book you will find that you can deal with your body with fewer drugs and more in line with Nature and Her laws.

Mark, bless you for your work and keep it up.
Didi Ananda Ruchira Director,
Abha Light Foundation, Kenya November 22 2004

Immune Restoration Handbook (IRH) the 2nd edition is the culmination of 15 years of grass-roots research, personal experience, searching thousands of past and present medical and health journals as well as testing and feedback from readers that have resulted from the efforts of Mark Konlee and Conrad LeBeau to find and keep alive the eternal flame of hope for safe and effective remedies for those who suffer from life-long chronic illness and immune dysfunction.

The first edition of Immune Restoration Handbook published in March 2003. The first edition was a major revision from 8 previous editions of *How to Reverse Immune Dysfunction*, the last edition of which was published in May of 2000. Previous to that there were 6 editions of another book he wrote titled "Aids Control Diet" that was first published in May of 1990. Mark Konlee also publishes the *Journal of Immunity* that is preceded by earlier newsletters, *Progressive Health News* and *Positive Health News*.

The authors' interest in health began in 1986, when after a period of prolonged stress, he was beset with deteriorating personal health problems including food allergies, hypothyroidism, hypoglycemia, digestive disorders, insomnia, fatigue, candidiasis and depression.

"It took two years before I emerged from a series of unending challenges to my health" and added: *"the essential elements to my recovery were the diet plan outlined in this book along with weekly colonics, raw vegetable juices and lots of prayer."*

Mark states: *"I would not wish on anyone such a prolonged period of misery, yet I know on this planet, there are millions who endure the daily torment of chronic illness and pain. It is my avowed purpose in writing this book to lead others on a path to recovery from conditions of ill health that their own physicians are often at a loss to diagnose and treat."*

This second edition has expanded information on the evolving role of Adrenal and Thyroid hormones in the balance and functional activity of the immune system. The facts presented here and the concepts that have evolved are no longer solely from the arena of immunology, but now include of necessity endocrinology – the science of the secretions of hormones by glands and how they inter-react with the immune system. So inter-related are the thyroid and adrenal hormones and chemical messengers of the immune system that without restoring normal adrenal and thyroid function, an immune system that functions optimally is not possible. This concept was neither understood nor appreciated as little as three years ago. Special mention and credit goes to Marty Zucker and Alfred Plechner DVM for their lifelong research on the connection between certain hormones and immune function and their impressive record of using these concepts and discoveries to successfully treat over 35000 pets in the past 30 years.

As a resource, **Immune Restoration Handbook** is a handy reference guide of self-help information for building and maintaining personal health. Over the years thousands of people have called or written to thank us the practical self-help that has changed and improved their lives and is now is your hands. We thank you for these kind words and hope that everyone will benefit from the use of these materials.

Enjoy.

Mark Konlee   *Conrad LeBeau*

by Ron Klatz MD:

"As a non-medical person, Mark Konlee has amassed an incredible amount of knowledge and understanding about human health, based on his very personal and often difficult medical experiences where he truly acted as his own and best patient advocate. IRH is the culmination of Mark's keen insights into the human condition, his compassionate and analytical mind and those "broad shoulders" that have shared the toils of others who have experienced similar health issues. These qualities make Mark an exemplary innovator who is truly interested in the well being of those around him. Marks' gift to all of us is the Immune Restoration Handbook that is richly endowed with new insights on immune function and self-help protocols that get you the medical attention you need – especially when you have exhausted all "conventional" options and it's time to "think outside the box."

Dr. *Ron Klatz* President – American Academy of Anti-Aging Medicine (A4M; www.worldhealth.net): Author, Infection Protection: How to Fight Germs That Make You Sick (Harper Collins, 2002)

1

The immune system

Louis Pasteur (1822-1895) is credited with discovering the "germ" theory of disease (1). Pasteur believed that most diseases were caused by airborne microbes that invaded the body. This theory has become the base on which "modern medicine" is established. New and stronger antibiotics are designed to "kill" the invading microbe, whether it be a virus, parasite, fungus or pathogenic bacteria. The treatments often work for their limited purpose, but then frequently leave the immune system in a weakened state.

Antoine Bechamp (1816-1908), a French professor, believed in the existence of "germs" but disputed that germs or "microbes" alone were the cause of disease. Bechamp believed that it takes the right conditions inside a person for disease to develop. Bechamp's view was that if the host has a weak defense (immune system) and other conditions favorable for the infection to take root, that it would. Are infections alone the cause of disease or are they opportunistic, invading the host whose immune defenses are weak or out of balance?

Two garden plots – health vs. disease

Bechamp's theory can be compared to two garden plots. In both garden plots are planted a mixture of seeds of grain and weeds. In one garden plot, the weeds grow and the grain doesn't, although the seeds of the grain are in the soil. In the other garden plot, the grain grows and the weeds do not, even though the soil has in it the seeds of the weeds. The garden plot that has only weeds growing in it is called "sick" while the other garden plot that has only grain growing is called "healthy." The only difference between the "healthy" garden plot and the "sick" garden plot is the soil, since they both contained the same seeds.

The theory of Bechamp makes good sense. In applying the analogy to humans, we see that two persons may be exposed to the same germs, virus or microbes – one gets sick while the other remains well. In many kinds of infectious diseases, we see this pattern consistently. The integrity of the skin and mucus membranes and mucosal immunity is often the dividing line between health and illness.

Dr. Alan Cantwell, Jr., M.D., summed up his feelings, and our feelings, about Bechamp and Pasteur in his book, "The Cancer Microbe" (1) when he wrote:

"My study of Bechamp had shattered the icon of Pasteur. The chemist made germs respectable and he was a genius at popularizing microbes as a cause of human disease. He gave the world "pasteurization," a monumental achievement. But he also put science on the wrong track. Pasteur's dogma transformed the art and science of medicine into a multibillion dollar biotechnical business in search of the perfect pill and a perfect vaccine to cure man of all his ills....In the process the physicians were blinded."

What is the immune system?

The "immune system" is the "Armed Forces" of our body. It is comprised primarily of white blood cells, that circulate alongside red blood cells, to defend us against infections, inflammations, cancer and foreign proteins. White blood cells (WBCs) do so by distinguishing self from non-self. Think of the white blood cells that circulate in your veins and arteries like Pac-men on a video machine. They circulate through the blood vessels and lymph system and eat things that don't belong there. Like red blood cells, the white blood cells originate in the bone marrow from stem cells. Stem cells divide and replenish our supply of red and white blood cells. An army of white blood cells is divided into about 130 subsets (T cells and B cells, neutrophils, monocytes, macrophages, Natural Killer cells, etc). These cells comprise most of what we call "the immune system." Components of the immune system have either the inherited ability or learned ability to distinguish what is part of our body from what is foreign (self vs. non-self).

Humoral immunity (antibody response)

The immune response that attacks infections outside of the cells is called "Humoral immunity." It is an antibody response (TH2) and involves interactions between B cells and CD4 helper cells in the lymph nodes. Dendritic cells and macrophages are sentry immune cells that pick up viruses and other foreign antigens and present them to the CD4 cells in the lymph nodes. The CD4 cells decide if and what type of immune response will be undertaken. If an antibody response is needed, the CD4 cells signal certain B cells to produce antibodies that tag viruses and bacteria for destruction by other immune cells. Once the infection is eliminated, certain cells retain memory about the invader and can mount a quick antibody reaction, if the invader returns. These white blood cells are called "memory cells." Persons who have these memory immune cells are said to be "immunized" against that particular infection. Vaccines that protect us against certain viruses create memory immune cells for those particular infections.

Cell-mediated immunity (CMI)

When a CD4 cell signals a Cell-Mediated Immune (CMI) response (TH1), it may signal a CD8 cytotoxic lymphocyte (CTL) to destroy a virus-infected cell or a cancer cell. CMI responses destroy infections inside the cells or destroy the infected cell, as well as cancer cells. Infections inside the cells are more effectively neutralized with a CMI response than with an antibody response. These include all the herpes family of viruses, cytomegalovirus, Epstein barr virus, HIV, cancer and most other chronic persistent intracellular infections (inside the cells).

Many kinds of infections stimulate chemical messengers and immune reactions that are not effective against the inherent infection. Candida albicans promote IL-6, a TH2 cytokine that will not promote an effective response against fungal infections. On the other hand, the Rhino-virus that causes the common cold will promote an IL-2 increase, a TH1 cytokine that is helpful in fighting cancer and intracellular infections, but not the common cold. Thus, people who get a good cold at least once a year are unlikely to ever get cancer, and people who are prone to get cancer never catch a cold or the flu.

The immune system – activated or anergic?

An Activated Immune System is like a fighting army that searches out and destroys what is foreign to the host (viruses, fungus, mycoplasmas, bacteria and cancer). The induction of a fever is one indication of an activated immune system. Skin tests can measure either Anergy or Activation called DCH (Delayed Cutaneous Hypersensitivity) by challenging the immune system with skin pricks and inserting a small amount of foreign proteins from dead viruses and bacteria (Candida, Diphtheria, Tetanus, TB etc). When non-specific effector cells cause a red welt to appear where the skin was pricked, it is considered an indication of an immune response. The bigger the welt, the stronger will be the immune response. An Activated immune system is said to be "functional."

In contrast, persons who do not respond to a skin test for Anergy or DCH are said to be Anergic. This also applies to persons who receive an organ transplant and are administered immunosuppressive drugs to prevent their immune system from rejecting the transplanted organ. When the immune system responds slowly or not at all, it is said to be "anergic," and the condition is called "Anergy." When the immune system is anergic, chronic infections, including candidiasis and cancer, can persist for months or even years. Chronic low body temperature and the inability to generate a fever are related to the condition of Anergy.

White blood cells

White blood cells (WBC), as a whole, comprise nearly all the immune cells in our body. WBCs are divided into three general categories: The first group linked to Humoral Immunity are the B cells. Some B cells mature into Plasma cells that produce antibodies. In herpes viral infections, the antibody response fails to neutralize the viral infections. Antibody or humoral immune responses are primarily effective against infections outside the cells, such as the common cold or the flu. Since HHV-6, herpes 1 and 2, Cytomegalovirus (CMV) and Epstein Barr virus (EBV) are all in the herpes family, the antibody response fails to get rid of the infection. HIV infection and Candida Albicans are also intracellular infections and get inside the cells.

The second group is linked to Cell Mediated Immunity (CMI) and comprises the T cells and other white blood cells with which they interact. These include the T cells subsets such as CD4 (Helper or inflammatory), the CD8 (Suppressor or Killer-T cells), neutrophils and macrophages. CD8 Killer T cells are very effective against herpes infections, and even cancer cells.

Neutrophils, free macrophages and Natural Killer (NK) cells are known as non-specific effecter cells, as they can independently eat infectious agent. Natural Killer (NK) cells, if they are functional, attack and destroy cancer cells and other foreign antigens. NK cells have an innate knowledge of what to attack or leave alone. NK cells are truly independent and do not need to consult with the CD4 helper T cells before taking out a target. Neutrophils and free macrophages can also eat infectious organisms without requiring a signal from the CD4 Helper cells.

Types of Immune responses

There are three major components of the immune system and they all inter-react. They are mucosal immunity, Humoral immunity and Cell-mediated immunity. Mucosal immunity is the foundation of a balanced and normal functioning immune system. The failure of mucosal immunity is frequently a direct cause of the humoral arm of the immune system becoming over active and the cell-mediated arm becoming anergic and non-responsive. The TH1 vs. TH2 arms of the immune system are on opposite ends of a teeter-totter. When one goes up the other goes down and vice versa. The integrity of the mucus membranes of the gastrointestinal tract is a must for the two arms of the immune system to be in balance. When mucosal immunity fails, it drives up the TH2 arm or antibody production (humoral immunity) that then suppresses the TH1 Arm.

Mucosal immunity

Mucosal Immunity, by its name, suggests it involves the mucus membranes. Mucus membranes line the nostrils, sinuses, lungs and the entire gastrointestinal tract from the mouth to the anus at the end of the colon (lower intestines). Having healthy mucus membranes is the foundation of mucosal immunity. During digestion, CD4 helper cells and other white blood cells line the gastrointestinal tract to survey the byproducts of digestion. If the byproducts are not of the size and shape that the body can use, the immune cells block, or try to block, their entry into the blood stream.

The immune cells (white blood cells) also try to stop foreign antigens (viruses, fungus, bacteria etc.) from entering the blood stream. Sixty to 80% of our immune cells are in the gastrointestinal tract during the digestive process. It is through the digestive tract primarily that new infectious diseases enter the body. Other ports of entry for new infections are the lungs, for air born diseases, and breaks in the skin (cuts, scratches, burns etc.). Our outer skin is designed to resist most infections from outside our body. The mucus membranes are our "inner skin," designed to protect us from infections entering through the gastrointestinal tract.

The mucus membranes of the gastrointestinal tract are vulnerable, as they are the ports-of-entry of nutrients, resulting from the digestion of food. They can also be the ports of entry for viruses, fungus, bacteria and other foreign antigens, when there is a failure of mucosal immunity, as in a condition known as "leaky gut syndrome."

Leaky gut syndrome linked to food allergies, Histamine and Acid-reflux

There are multiple causes in the development of food allergies. One is "leaky gut syndrome," a condition where the intestinal wall is compromised with tiny pinholes that allow partially digested particles to enter the blood stream. When this happens it promotes an antibody response against the particles (usually foreign proteins) or an increase in histamine production, or both. Food allergies, by stimulating histamine production, are a direct cause of acid reflux syndrome. This is because an allergic reaction to food causes an inflammatory reaction — an increase in histamine production that, in turn, is a powerful inducer of hydrochloric acid production in the stomach.

Based on the amount of anti-acids and histamine blockers being advertised and sold, there must be millions of people with acid-reflux syndrome, all of whom have underlying food allergies and leaky gut syndrome, although most have never been told of this associated condition. There is a chain of events that leads to food allergies and a chronically acid stomach, and it is this:

Failure of mucosal immunity is caused by a long-term absence of friendly flora and butyrate

Any combination of the following, when used over a long period of time, will lead to damage of the mucosal lining of the gastrointestinal tract: antibiotics, steroids, salt, MSG, hard liquor, foods deep fried or cooked at high temperatures, refined carbohydrates (white bread, pasta, candy, white sugar, corn syrup etc) food preservatives (found in all lunch meats — ham, salami etc, in cheese, diet drinks and soda and many other processed foods). There is an absence of fiber in the diet — whole grains, sprouted seeds, raw nuts, fresh fruits and vegetables, boiled or simmered high quality proteins, like fish, legumes, organic grass-fed beef and poultry. Eating foods with preservatives daily is like eating antibiotics each day. Sooner or later, they will destroy or suppress the growth of friendly flora in the intestines.

IL-12 & IgA for Mucosal Immunity (IgE linked to allergies) L-Plantarum for IL-12 - B-Longum for IgA

Il-12 stimulates a CD8 Killer T cell response. The Killer T cells (cytotoxic lymphocytes) in the mucus membrane stop viral invasions before they get inside the cells. The skin outside the body and the mucus membranes inside are nature's protective envelope to keep out unwanted pathogens. An open cut and/or a leaky gut with small pinholes in it is like a fortress with an open door. The enemy (viruses, fungus bacteria, parasites, etc) have an easy access to get inside. Restoring normal Immunoglobulin type A (IgA) in the mucus membranes is also critical to help reduce excessive IgE (linked to food and chemical allergies) and to restoring mucosal immunity. Research has indicated that B Longum, a type of bifido bacteria increases IgA levels in the mucus membranes

Seven Researchers from Japan, Murosaki S et al, report in the July, 1998 Journal of Allergy and Clinical Immunology (1) that "Heat-killed Lactobacillus plantarum L-137 suppresses naturally fed antigen-specific IgE production by stimulation of IL-12 production in mice." They report that L. Plantarum directly increased Il-12 and IFN-gamma in mice in vitro in peritoneal macrophages and spleen cells. They report that production of IgE against dietary antigens is a common cause of food allergies, and that L plantarum, by increasing IL-12, suppresses IgE production. They obtained these effects with heat-killed L plantarum.

They also found that IgE can be suppressed by directly giving IL-12 to mice. They also report that giving L plantarum to mice in vivo (in the living mouse) increased plasma levels of IL-12 and that Il-4 (a Th2 cytokine) was suppressed. Their research found that L plantarum increased IL-12 production in mice in both vitro and vivo (in the lab and in the mouse). They concluded that L-plantarum is "a potent inducer of IL-12 and is useful for the prevention and treatment of food allergy."

1. Murosaki S et al; J. Allergy Clin Immunol 1998 Jul;102(1):57-64

The role of food preservatives and salt

Table salt, (sodium chloride), considered to be a safe flavor enhancer, is not so safe at all, when used in excess. Salt is a food preservative, and for thousands of years before the discovery of electricity and refrigerators, was used to preserve meats. The meats were packed in pure salt or in a brine of salt and water. If you want to see for yourself how salt prevents the growth of bacteria and all other forms of life, go to the Middle East to a place called the Dead Sea.

It is called the "Dead Sea" because it contains no life, no fish, no algae, and no bacteria - nothing. What is in the Dead Sea that is hostile to all life forms? The answer: Salt and lots of it - so much, in fact, that you cannot drown in the Dead Sea. You will just float in this brine. It is not a healthy place to stay in this water for any length of time. Plain and simple, salt is a poison, when used as it is used today, on and in every kind of processed food.

Excess salt stresses the kidneys, adrenals, contributes to insulin resistance, high blood sugar, diabetes, obesity, high blood pressure and suppresses the growth of friendly flora. Add regular food preservatives to salt in food and include only refined carbohydrates in the diet, you end up, eventually, with a wide range of gastrointestinal problems, ranging from food allergies to acid reflux to ulcers to ulcerated bowels to colitis to candidiasis, indigestion, stomach gas, aches and pains and even cancer of the stomach, small or large intestines. Salt, food preservatives, hard liquor (but not beer), and refined carbohydrates, all contribute to an internal environment that is hostile to the growth of friendly flora. Researchers and most physicians know that when butyrate levels in the stools are low, a person is more likely to develop colon cancer. Butyrate is produced by bifido bacteria and promotes a healthy intestinal mucosal lining.

Friendly flora produce butyrate, acetic and lactic acid. Butyric acid is required to promote the growth of the epithelial lining of the intestines and an intestinal lubricant called "mucin" that helps prevent and heal a leaky gut. The presence of mucin acts like a lubricant to move food through the intestines and prevent constipation. Fiber and other forms of indigestible carbohydrates are fuel that supports the growth of the friendly flora, that in turn produce butyrate which prevents leaky gut syndrome and the resulting food allergies and eventual acid-reflux syndrome, not to mention colon cancer.

Thus we see a step-by-step process from a flawed diet to a failure of mucosal immunity and eventual illnesses and an imbalanced immune system that promotes the TH2 arm (Humoral immunity) to excess. Vitamin A, carotenoids, silica and selenium from whole food sources (fish liver oil, carrots, horsetail herb and high-selenium mustard greens or yeast) support a healthy intestinal tract and mucus membranes. There is no evidence that synthetic forms of these nutrients (cheaply made amino acid chelates and synthesized vitamins etc), which are sold as dietary supplements, have the same benefits for the consumer as natural plant-based nutrients. Supplements in pill form, unless derived exclusively from whole food sources, should usually be avoided.

Humoral immunity (TH2)

Persons with poor mucosal immunity usually have an overgrowth of yeast and Candida Albicans in the intestines. They will also often develop allergies to chemicals and environmental factors. Leaky gut syndrome (LGS) is an underlying cause of excess antibody production, and thus an overactive humoral immunity. Health conditions associated with a failure of mucosal immunity and an excess of TH2 cytokine production, include autism, food allergies, candidiasis, chronic fatigue syndrome, ulcers, crohns, multiple chemical sensitivities, Lyme, hepatitis, high blood pressure, AIDS and cancer. LGS is not considered to be the sole contributing factor but a contributing factor, in most of these conditions.

The humoral (B cells) try to quickly wipe out the invading enemy. The inflammatory responses include fevers and the massive production of new B cells. Some B cells evolve into Plasma cells that produce the antibodies. The B cells are like foot soldiers that tag enemies for future destruction. Once the virus is tagged with an antibody, the CD4 cells signal other immune cells (macrophages, monocytes and neutrophils) to come in and devour them. In AIDS, CFIDS, HHV-6A infection, inflammatory immune responses result in swollen lymph nodes and unfortunately, an ineffective immune response to the infection. The antibody response alone fails to neutralize the infection.

Humoral immunity involves certain chemical messengers (cytokines) and a group of white blood cells called B cells, that mature into Plasma cells and produce antibodies. CD4 cells of the TH2 type control the B cells. Antibodies bind with viruses and other pathogens that live outside of the cells and tag them for destruction by other types of white blood cells. Persons with strong humoral immunity rarely get the common cold or the flu. Humoral immunity targets infections outside of the cells. Cytokines that support humoral immunity are Interleukin 4, 5, 6 and 10, and are known as TH2 type cytokines.

Getting a good nights sleep is important to keep the immune system in balance and prevent an overactive humoral immunity. Persons with chronic insomnia will have elevated IL-6 levels the following day. IL-6 is an exclusive TH2 cytokine, whereas IL-10 has cross-regulatory roles that involve TH1 cytokines as well. IL-6 levels are predominantly elevated in persons with overactive humoral (TH2) immune systems. When humoral immunity is over-active, Cell Mediated Immunity (CMI) is underactive and suppressed – the teeter-totter effect.

Cell-mediated immunity (CMI)

TH1 cytokines that support CMI and mucosal immunity include Interleuken 12 (IL-12), gamma interferon (IFN-gamma) and Immunoglobulin type A (IgA). Friendly intestinal flora (acidophilus and bifido bacteria) support mucosal immunity by producing butyrate and other short chain fatty acids that rebuild the mucus membranes of the intestines. Diets high in fiber support the growth of the friendly flora. Researchers have found that B Longum is one strain of friendly flora that increases mucosal IgA levels, while L. Plantarum increases IL-12 and IFN-gamma levels.

Cell-Mediated Immunity (CMI) targets infections inside the cells and involves a group of white blood cells known as CD8 Cytotoxic Lymphocytes (CTLs) and also the Natural Killer (NK) cells. The CD8 CTLs are under the influence of CD4 cells of the TH1 type.

Persons with weak CMI are susceptible to cancer and a wide range of infections inside the cells (mycoplasmas, herpes, HHV-6, HIV, hepatitis, CMV, EBV etc.). Persons with strong CMI have natural immunity from cancer and can reduce infections inside cells to a level where they are free of symptoms. Occasionally, persons with exceptionally good CMI eradicate some types of viruses completely. Cytokines that support CMI are IL-12, IL-2 and IFN-gamma. IL-12 and IFN-gamma also support mucosal immunity. These cytokines are known as the TH1- type. (TH refers to T Helper (CD4) cells. TH1 means T cell Helper Type 1, while TH2 means T cell Helper Type 2. The "Type" refers to whether they produce TH1 or TH2 type cytokines).

CD4 Helper cells work with all types of white blood cells in the immune system and can be either of the TH1 type or the TH2 type. The immune response to a challenge can be either TH1 or TH2 or both. When both kinds of responses become active, the TH1 response usually follows the TH2 (antibody) response. Some research points to the intracellular levels of Glutathione as a controlling factor in determining whether the immune response is TH2 or TH1. When Glutathione levels are low, the immune response is of the antibody type (TH2). When levels of Glutathione in the immune cells are high, the response is TH1 (CMI). Apart from this, the Natural Killer cells work independently of any influence from the CD4 Helper cells.

In restoring mucosal immunity, CMI and Natural Killer cell function is critical in an immune-based therapy for Cancer, CFIDS, Candidiasis and AIDS. Just as you cannot restore CMI, unless you first restore mucosal immunity, rebuilding the mucus membranes of the intestinal tract is the foundation of any program to successfully restore a normal and balanced immune system.

L-Glutathione – reduces viral replication

Glutathione is important for the immune system for three reasons: (1) Cells use Glutathione to remove heavy metals and other toxins; (2) Glutathione is a powerful antioxidant. (3) intracellular Glutathione helps individual cells process antigen. The processing and presenting of viral antigen on the cell surface stimulates a Th1 CD8 cytotoxic lymphocyte response to kill virus-infected cells.

There is a significant amount of published research on the anti-oxidant L-Glutathione. J.D. Adams et al, writing in J. Med. 1993;24 (6):337-52 states that Glutathione (GSH) "is essential for lymphocyte proliferation and inhibits HIV replication."

In an article published in Cell Immunol. 1991 Nov.; 138 (1) 229-37 H. Gmunder and W Droge state that "Depletion of intracellular GSH (Glutathione)....decreases the proportion of CD8+ cells (i.e. increases the CD4/CD8 ratio) ...and inhibits ....cytotoxic T lymphocyte (CTL) activity." He adds: "The results of these studies suggest that the decreased intracellular GSH levels in HIV-1 seropositive persons are probably not (directly) responsible for the selective depletion of the CD4+ T cell subset but may be responsible for a cellular dysfunction of the CD8+ subset and for the ultimate failure of the CTL to control the viral infection in these patients."

In plain English, Gmunder is saying that low levels of Glutathione in the cells not only decreases the total CD8 counts, but decrease the functioning of the CD8 Cytotoxic T cells, that is, their ability to control the viral infections by killing the virus-infected cells. Research also shows that increasing Glutathione levels reduces Tumor Necrosis Factor (TNF)(1). High TNF levels have been linked to wasting syndrome and increased viral replication.

An immune response requires antigen presentation

An effective immune response in AIDS, Chronic Fatigue Immune Dysfunction Syndrome (CFIDS), Gulf War Syndrome (GWS), chronic candidiasis, Epstein barr virus (EBV), other persistent chronic infections, and possibly even cancer, begins with restoring the ability of the individual cell to process and present foreign antigens on the cell's surface. Certain subsets of white blood cells (i.e CD8 CTL's, macrophages, natural killer) respond to the presentation of a foreign protein (antigen) on the cell's surface, and, in a series of events that follow, move to either destroy the infectious agent (virus, fungus, mycoplasma, bacteria etc.) on or near the surface of the cell's membrane, or to destroy the infected cell. In other words, before the white blood cells can attack and eliminate an infection from the host, the white blood cells must see, identify and locate which cells are infected with viruses, fungus, bacteria etc. Only the presentation of antigen on the cell's membrane enables the immune system to see the foreign invader and locate the source of the infection (the infected cell). You could call this process microsurgery.

Unless antigen presentation takes place in every single infected cell, the complete elimination of an infection from the host by an immune response will not be possible and a chronic infection will persist at some level of activity. If complete elimination of the infection is not possible, but the level of the pathogen (i.e virus) activity is low enough, the patient will have no symptoms and will feel normal and functionally healthy. The key to complete viral eradication depends on healthy cells that can process and present antigen.

What is a "foreign antigen"?

A "foreign antigen" is a protein that is "not self" but is part of a virus, fungus or bacteria that invades a cell. In contrast to a foreign protein is a usable protein like an amino acid that results from the digestion of meat. When you eat a hamburger, you are eating foreign protein that comes from a cow. When meat is digested, it is broken down into amino acids, the building blocks of human muscle and other tissues. Thus, what was once foreign protein (hamburger) eventually becomes "self" (human muscle). If a hamburger is not completely digested, and some of the meat proteins that are not usable are absorbed into the blood supply through a leaky gut, the immune system will attack the unusable proteins as "foreign" and this will turn on an antibody response from the B cells that will tag the foreign protein with an antibody.

Cell-mediated immunity depends on antigen presentation

In an article written by R. Ehrlich in Human Immunology – 1997 May;54(2):104-16], titled "Modulation of Antigen Processing and Presentation by Persistent Virus Infections and in Tumors," Ehrlich writes:

"Cell-mediated immunity is effective against cells harboring active virus replication and is critical for the elimination of ongoing infections, opposing tumor progression, and reducing or preventing the reactivation of persistent viruses and tumor metastasis.......By suppressing the expression of molecules associated with antigen processing and presentation, abrogation of the major immune mechanism that deals with the elimination of infected and transformed (cancer) cells is achieved....This is accomplished...in cells expressing viral proteins by interfering with peptide transport and the assembly/transport of (MHC) class I complexes."

MHC stands for "Major Histocompatibility Complex." There are two types - type I and type II. All cells present MHC type I on their cell surface. This is like an identification card that says to the immune system, "I am self ...do not attack me." Natural Killer cells will normally attack and destroy any cell not presenting MHC class I molecules on the cell surface. MHC class II molecules are presented only by some subsets of white blood cells like macrophages. Antigen presentation occurs after a piece of the virus is processed inside the cell and transported to the cell membrane and is locked inside the folds of the MHC class I molecule. A transporter called TAP does the transportation of the antigen from inside the cell to the cell surface. One type of transporter is called TAP-A and is ATP-dependent. ATP stands for "adenosine tri-phosphate," which is stored energy for the cells.

1. Nature 1995 Jun 1;375(6530):411-5

Factors that affect antigen presentation

Two factors that adversely affect antigen processing and presentation are low ATP (adenosine tri-phosphate) and decreased levels of the anti-oxidant - L-Glutathione. Scientific studies also indicate that a lack of gamma interferon (IFN gamma) impairs the presentation of MHC class I molecules. IFN gamma is a TH1 type cytokine that, along with Interleuken II and Interleuken 12, increases CD8 cytotoxic lymphocyte activity, and especially when TH2 cytokines, like Interleuken 6 and 10, are down-regulated. While the antibody response is effective against the common cold and flu (infections outside of the cells), it is not effective in conditions of chronic intracellular infections that occur in AIDS, CFIDS, candidiasis and cancer where a TH1 or cell mediated immune response is needed.

An article titled "Defective Antigen Processing Correlates With a Low Level of Intracellular Glutathione," (by S. Short, BJ Merkel, R Caffrey and KL McCoy of the Department of Microbiology and Immunology, Virginia Commonwealth University, Richmond, VA and published in Eur J Immunol 1996 Dec: 26(12):3015-20), the authors report on the results of an experiment with Chinese hamster ovary cells that exhibit a defect in processing Antigen with disulfide bonds. They state: "Low intracellular glutathione levels in antigen-presenting cells, correlated with defective processing of AG with disulfide bonds, indicating that this thiol may be a critical factor in regulating Ag (antigen) processing."

Selenium increases glutathione, lowers beta 2 microglobulin

A study done of 125 HIV+ persons at the Center for Disease Prevention, University of

Miami's School of Medicine, showed that persons with below-normal levels of selenium were 20 times more likely to die of AIDS-related opportunistic infections than those with normal levels. The study also showed that maintaining normal levels of vitamin A, B12 and zinc produced a lower rate of mortality and improved survival.

The Natural Killer cells

NK cells can operate totally independent of any other immune cells and do not need their assistance to locate and destroy foreign invaders. NK cells are effective against viruses, fungus, bacteria and cancer cells. NK cells can do more than just reduce viral load in the blood, they can locate and destroy cells infected with viruses. While the antibody (inflammatory) humoral responses are active, the NK cell activity is suppressed.

In a fax sent to me from Specialty Labs (Santa Monica, CA), 11/18/96, here is what was reported about NK cell function:

"Individuals with abnormally low NK activity levels are particularly susceptible to viral infections, including cytomegalovirus (CMV) and varicella. Abnormally low NK activities have been reported in AIDS and several other viral infections, solid tissue malignancies, autoimmune diseases, congenital immunodeficiencies, chronic fatigue immune dysfunction syndrome (CFIDS), protein calorie malnutrition...and in chemotherapy of cancer patients."

NK cell activity is considered part of the TH1 arm of the immune system. Significant amounts of published scientific research on the importance of NK cell activity and CD8 cells in immune function can be found through a computer search at the National Library of Medicine at http://igm.nlm.nih.gov/

TH1 Summary

1. Low-dose Hydrocortisone (10 to 20 mg daily) – a natural Adrenal hormone that lowers IL-6 and TNF – improves cellular immunity and Natural Killer cell function.
2. L-Glutathione – Researchers have found that high or low Glutathione levels inside immune cells are a switch to determine the preferential immune response – TH1 or TH2. Sufficient Glutathione inside immune cells strongly promotes a TH1 cytokine response that is the most effective immune response against cancer and most chronic intracellular infections. It stimulates antigen presentation and CD8 CTL's, macrophage and neutrophil activity. Glutathione reduces tumor necrosis factor (TNF), a main cause of wasting syndrome. As an antioxidant, Glutathione also neutralizes free radicals.

On the other hand, low Glutathione levels cause a TH2 immune response (antibody) that is not effective against cancer and intracellular infections (i.e. Herpes, HHV-6, candidiasis, parasites, mycoplasma, EBV, CMV, HIV, HPV, HCV, HBV and many others), but a strong antibody (TH2) response will prevent the flu and the common cold.

Selenium sources from food – Brazil nuts, fish and sea vegetables.

Best supplements: high-selenium mustard greens and high-selenium. Preventative amounts - 400 mcg daily. Therapeutic amounts: 800 to 1200 mcg or more daily.

For undenatured L-cysteine: cold processed whey proteins (Immunocal or Immunepro), Aged Garlic extract (Kyolic), raw or sprouted seeds and nuts, raw onions and garlic. Horseradish contains significant amounts of Glutathione peroxidase. Smaller amounts are in winter squash and avocados. Silymarin also help increase Glutathione levels. Riboflavin (B2) recycles oxidized Glutathione back to its reduced form.

3. Omega-3 fatty acids (DHA & EPA) found in cold-water fish, salmon, sardine and cod liver oil (improves DTH, lowers triglycerides, TNF and IL-6) - helps prevent heart disease and cancer. Flaxseed also contains some omega-3 fatty acids. Dietary supplement: Seacure

4. Olive Oil – increases IL-2* Monounsaturated fats are found in olive, macadamia, avocado and hazelnut oils and to a lesser extent in peanut oil. (reduces TNF and increases IgA - supports mucosal immunity). Adult therapeutic dose: 4 tablespoons daily.
   *Cytokine. 1995 Aug;7(6):548-53

5. Vitamin A (increases transport of IGA - supports mucosal immunity). Cod liver oil one to three teaspoons daily.

6. Vitamin K – reduces interleuken 6 (IL-6) and prostaglandin E2. (Source – parsley)

7. Silica - reduces IgG and improves NK function. (Food sources: Horsetail herb and/or Oatmeal).

8. Vegetarian digestive enzymes - improves digestion and assimilation of proteins and other nutrients, reduces circulating immune complexes that cause antibody and auto-antibody formation. Increases albumin levels. Protein digestive enzymes are found naturally in fresh ginger root, raw pineapple and kiwi fruit. . Additional factors that support digestion are:
   a. Cayenne - 1 or 2 capsules taken before meals stimulates hunger and digestive enzymes. (lowers IL-6, supports digestion of nutrients – heals ulcers)
   b. Lemon juice or apple cider vinegar - taken with meals stimulates hydrochloric acid for protein digestion. (support digestion of nutrients for mucosal membrane integrity).
   c. Magnesium - needed by pancreas to produce pancreatin - used to digest proteins.

9. Friendly intestinal flora
   a. Lactobacillus Plantarum and L casei - potent inducers of IL-12 and IFN-gamma. Supports mucosal immunity. Reduces IgE and food allergies.
   b. Bifidobacterium Longum - increases IgA - supports mucosal immunity - reduces candida albicans - improves lactose tolerance.
   c. Acidophilus - promotes resistance to colonization of candida albicans.
   d. Fiber/pectin/probiotic blend (Very important)
   e. Slippery elm tea or powder – helps rebuild the intestines, or try Ojibwa tea.

10. Chlorella- broken cell wall or Spirulina - use liquid, granules or capsules. Increases IL-12, GM-CSF and activates macrophages.

11. L-Thyroxine (T4) a thyroid hormone that is a potent inducer of IFN-gamma. Sources: Am J Physiol 1997 Oct;273(4 Pt 1):C125-32 and J Immunol 1998 Jul 15;161(2):843-9

12. Garlic - raw or aged extract - promotes NK function and IL-2. Never eat raw garlic alone – eat only with whole grain crackers or bread.

13. DHEA - increases IL-2, IFN-gamma and decreases IL-6 and IL-10.

14. Acupuncture (points ST36, LI11 and RN6) increase IL-2, IFN-gamma and NK function.

15. UVA light - promotes IL-12. (indoor tanning)

16. Vitamin E (natural) - increases IL-2, NK function and IFN-gamma. Reduces NF-kappa B. Use only natural vitamin E with its various tocopherol forms for best results.

17. Transfer factor - protein immuno-modulators extracted from colostrum from immunologically stimulated animals that promotes DTH and specific immunity to certain antigens (viruses etc).

18. Colostrum - contains IgA - promotes mucosal immunity and immunity to specific antigens to which the animal was exposed.
19. Naltrexone - promotes NK function and resistance to candida albicans. Reduces IL-6 levels, promotes deep restful sleep.
20. IP6 - found in brown rice and corn - promotes NK function.
21. Lentinian, Shiitake, Maitake and certain other mushrooms - promote TH1 cytokines and NK function.
22. BioPro Thymic Protein A - increases platelets, IL-2 and T cell counts. Laboratory grown thymus from a single healthy calf over 10 years ago.
23. DNCB - promotes DTH (antigen presentation) and CD8 CTL activity
24. Beta 1, 3 glucan - found in the common yeast and in oats and oat sprouts/rye sprouts - stimulates macrophage and neutrophil function.
25. Noni -Tahitian - 2 tablespoons twice daily - promotes NK function and immunity against cancer.
26. Neem - promotes IFN-gamma and increases CD8s - also, a powerful antiviral, antifungal and antibacterial herb.
27. Gingko Biloba - improves memory.
28. Exercise - aerobic - light and fun. Walking, gardening, dancing, sports. increases endorphin levels - improves NK function - removes toxins from body.
29. Water- Drink 8 to 12 glasses daily - removes toxins - reduces stress on adrenals, liver and kidneys. Miraculous water from San Damiano, Italy.
30. Positive attitude, prayer, classical music. - ability to forgive, compassionate, willingness to help others. Reduces stress on the adrenal glands.

Fiber/pectin/probiotic blend (stool formula)

A good blend is L. Acidophilus, B Bifidum, B Longum, L. Plantarum and L Salivarius (consider Green Probiotics from 414-329-0648 or something equivalent)). Mix 1/4 cup of this probiotic blend, with 1/2 cup pectin (citrus or apple) and 1 cup of fiber (freshly ground flax seed or psyllium husk powder). Refrigerate and use 1 tsp in a glass of water or carrot juice with each meal 3 times daily. If you are sensitive to the sugars in the carrot juice, mix 2 tablespoons of cooked winter squash or canned pumpkin in a glass of water and mix in a blender along with the fiber/pectin/probiotic blend. Note: if maltodextrin is a problem, find a probiotic blend with some other filler, like a vegetable powder or buy the pure strains. These may also be sprinkled directly over your food with each meal or mixed with a small glass of water.

When the friendly flora in your intestines reach therapeutic levels, your stools will be large diameter, medium brown in color and will float on water. If you have stools that sink to the bottom of the toilet bowl, you have more unfriendly flora than friendly and most likely have weak mucus membranes and poor mucosal immunity. Note: Persons with AIDS, cancer, candidiasis, CFS and other chronic conditions usually report they have sinkers. When digestive health improves, the stools will start to float.

TH2 Summary

1. Leaky Gut Syndrome (LGS) – caused by long-term use of any combination of the following: antibiotics, food preservatives, refined carbohydrates (no fiber, very little fruits and vegetables in the diet). A lack of fiber causes low bifido bacteria counts in the colon and thus low butyrate levels. Butyrate, produced by bifido bacteria, is an essential fuel for colonic cells to produce mucin, the mucus membranes and rebuild the cell walls of the intestines. LGS allows foreign protein particles of indigestion to enter the blood and provoke an antibody response and increased levels of IL-6.
2. Processed vegetable oils high in trans-fatty acids and polyunsaturated fatty acids (safflower, soy, canola, corn and sunflower). Unless they are cold-processed or expeller pressed, they are already damaged goods by the time they reach grocery shelves and very immunosuppressive. They can also cause heart disease and cancer.
3. Glucose (white sugar) -candy bars, pastry, soda etc - suppresses function of all white blood cells, particularly macrophages.
   1. Foods cooked at very high temperatures (deep fried) contain acrylamides (cancer causing agents)
5. HIV, Candida Albicans, HCV, E Coli and many other pathogens.
6. Stress (continuous) - emotional, financial, fear and worry
7. Pesticides, asbestos. air and water pollutants
8. Adrenal exhaustion – subnormal levels of cortisol and DHEA.
9. Prednisone or Prednisolone (synthetic antiflammatory steroids)
10. Morphine
11. Tobacco
12. Lead, mercury and other heavy metals
13. Anal sex leading to discharge of semen
14. Thalidomide
15. UVB
16. Pregnancy - A Th2 cytokine predominant profile is needed. A strong Th1 cytokine profile including TNF can cause a miscarriage. Immune system may reject fetus.
17 Alcohol - Note: Studies on animals show that ethanol (alcohol) definitely suppresses Th1 cytokines and induces Th2. Note: Beer has beta glucan in it that may cancel the alcohol effects
18. Candidiasis (systemic candida albican infection) - stimulates Th2 cytokines.
19. Circulating immune complexes (CIC's) - caused by a combination of leaky gut syndrome and poor digestion of proteins due to a lack or HCL and digestive enzymes. Also caused by semen ejaculation during anal sex in persons with impaired mucosal immunity.
20. Sedentary life - lack of exercise contributes to a build-up of toxins that weaken CMI.
21. Water consumption inadequate to remove toxins inside the cells and organs.
22. Negative attitudes - suppressed anger/rage - inability to forgive, resentful
23. Low body temperature
24. Acid saliva pH
25 Chronic insomnia - inability to dream and get restful sleep. Insomnia increases IL-6.
26. Weight lifting - muscle tearing may stress cortisol reserves.
27. Steroids used for muscle gain - some are very hard on the liver and adrenals.

2

Selenium in the prevention and treatment of chronic illness

Selenium is a trace element that is well known for its antioxidant properties. It has a physical structure similar to sulfur. In plants, it has an affinity to bind to sulfur-based proteins like methionine or cysteine. Selenium is a key component and controlling factor in the body's main antioxidant and immune stimulant - L glutathione.

From June through August 2001, extraordinary lab results came to my attention in two cases where persons, who had hepatitis C, credited selenium with reducing their viral load by 87% in one case and 94% in another. What makes these two cases unique is the dosage used, 1200 mcg daily in the first case and 1000 mcg daily in the second of a high-selenium yeast supplement. These amounts are higher than the usual RDA of 70 mcg. Most dietary supplement manufacturers advise consumers not to use over 200 mcg or 400 mcg daily, due to concerns of side effects or adverse effects from too much selenium. Using over 800 mcg daily has caused side effects, if the types of selenium used are either sodium selenite or a laboratory-made synthetic-form called L-selenomethionine.

Researchers have found that Glutathione is a crucial antioxidant that inactivates many kinds of free radicals, but also supports antigen processing inside cells, and thus helps with cell-mediated immune responses. Selenium along with Cysteine are the best known precursors to increasing Glutathione production in the body. Selenocysteine and L-selenomethionine are two forms found in Brazil nuts, fish, yeast and other natural sources. Riboflavin, or Vitamin B2, is reported to help recycle oxidized glutathione back to its reduced form. Vitamin E is reported to help with the assimilation and utilization of selenium. Over the course of the past 14 months, other than food sources, only high-selenium yeast and high-selenium mustard greens (Phytosel) by Nucycle or selenium broccoli (SeBroc®) have proven to be safe and effective.

According to Regina Brigelius-Flohe of Potsdam, Germany, the family of glutathione peroxidases consist of 4 distinct selenoproteins. They are cGPx, GI-GPx, pGPx and PHGPx. All 4 types of Glutathione are called selenoproteins because they incorporate selenium into their molecular structure. Selenium is also involved in several other proteins in people and has various functions other than as an antioxidant. About 30 types of selenium-bound proteins have been detected in mammals, and may well exist in humans as well.

Selenium, used at 1200 mcg daily, reduces Hepatitis C viral load by 87% in 6 weeks

July 2001
San Paulo, Brazil

"I had a viral load of 1.5 million or log 6 when I was first diagnosed 3 years ago. I started on a high selenium dose intake of 1200 mcg daily that I did for 45 days. The viral load dropped from 1.5 million to 200,000 and has stayed there since. 200,000 is low for HCV by NIH Hepatitis Consensus Conference.

I haven't taken the viral load very often for HCV as I consider the enzyme levels to be a more important indicator of the health of my liver. No elevated enzymes means no inflammation and no damage to the liver regardless of the viral load. I have seen people with HCV viral loads over 5 million and with normal liver enzymes. Also, I have seen people with low viral loads and high enzymes and resulting damage to the liver.

Jose

Update: Jose sent an e-mail message in which he stated that after 45 days of using 1200 mcg daily of selenium, he reduced the dose to 200 to 400 mcg daily for the past two years. Recently, he increased the dose to 600 mcg daily.

The following month, August, I received an e-mail from another reader with hepatitis C who shared his experiences with 1000 mcg of selenium daily for one year. This time, his message and the results he obtained captured my attention - big time.

High-selenium yeast reduces Hepatitis C (HCV) by 94%

"Let me preface my thoughts by saying that the current minimum RDA for Selenium in the US is around 70 mcg daily for adults. The typical dose in dietary supplements is about 200 mcg daily. I have read that selenium from dietary sources alone ranges from near zero to a high of 1100 mcg daily, depending on where you live and the amount of selenium found in the soil and eventually in the food. So far, we can assume that selenium levels vary widely among the populations of the world."

While in normal individuals, over exposure to selenium may be toxic causing gastrointestinal problems, hair loss and nerve damage, in persons with AIDS or hepatitis whose selenium levels are usually depleted because of the disease process, the normal and safe levels are thought to be much higher than the 200 to 300 mcg used daily by normal healthy individuals.

Contrary to conventional wisdom, I have supplemented with selenium at 1000 mcg daily with occasional lapses for over a year now without any noticeable ill effects, other than faster than normal hair and nail growth. During this time, I've seen my viral load for HCV drop from over 10,000,000 to around 600,000 along with a corresponding improvement in my overall condition."   *Cliff*

The letter from Cliff arrived a few weeks after the letter from Jose. It was the letter from Cliff that caused me to sit up and take notice. The decline of HCV from 10 million to 600,000 is a 94% drop in viral load. These kinds of results are impressive, as no side effects have been reported either. The cost is low and no prescription is needed.

Published literature indicates that as the Glutathione levels increase, the HIV and hepatitis viral loads decrease. The extent of the decrease in viral load may well depend on how much Glutathione is available inside the cells. Understanding the subject of "Glutathione" can become complex, as medical writers refer to various Glutathione compounds.

Besides selenium, Alpha Lipoic Acid (ALA), Silymarin (Milk Thistle), L-glutamine and IP6 are additional dietary supplements that support glutathione activity and protect the liver. Cold processed whey proteins like ImmunePro or Immunocal enhance Glutathione activity due to the undenatured L cysteine contained in these products. Lab results indicate that ImmunePro, a cold processed whey protein, also contains 170 mg of Lactoferrin per 5 gram serving, a significantly high lactoferrin content. Lactoferrin binds to iron and thus blocks viruses from using iron to replicate.

Selenium against AIDS and Cancer

Richard Passwater first published his research on selenium in the December, 1971, issue of "Prevention" magazine, and has been researching the benefits of selenium ever since. His 48-page book "Selenium Against Cancer and Aids" is published by Keats Publishing and is found in health food stores. In reading through his book and in a partial review of hundreds of scientific abstracts and references to over 600 scientific studies, here is a useful but incomplete summary of what I have learned.

Selenium -

1. Reduces mutations among viruses and other pathogens.
2. Increases glutathione peroxidase levels, the main antioxidant that our cells use to protect us from free radicals.
3. Helps prevent most types of cancer including prostate cancer.
4. Is used to produce an enzyme that helps the thyroid convert the hormone T4 to T3. (may help normalize body temperature)
5. Low levels have been associated with depression and schizophrenia.
6. Reduces the toxic effects of mercury and cadmium in the body.
7. Protects the liver
8. Improves cell-mediated immune responses by helping with antigen processing inside cells.
9. Helps cellular respiration.
10. Works synergistically with vitamin E in preventing cancer.
11. At therapeutic doses, reduces HIV and Hepatitis viral replication and helps shrink cancers.
12. Levels of selenium have been found to be subnormal for all types of cancer tested.

Ref.:
1. J Infect Dis. 2000 Sep;182 Suppl 1:S69-73
2. J Assoc Nurses AIDS Care. 2000 Mar-Apr;11(2):103
3. J. Neurovirol. 1998 Jun 3-6;4(suppl):343
4. Conf Retroviruses Oppor Infect. 1996 Jan 28-Feb1;3rd:122
5. Annu Conf Australas Soc HIV Med. 1997 Nov. 13-16;9:133
6. Lancet. 2000 Jul 15;356(9225):233-41
7. Int Conf AIDS 1996 Jul 7-12;11(1):124

Selenium deficiency linked to cancer, AIDS and heart disease

A substantial amount of published scientific research has linked selenium deficiency to AIDS progression, increased HIV replication, weight loss, heart disease and elevated beta2 microglobulin levels. Supplementation with selenium has been reported to increase interleuken 2 levels, increase T cell counts, reduce tumor necrosis factor, reduce the risk of cancer, reduce HIV replication, reduce beta2 microglobulin levels (measures rate of cell destruction), reduce depression and decrease the risk of death from HIV infection. (1, 2, 3, 4, 5). Selenium also is reported to help increase thyroid hormone production. (6). In AIDS, selenium deficiency has been linked to weight loss, heart disease and poor prognosis for toxoplasmosis. (7).

Selenium - questions and answers

Q: What is the normal level of selenium in the blood?
A: Every laboratory that tests for selenium has its own "normal" reference ranges and they vary. Cancer, AIDS and hepatitis patients usually have low levels - less than 150 mcg/liter of selenium in the blood. In HIV cases, researchers have found that, when selenium levels in the blood are less than 135 mcg/l, that the chances of developing a mycobacteria infection increase 13 fold. (Researchers have also found that persons with less than 45 mcg/liter are at high risk to get a stroke or heart attack.). From our perspective, the normal range for selenium in blood serum for basically healthy persons should be between 135 mcg/l and 200 mcg/l for preventive purposes. For therapeutic purposes, blood serum levels should start at 200 mg/l and safely goes up to 600 mcg/l. Chinese researchers have found that when consuming only plant-based selenium foods, side effects did not occur until blood serum levels of selenium went over 1000 mcg/l.

Q: What is the RDA for selenium?
A: The RDA is rated at 70 mcg per day for adults, but this is way too low an amount for preventing cancers or to stop hepatitis, candidiasis or AIDS progression. In the United States, diet alone provides about 100 mcg daily. In the UK, the average daily intake is 60 mcg. In Japan, where selenium rich seafoods are consumed, and cancer and AIDS are substantially lower than in the US, and the life span is considerably longer, the average intake of selenium from diet is 600 mcg daily.

Q: Is it important to take iodine supplements, when consuming selenium at higher dosage levels?
A: Organic selenium helps convert the thyroid hormone T4 to T3. Ocean fish are a rich source of selenium and are also high in iodine. Taking 2 or more kelp capsules daily, as a source of iodine is recommended when using natural selenium supplements like high-selenium yeast or mustard greens. Persons with low body temperature should also use kelp along with selenium.

Q: What about toxicity?
A: Passwater states that organic forms of selenium (high-selenium yeast, mustard greens etc) may have side effects at a dose over 3,500 mcg daily, while inorganic forms like sodium selenite may have side effects at 1200 mcg or more daily. The most common symptom is hair falling out, followed by loose toe and fingernails. The symptoms are reversible when dosage is reduced or stopped temporarily. More advanced side effects from higher doses of selenium include gastrointestinal problems and nervousness. Based on animal studies, an adult would have to consume over 100,000 mcg daily for 3 or 4 weeks to have a fatal overdose. A very detailed report on selenium and research on toxicity can be found on

Toxline at http://toxnet.nlm.nih.gov (3). Conclusion: Selenium is a very safe dietary supplement providing you only use plant based products and not the synthetic forms (amino acid chelates (actually complexes) i.e. L-selenomethionine or selenium aspartate).

Q: If a person is healthy, how much organic selenium should be taken daily as a supplement to prevent selenium deficiency?
A: I think the Japanese consumption level of 600 mcg daily would be good to emulate. Passwater reports that in Greenland, many residents consume 1,300 mcg daily with no known side effects.

Q: How much selenium and vitamin E is needed to have a therapeutic effect if you have AIDS, hepatitis or cancer?
A: Our two readers who reduced their HCV viral load up to 94% did it by taking 1000 to 1200 mcg daily or about 100 to 200 mcg of selenium per 20 pounds of body weight daily. Note: for therapeutic effects, a person weighing 160 lbs should take from 800 to 1600 mcg daily of natural organic selenium. A good mix is 2 capsules of Phytosel (Natural Selenium) twice daily for a total of 800 mcg of organic selenium plus 4 Brazil nuts for another 400 mcg of natural selenium. Total 1200 mcg daily. Vitamin E is known to help with the assimilation of selenium. Use about 30 to 50 mg of vitamin E for each 200 mcg of selenium you take to help with absorption.

Q: What foods are highest in selenium?
A: Brazil Nuts have the highest concentration of natural organic protein-bound selenium of any food on the planet.(about 100 mcg per nut). Other sources are brewers yeast, fatty fish (salmon, tuna, sardines), oysters, clams, wheat germ, mushrooms and whole grains. Note: If you weigh 180 lbs, eating 3 Brazil nuts 3 times daily would give you 450 to 900 mcg of selenium and a therapeutic dose that could be increased under a physician's supervision and monitoring of blood levels. The selenium content of Brazil nuts is not standardized and depends on the selenium content of the soil where the nuts are grown.

Note on blood levels: Reduce selenium intake if blood levels go above 600 mcg per liter or if your hair gets thin or starts falling out. Based on current available information, an immediate target goal is to raise selenium blood levels to 200 mcg per liter and then to increase the level up to 600 mcg/liter, or until side effects start to occur; then back off a bit until the side effects stop. This should give you the best therapeutic effects in treating AIDS, Candidiasis, Lyme disease, hepatitis, Cancer, Lou Gehrigs, Chronic fatigue syndrome and other similar conditions.

Selenium taken at 200 mcg daily reduces risk of prostate cancer by 50% and reduces the risk for breast cancer

Stanley Brosman MD and Mark Moyad MD write about Nutrition and Prostate Cancer in the eMedicine Journal (1). Dr Brosman is a Professor at the Department of Urology at the University of California Los Angeles Medical School. The authors have found that the risk of developing prostate cancer in the United States is 204 times greater here than in China. In a population of 200,000 men, one person will develop prostate cancer in China annually, while in the US the number would be 204 each year. The physicians looked for dietary factors that contribute to this difference. They found a higher risk for prostate cancer among persons who eat red meat, are on diets high in fat and/or are obese. The researchers found a relationship in the protective effects of selenium peroxidases that repaired oxidized phospholipids and the prevention of oxidation of lipids by vitamin E; hence a synergistic relationship between vitamin E and selenium.

A study by Clark et al (2) demonstrated a 50% decrease in cancer mortality and in the incidence of prostate cancer in men who took 200 mcg daily of selenium, versus a control group taking a placebo. Another study on the effects of 200 mcg of selenium found no effects on skin cancer, but found a reduction in breast cancer and prostate cancer.

Ref:
1. eMedicine Journal, July 19, 2001 Vol 2, No 7
2. Clark LC et al; Decreased incidence of prostate cancer with selenium supplementation... Br J Urol 1998 May;81(5): 730-4 (Medline)
1. WHO working group: TA: Environmental Health Criteria PG:306 p YR:1987 IP: VI:58. Can be downloaded from www.toxnet.nlm.nih.gov. Search the phrase "selenium toxicity"

Doctor uses selenium, alpha lipoic acid and silymarin to treat 3 patients in need of liver transplants.

Dr. B.M. Berkson, of the Integrative Center of New Mexico, reported in a German medical journal (Med Klin) in October 1999, the results of treating 3 patients, who needed liver transplant surgery, with a triple antioxidant therapy. The therapy consisted of therapeutic doses of alpha lipoic acid, silymarin and selenium. Dr. Berkson stated that interferon therapy works about 30% of the time, and that, even with liver transplant surgery, residual hepatitis C virus will infect and damage the new liver.

Dr. Berkson states that the antioxidants, alpha lipoic acid, silymarin and selenium have antiviral, antioxidant and free radical scavenging properties. Berkson treated 3 patients who had cirrhosis of the liver and portal hypertension, and reported that they recovered quickly, did not need the liver transplants, and have all returned to work and are feeling healthy. A major factor in the success of this therapy probably was the dosage that was used, which consisted of 600 mg of Alpha Lipoic Acid, 400 mcg of food-based selenium and 900 mg of silymarin (milk thistle extract) daily, in two or three divided doses. Dr. Berkson can be reached in NM at his clinic at 505-524-3720. The full article can be found at www.nationalhepatitis-c.org/newswinter2000

In researching the published medical literature, I found other sources recommending 600 mg daily of ALA for chronic liver disease and no reports of side effects from this much Lipoic acid. Raw white potatoes are a source high in natural alpha lipoic acid. Also, for Silymarin (milk thistle), no reports of side effects from high doses of 900 mg daily for adults.

Persons with HCV and HIV have severe selenium deficiency

Selenium and glutathione levels decline as AIDS progresses, according to Look MP et al in the 1997 European Journal of Clinical Nutrition (1). In stage I of HIV infection, selenium levels in the blood were an average of 82 mcg per liter. Even in Stage I, the selenium levels are below the minimum of 85 mcg/l, considered the least amount needed to maintain health. In Stage II, the selenium levels dropped to an average of 68 mcg and in Stage III, selenium levels dropped to 51 mcg/liter. Researchers found that selenium levels correlated positively with CD4 counts, and inversely with levels of tumor necrosis factor receptors type II. They found that in persons with both HIV and HCV, the selenium levels were the most depressed. Hence, this latter group is in urgent need of selenium supplementation.

In a study published in The Lancet (3), it was found in Finland that when selenium levels were less than 45 mcg per liter of blood, there was an increased risk for strokes and heart attacks. In another study in men, the risk factor was 3.7 times higher for strokes and heart attacks in men whose selenium levels were less than 45 mcg/l. (4)

Selenium deficiency is associated with a 3-fold increase in shedding of HIV-1 infected cells in the female genital tract

Baeten JM et al, from the Univ. of Washington in Seattle, report of a study done in Kenya (2) with 318 HIV positive women, to assess the relationship between selenium deficiency and HIV-1 shedding in the vaginal tract. HIV+ women can infect HIV negative men, if HIV viruses are shed in the vaginal tract. The study classified a deficiency of selenium as blood levels less than 85 mcg of selenium per liter. 11% of the women in the study were observed to have less than 85 mcg/l. The researchers found that selenium deficiency was associated with HIV-1 shedding in the vagina that was three-fold higher than women whose selenium blood levels were greater than 85 mcg/l. The implications are that, in sex without condoms, women who are deficient in selenium are 3 times more likely to pass the infection on to a man than women who are not deficient in selenium. Hence, selenium supplementation may reduce HIV transmission in persons who do not take preventive measures, such as using a condom.

Ref:
1. Look MP et al; Eur J Clin Nutr. 1997 Apr;51(4):266-72
2. Baeten JM et al; J Acquir Defic Syndr. 2001 Apr 1;26(4):360-4
3. Lancet, 2 (8291):175-9 1982 Jul 24
4. Am J Epidemiol, 122(2):276-82 1985 Aug

Ma Lan and Wallach on Illnesses linked to selenium deficiency

An excerpt from a book published in 1994, titled RARE EARTHS: FORBIDDEN CURES, has some intriguing information on selenium.

"The School of Pharmacy from the University of Georgia released a report in August of 1994 that concludes a human selenium deficiency is related to the onset of full blown AIDS in chronically infected HIV patients.....The HIV patient actually dies of selenium deficiency encephalopathy, liver cirrhosis or cardiomyopathy. Long term HIV patients (20 years or more), that never developed full blown AIDS, had supplemented with relatively large amounts of selenium."

Drs. Ma Lan and Wallach cited a long list of illnesses linked to selenium deficiency and backed it up with a litany of references to published medical literature. Here is their list:

Selenium deficiency diseases

HIV progression to AIDS
Anemia (RBC fragility)
Age spots and Liver spots
Fatigue
Muscular weakness
Myalgia
Scoliosis
Muscular Dystrophy
Cystic Fibrosis (congenital)
Cardiomyopathy
Multiple Sclerosis (linked to mercury poisoning)
Heart palpitations
Irregular heart beat
Liver cirrhosis
Pancreatitis
Pancreatic atrophy
Lou Gehrig's disease (ALS)
Parkinson's Disease (associated with mercury poisoning)
Alzheimer's (associated with high vegetable oil consumption or poly unsaturated fatty acids)
Adrenoleucodystrophy (ALD)
Infertility
Low birth weight
High infant mortality
Sudden Infant Death Syndrome (SIDS)
Cancer
Sickle Cell anemia

The authors state that "high intakes of vegetable oils including salad dressing, margarine and cooking oils concurrent with a selenium deficiency is the quickest route to a heart attack and cancer....The clinical diseases associated with selenium deficiency are diverse and to the uninformed allopathic physician shrouded in mystery. Selenium deficiency is one of the more costly mineral deficiency complexes affecting embryos, the newborn, toddlers, teens and adults."

A list of their references in the medical literature follows. The complete article can be found at http://www.cc.nih.gov/ccc/supplements/selen.html
1. National Research Council. Food and Nutrition Board. Recommended Dietary

Allowances. 10th ed. Washington, DC: National Academy Press, 1989
2. Combs GF, Jr and Gray WP. Chemopreventive agents: Selenium. Pharmacol Ther 1998;79:179-92.
3. Levander OA. Nutrition and newly emerging viral diseases: An overview. J Nutr 1997;127:948S-950S.
4. Arthur JR. The role of selenium in thyroid hormone metabolism. Can J Physiol Pharmacol 1991;69:1648-52.
5. Corvilain B, Contempre B, Longombe AO, Goyens P, Gervy-Decoster C, Lamy F, Vanderpas JB, Dumont JE. Selenium and the thyroid: How the relationship was established. Am J Clin Nutr 1993;57 (2 Suppl):244S-248S.
6. Longnecker MP, Taylor PR, Levander OA, Howe M, Weillon C, McAdam PA, Patterson KY, Holden JM, Stampfer MJ, Morris JS, Willett WC. Selenium in diet, blood, and toenails in relation to human health in a seleniferous area. Am J Clin Nutr 1991;53;1288-94.
7. Pennington JA and Schoen SA. Contributions of food groups to estimated intakes of nutritional elements: Results from the FDA total diet studies, 1982-91. Int J Vitam Nutr Res 1996;66:342-9.
8. Pennington JA and Young BE. Total diet study nutritional elements. J Am Diet Assoc 1991;91:179-83.
9. Institute of Medicine, Food and Nutrition Board. Dietary Reference Intakes: Vitamin C, vitamin E, Selenium, and Carotenoids. National Academy Press, Washington, DC, 2000.
10. Pennington JA. Intakes of minerals from diets and foods: Is there a need for concern? J Nutrition 1996;126:2304S-2308S.
11. Levander OA and Beck MA. Interacting nutritional and infectious etiologies of Keshan disease. Insights from coxsackie virus B-induced myocarditis in mice deficient in selenium or vitamin E. Biol Trace Elem Res 1997;56:5-21.
12. Levander OA. Scientific rationale for the 1989 recommended dietary allowance for selenium. J Am Diet Assoc 1991;91:1572-1576.
13. Itokawa Y. Trace elements in long-term total parenteral nutrition. Nippon Rinsho 1996;54:172-8.
14. Abrams CK, Siram SM, Galsim C, Johnson-Hamilton H, Munford FL, Mezghebe H. Selenium deficiency in long-term total parenteral nutrition. Nutr Clin Pract 1992;7:175-8.
15. Gramm HJ, Kopf A, Bratter P. The necessity of selenium substitution in total parenteral nutrition and artificial alimentation. J Trace Elem Med Biol 1995;9:1-12.
16. Rannem T, Ladefoged K, Hylander E, Hegnhoj J, Staun M. Selenium depletion in patients with gastrointestinal diseases: Are there any predictive factors? Scand J Gastroenterol 1998;33:1057-61.
17. Rannem T, Ladefoged K, Hylander E, Hegnhoj J, Jarnum S. Selenium status in patients with Crohn's disease. Am J Clin Nutr 1992;56:933-7.
18. Bjerre B, von Schenck H, Sorbo B. Hyposelaemia: Patients with gastrointestinal diseases are at risk. J Intern Med 1989;225:85-8.
19. Russo MW, Murray SC, Wurzelmann JI, Woosley JT, Sandler RS. Plasma selenium levels and the risk of colorectal adenomas. Nutr Cancer 1997;28:125-9.
20. Patterson BH and Levander OA. Naturally occurring selenium compounds in cancer chemoprevention trials: A workshop summary. Cancer Epidemiol Biomarkers Prev 1997;6:63-9.

21. Knekt P, Marniemi J, Teppo L, Heliovaara M, Aromaa A. Is low selenium status a risk factor for lung cancer? Am J Epidemiol 1998;148:975-82.
22. Fleet JC. Dietary selenium repletion may reduce cancer incidence in people at high risk who live in areas with low soil selenium. Nutr Rev 1997;55:277-9.
23. Shamberger RJ. The genotoxicity of selenium. Mutat Res 1985;154:29-48.
24. Young KL and Lee PN. Intervention studies on cancer. Eur J Cancer Prev 1999;8:91-103.
25. Burguera JL, Burguera M, Gallignani M, Alarcon OM, Burgueera JA. Blood serum selenium in the province of Merida, Venezuela, related to sex, cancer incidence and soil selenium content. J Trace Elem Electrolytes Health Dis 1990;4:73-77.
26. Combs GF, Jr., Clark LC, Turnbull BW. Reduction of cancer risk with an oral supplement of selenium. Biomed Environ Sci 1997;10:227-34.
27. Garland M, Morris JS, Stampfer MJ, Colditz GA, Spate VL, Baskett CK, Rosner B, Speier FE, Willett WC, Hunter DJ. Prospective study of toenail selenium levels and cancer among women. J Natl Cancer Inst 1995;87:497-505.
28. Hercberg S, Galan P, Preziosi P, Roussel AM, Arnaud J, Richard MJ, Malvy D, Paul-Dauphin A, Briancon S, Favier A. Background and rationale behind the SU.VI.MAX Study, a prevention trial using nutritional doses of a combination of antioxidant vitamins and minerals to reduce cardiovascular diseases and cancers. Supplementation en VItamines et Mineraux AntiXydants Study. Int J Vitam Nutr Res 1998;68:3-20.
29. Gey KF. Vitamins E plus C and interacting conutrients required for optimal health. A critical and constructive review of epidemiology and supplementation data regarding cardiovascular disease and cancer. Biofactors 1998;7:113-74.
30. Ozer NK, Boscoboinik D, Azzi A. New roles of low density lipoproteins and vitamin E in the pathogenesis of atherosclerosis. Biochem Mol Biol Int 1995;35:117-24.
31. Lapenna D, de Gioia S, Ciofani G, Mezzetti A, Ucchino S, Calafiore AM, Napolitano AM, Di Ilio C, Cuccurulo F. Glutathione-related antioxidant defenses in human atherosclerotic plaques. Circulation 1998;97:1930-4.
32. Neve J. Selenium as a risk factor for cardiovascular diseases. J Cardiovasc Risk 1996;3:42-7.
33. Kose K, Dogan P, Kardas Y, Saraymen R. Plasma selenium levels in rheumatoid arthritis. Biol Trace Elem Res 1996;53:51-6.
34. Heliovaara M, Knekt P, Aho K, Aaran RK, Alfthan G, Aromaa A. Serum antioxidants and risk of rheumatoid arthritis. Ann Rheum Dis 1994;53:51-53.
35. Stone J, Doube A, Dudson D, Wallace J. Inadequate calcium, folic acid, vitamin E, zinc, and selenium intake in rheumatoid arthritis patients: Results of a dietary survey. Semin Arthritis Rheum 1997;27:180-5.
36. Grimble RF. Nutritional antioxidants and the modulation of inflammation: Theory and practice. New Horizons 1994;2:175-185.
37. AasethJ, Haugen M, Forre O. Rheumatoid arthritis and metal compounds-perspectives on the role of oxygen radical detoxification. Analyst 1998;123:3-6.
38. Patrick L. Nutrients and HIV; Part One--Beta carotene and selenium. Altern Med Rev 1999;4:403-13.
39. Baum MK, Shor-Posner G, Lai S, Zhang G, Lai H, Fletcher MA, Sauberlich H, Page JB. High risk of HIV-related mortality is associated with selenium deficiency. J Acquir Immune Defic Syndr Hum Retrovirol 1997;15:370-4.

40. Campa A, Shor-Posner G, Indacoche F, Zhang G, Lai H, Asthana D, Scott GB, Baum MK. Mortality risk in selenium-deficient HIV-positive children. J Acquir Immune Defic Syndr Hum Retrovirol 1999;15:508-13.
41. Baum MK and Shor-Posner G. Micronutrient status in relationship to mortality in HIV-1 disease. Nutr Rev 1998;56:S135-9.
42. Koller LD and Exon JH. The two faces of selenium-deficiency and toxicity-are similar in animals and man. Can J Vet Res 1986;50:297-306.
43. Hathcock J. Vitamins and minerals: Efficacy and safety. Am J Clin Nutr 1997;66:427-37.
44. Raisbeck MF, Dahl ER, Sanchez DA, Belden EL, O'Toole D. Naturally occurring selenosis in Wyoming. J Vet Diagn Invest 1993;5:84-87.
45. Pennington JA, Young BE, Wilson DB, Johnson RD, Vanderveen JE. Mineral content of foods and total diets: The Selected Minerals in Foods Survey, 1982-1984. J Am Diet Assoc 1986;86:876-91.
46. U.S. Department of Agriculture, Agricultural Research Service. Nutrient Database for Standard Reference, Release 12. : Nutrient Data Lab Home Page. URL http:://www.nal.usda.gov/fnic/foodcomp 1998.

L-Selenomethionine (made in a laboratory) is dropped from our list of recommended supplements.

Mark Konlee (July, 2002, monthly report)

The issue of what kind of selenium compound is safe and effective, in helping to restore immune function, has been an open question for several years. In this issue, I believe we are making some real progress toward resolving this outstanding question.

Since beginning this series of articles on selenium, in September of 2001, I have consistently recommended food sources of selenium, especially Brazil Nuts, along with selenium bound to either Methionine or Cysteine, and to avoid sodium selenite, because of toxicity issues. With this month's report, we are no longer recommending L seleno-methionine (laboratory made) as a source of selenium, because of reported side effects and the absence of any noticeable benefits. Yes, we have changed our mind about this manufactured source of selenium.

L-selenomethionine (SeM), as an amino acid chelate, is the most widely sold source of selenium available in health food stores, the other being sodium selenite. SeM is made in a laboratory under proprietary methods that bond selenium to the amino acid L-methionine. Albion is a manufacturer of L-selenomethionine and other amino acid chelates, and wholesales its products to dietary supplement manufacturers.

With daily usage of L-selenomethionine as high as 1800 mcg over a period of several weeks and months, there is no evidence that fungal and staph infections are decreasing, no evidence that white blood cell counts or CD4 counts are increasing, and no evidence of other tangible benefits, except for a few published studies that indicate a small decline in mercury levels for a dose as low as 100 mcg daily.

In contrast, the use of Brazil Nuts, the world's richest natural source of selenium, or supplements made from high selenium mustard greens or high selenium broccoli, we are getting reports of increasing WBC and CD4 counts, the disappearance of fungal and staph infections, greater energy and well being, and in one case reported in this issue, an end to chronic fatigue syndrome. Most of these results are occurring very rapidly - often within the first week of use.

In five cases, where the Albion source of seleno-methionine was consumed in high daily doses, ranging from 1200 to 1600 mcg, there are no beneficial results to report. Two of the cases were CFIDS related and 3 HIV related, with two of the three HIV+ persons also using drug cocktails. Nothing in the lab results of any of these three cases indicates any increase in WBC counts, CD4 or CD8 counts, or even a decrease in the viral load. In all five cases, none of the participants used any other form of selenium, other than the synthetic L-selenomethionine that is made in a laboratory.

Only one of the five persons using the Albion source of L-selenomethionine reported using foods rich in selenium, like Brazil nuts, ocean fish or seaweed nor did any of the five persons have blood serum levels of selenium tested after using the methionine bound selenium for several weeks.

Adverse effects from high doses of "L-selenomethionine"

Granted that the usual dosage range of methionine bound selenium is 100 to 400 mcg daily, and side effects are quite unlikely to show up at these low levels; yet if this compound is not what the body wants, it should not be used in any amount.

One reader with CFIDS took 1600 mcg daily of L-selenomethionine for several weeks and then had a numbing sensation on the right side of his body. He stopped using the selenium and fully recovered in a few days. After contacting me with this report, I initially was not convinced that the methionine bound selenium had anything to do with his symptoms, but suggested he switch to a food source of selenium and start with a low dose, 200 to 400 mcg daily, and gradually increase it. I also suggested he have his blood serum levels tested for selenium before starting on any new supplement. A second person using just 800 mcg daily of L selenomethionine noticed pain in the kidney area and stopped using it.

Note: Alternatives to L selenomethionine are high selenium yeast (Selenomax – available from Source Naturals), high selenium broccoli (Activated Selenium by Jarrow Formulas), high selenium mustard greens (Phytosel) or Selenium Cruciferate by Ecological Formulas). At this juncture, I am of the opinion that the Brazil nuts, high selenium mustard greens and broccoli, plus the high-selenium yeast, are the safest and most efficacious of all the selenium supplements.

With high doses of selenomethionine, persons have also reported lung congestion, dermatitis and other skin conditions. Simon and Vale both reported adverse side effects from high doses of sodium selenite and selenomethionine. In an e-mail from Simon in the UK, he said that at 1000 mcg daily of sodium selenite, his hair started falling out, but this stopped when he reduced the dose to 500 mcg daily. With equally high doses of selenomethionine, he reported big flare-ups of dermatitis. Both Vale and Simon reported the symptoms going away in a few days after stopping these selenium supplements. Another person, Del, also reported problems with high doses of selenomethionine. No one has reported any benefits.

All the reports of adverse effects are coming from the synthetic or laboratory made L-selenomethionine (amino acid chelates) and not from any known natural plant source of seleno methionine. The problem may be defects in the product, resulting from flaws in the manufacturing process.

Message Board Reports

Several reports on experiences, both good and bad, of using various types of selenium can be read on the Message Board at our website (keephopealive.org). Here is one of them:

Posted June 21, 2002.

Mark, I just picked up my new supply of Selenium from Solaray. It is called Bio-Active Selenium. It is from the Indian mustard plant that is grown in a greenhouse and no soil. They call it hyper-accumulation. Their label does not list the type of Selenium, however it must be a mix like the one you mentioned. This product is actually manufactured by Nutraceutical Corp. I'll let you know if this product causes the same side effects as the others.   Vale

Regarding the Bio-Active Selenium from Solaray made from greenhouse grown mustard greens, Vale reports no side effects after using 1800 mcg daily for several days. He reports that so far this is the only selenium supplement that he can take in high doses without side effects although he has not reported trying high selenium yeast.

My Message Board comments on selenium

July 5th, 2002.

"Within the past few weeks I have reached a conclusion that there is a problem with L selenomethionine. Two HIV + and two persons with immune problems not HIV related used high doses of selenomethionine with no apparent good results. They used the amino acid chelate, Albion brand. No resolution of symptoms was reported by any of these 4 cases and no increases in T cell counts or white blood cells.

On the contrary, concerning Jarrow Formulas "Activated Selenium" that has selenocysteine plus methionine also includes Vit. E, Riboflavin, broccoli and garlic - I have had two good reports from persons with long standing candidiasis (not HIV related). Both reported significant improvements in resolving candida infections after a week or two. The dose was around 900 mcg daily or 9 capsules a day.

I was aware that Ecological Formulas had a mustard green source of selenium that had 200 mcg per capsule. Right now, I am taking 2 Activated Selenium by Jarrow Formulas with one Selenium Cruciferate by Ecological Formulas but will probably go with the Solaray brand in place of Ecological Formulas later on. I do this once or twice a day. I personally like this combination very much. Thanks for sharing your results with me. It is time to send L selenomethionine down the pike, after the disappointing results of these 4 cases, and now the side effects that several of you have reported on this message board. Take Care."   Mark Konlee

Good reports on Brazil nuts

Kansas City, KS. Al, who has Gulf War Syndrome, reports very good results with eating about 10 Brazil nuts daily as his main source of selenium for the past 6 months although he also eats ocean fish 5 times a week. He reports his selenium blood serum levels are 240 mcg/l in a reference range that goes from 60 to 160.

Note: Our goal is to increase the blood serum selenium levels to 300 to 600 mcg/l. Our normal reference range for selenium in blood serum is from 150 to 300 mcg/l. For now, we are disregarding the various low reference ranges given by different testing labs. Al reports that after consuming about 10 Brazil nuts daily for the past several months, his white blood count has increased from 3.1 to 4.3. Significantly, a chronic staph infection that he has had in his thumb for the past several years has completely healed. Previously, there was a flare-up of the infection with pus every 2 or 3 months. Several prescriptions of antibiotics failed to permanently eradicate the infection during the past 5 years. Al reports his thumb is now totally healed, he has no fungal or yeast infections, and feels basically normal.

Sterilization of Brazil nuts

Brazil nuts, like peanuts, can become contaminated on the surface with molds and mildew. This can happen, when the nuts stay on the ground for too long before being harvested. Here is how you can remove most of the mold and toxins that may be present:

Place one or two pounds of Brazil nuts into a large sieve or strainer. Pour either of the following solutions over the nuts

a. Two quarts of ozonated water or

b. add 1/4 cup of 3% hydrogen peroxide to 2 quarts of warm water.

Pour either solution over the nuts, stir and mix. Let stand one minute.

Then, pour two quarts of hot tap or boiling water over the nuts to rinse them. Let them drain for two minutes, then -

1. Spread the nuts single layer on a towel on a table. Place a second towel over the nuts to absorb excess moisture. Remove this towel and let air dry for 30 to 60 minutes, or use a hair dryer to dry them in about 5 minutes.

2. Store the nuts in a glass jar in the freezer until ready to use.

June Wiles on selenium (removes tumors)

June Wiles, who teaches the Carey Reams method of diagnosis, writes in a December newsletter that ...

"Selenium will remove ferritin from white blood cells (ferritin helps gobble up asbestos). With ferritin gone asbestos can be gone too - but more importantly, with ferritin gone, phenol and ascaris parasites will be disabled and discarded as well as flushing bacteria and toxins. It may require up to 3000 mcg of (plant-based) selenium daily to unload the enemy. Fresh coconut meat for four days will help with removal of all ascaris. Using 1000 mcg of selenium per day for 3 to 6 months may also assist removal of tumors."

June Wiles - ph no. 813-977-1000

Animal studies that used the equivalent of 3700 mcg of selenium daily in humans stopped several types of cancer.

A book by John Boik, "Natural Compounds in Cancer Therapy," is, in my opinion, one of the most carefully researched books on natural cancer treatments ever written. It is published by Oregon Medical Press LLC., 315 10th Ave N, Princeton, MN 55371 763-389-0768. www.ompress.com.

The book has the endorsement of six medical doctors, five of whom are oncologists who specialize in cancer therapy. This book likely has more scientific analysis of natural therapies for cancer than any other that has been published to date. The 500 plus pages covers a wide range of topics and is supported by good clinical and scientific data. What a great treasure house of information. I highly recommend it for the health care professional, the informed public, and certainly friends of cancer victims. In a nutshell, here is what Boik states about the action of selenium in preventing or treating cancer:

"Selenium induces apoptosis at the cellular level, inhibits PKC, inhibits NF-KB/AP-1 activity, improves cell to cell communication, inhibits angiogenisis, inhibits histamine, inhibits tumor necrosis factor, inhibits VEGF effects, inhibits insulin resistance, inhibits invasion and metastasis, inhibits collagenase effects and supports the immune system."

At the average equivalent of 3700 mcg daily, Boik cites scientific studies that, in animals, selenium inhibited metastasis of melanoma cells, Ehrlich ascites cells in mice, several different cancer cell lines, brain cancer, some types of leukemia, breast cancer and lung cancer. Other researchers have found selenium inhibits prostate cancer.

In support of the position that sodium selenite, the inorganic form, should not be used as a dietary supplement, Boik states that the sodium selenite has been "reported to cause DNA strand breaks in cancer cells in vitro, probably via free radicals and/or SAM deficiency, and to induce p53 dependent apoptosis. In contrast, methylselenocysteine and organic related forms act through a different means: they appear to induce apoptosis, independent of DNA damage and p53 activity."

Boik also states: "Of the organic forms, methylselenocysteine, and selenomethionine are among those causing the least adverse effects at high doses, since they can be converted directly to methylselenol without methyl donors......Methylselenol is of prime importance to us, since this form seems to be responsible for selenium's anticancer effects in vivo."

Our caveat on buying any product that is called "Selenium"

Update: September, 2002: We now have 14 cases, where "Selenium" dietary supplements claiming to contain L-selenomethionine, have failed to provide any benefits, with half the persons using it reporting adverse side effects. One source told us that to sell selenium for under $2 a bottle, manufacturers have resorted to using the cheapest raw materials they can find and mixing in inorganic selenium and water and then spray drying it. No wonder these "amino acid chelates" are not working because they really are not what they claim to be – amino acid chelates. The real amino acid chelates are produced by nature and found only in plants. The synthesized versions made in labs are not only ineffective, they are not safe to use.

Unfortunately, the vitamin discount houses are peddling this junk to the public on television and on the Internet, and telling people how much money they are saving. Saving money they are, but getting a selenium supplement that is safe and effective they are not. So far, two persons, who have used man-made L-selenomethionine, have had transitory strokes. These serious side effects occurred with doses ranging from 900 to 1600 mcg daily. Fortunately, both have recovered completely and are now using plant-based selenium supplements with no side effects.

In well over 20 recent cases, the plant based sources of selenium (Bio-Active Selenium and SelenoMax) have completely resolved many cases of long standing of candidiasis, have reduced fatigue, increased T cell counts and WBCs, restored the ability to sweat and restored pure whiteness to the whites of the eyes. Not one case of adverse effects has been reported in the past year from using plant based selenium supplements at dosages up to 1800 mcg daily.

An Albion employee admission on their selenium product

Nov 19, 2002. I found an advertisement for Albion Amino Acid chelates in a Health Supplement Retailer magazine (Vol 8, No 12). The ad stated "Nobody talks CHELATES like Albion CHELATES" and goes on to make the following claims: "Albion's patented chelation processes form mineral compounds that have a multitude of advantages! Nutritionally functional, Kosher-Parve, Chemically Validated, CAS Registered and Clinically Proven." I went to their website at www.albion-an.com and looked for the clinical data and test results on their selenium amino acid chelate (L-selenomethionine). There was data on iron, zinc and some of the other amino acid chelates but I could find nothing on selenium so I called them at 1-586-774-9055. A female employee answered the phone.

She, herself, did not know where to find the information about selenium on the company website, but said a company technician who could help me was at a meeting. I told her I wanted to see the test results and clinical data on L-selenomethionine, an amino-acid chelate that they manufactured. She then said that it was not actually an amino acid chelate but a "complex." She added: "For various technical reasons, we have not been able to make amino acid chelates with selenium, boron or potassium." I said: "That is interesting. I understand that a "complex" is a mixture of an inorganic mineral with an amino acid." She replied: "that is correct." I was so stunned by her admission that I forgot to ask her name before I hung up the phone. In fact, one place on the Albion website they boast that they do not make proteinates or "complexes" (mixtures of inorganic minerals and amino acids) but true structural amino acid chelates.

I am aware of at least one major dietary supplement manufacturer (Futurebiotics) that sells selenium as an "amino acid chelate" made by Albion labs and calls it L-selenomethionine and not what it really is – an inorganic selenium in a base of L-methionine. Right now, there are millions of bottles of selenium described as L-seleno-methionine, from numerous dietary supplement manufacturers on store shelves that are mislabeled and misbranded. In December 2002, I even sent the company an e-mail about the safety questions raised from the use of their product and reported on the two persons who claim it caused them to get a transitory stroke. Albion has not replied to my e-mail.

3
The immune system cure for candidiasis

Selenium + cysteine restores glutathione and neutrophil function leading to destruction of candida albicans

Candidiasis is an invasive colonization of a type of fungal infection called "candida albicans." Symptoms of Candidiasis are sore or burning tongue, sore or white spots in the mouth, indigestion, flatulence (gas) with a strong cheese odor, bloating, insomnia, night sweats, diarrhea, uncontrollable sugar cravings, lactose intolerance, food allergies, a feeling of sickness all over the body, fatigue, mental depression, flaking or peeling skin, thick throat sensation or difficulty in swallowing, athlete's foot, jock itch and vaginitis.

Causes of Candidiasis, or contributing factors are recurring yeast infections, which commonly occurs in persons with chronic infections that deplete glutathione levels; use of antibiotics and steroids, prolonged stress, malnutrition, malabsorption, and low Neutrophil, macrophage and Natural Killer function. This could indicate a chronic underlying infection with HHV-6A, or any other viral infections that steal selenium from the host and binds it to viral receptors. Note: HIV has one selenium receptor.

Food preservatives, sugar and alcohol consumption and lack of exercise are also contributing factors. The depletion of selenium levels weakens the cell-mediated immune response of the host against 0invading pathogens. The B vitamin Biotin is helpful in treating candidiasis as it keeps candida albicans in a single cell state.

Do you have candidiasis?

(Score Points)
1. Have you taken antibiotics within the past year?..20
2. Do you presently have any of the following symptoms – athlete's foot, jock itch or vaginitis?...20
3. Do you have a sore or burning tongue?..20
4. Do you have small white spots or patches in the mouth area with swollen and sore tissue around them?..40
5. Do you have almost continuous foul smelling lower intestinal gas?...............................20
6. Do you have bloating and/or upper intestinal gas?..10
7. Do you have indigestion frequently?...10
8. Do you have severe insomnia? (can't sleep for more than a few hours at a time)............20
9. Do you wake up sweating at night?...10
10. Do you have strong cravings for sweets or lactose containing dairy products like milk, cheese and ice cream?..20
11. Do you frequently get hives or rashes?..10
12. Do you have a lot of allergies?...20

13. Do you usually find it difficult to breathe through your nose?..10
14. Do you feel sick all over and don't know the cause?...20
15. Do you feel tired and fatigued most of the day?...20
16. Do you feel severely depressed at times?...10
17. Do you find your memory failing you frequently?...10
18. Do you have visual disturbances?...10
19. Do you crave alcoholic beverages?..10
20. Does tobacco smoke really bother you?...10
21. Do you have a loss of sexual drive?...10
22. Do you have crying attacks?..10
23. Do you have rectal itching or nasal itching?..10
24. Do you have severe itching skin?..20
25. Do you feel a burning sensation when you urinate?...10

The total grand score is 350

If your score is less than 60, yeast infection is most likely not a problem for you at this time. If your score is over 60 and less than 90, yeast overgrowth may be a problem. If your score is over 90, yeast overgrowth most certainly is a problem that must be addressed. The higher your score over 90, the more serious the problem.

Selenium and glutathione levels linked to neutrophil function and Candidiasis

From an immunological perspective, we have learned several factors that adversely affect candida and fungal overgrowth. They are CD4's with a TH2 response; lack of neutrophil function; lack of CD8 Cytotoxic Lymphocytes, and lack of Natural Killer (NK) cell function.

Some people have spent several years on a diet of meats and vegetables and avoiding grains and fruit as it causes a flare-up of candida albicans, food allergies and environmental sensitivities. In plain English, these normal wholesome foods are making people sick. These people are deprived of carbohydrates for years, and also suffer from intestinal dysbiosis and depression, due to low serotonin and endorphin levels. Carbohydrates are needed to support serotonin and endorphin levels in the brain. Fatigue, intolerance to carbohydrates and chronic insomnia are all part of the syndrome of chronic candidiasis and chronic fatigue syndrome. Restoring the health of the immune system runs parallel to restoring intestinal health and normal levels of ionic calcium and trace minerals that will resolve other problem areas.

Researchers have found an immune system defect that allows Candidiasis and fungal infections to multiply, with little opposition from the immune system. This defect is caused by Neutrophil inactivity (Anergy). Normally, Neutrophils keep yeast and fungal infection under control. The anergy of this non-specific effector white blood cell is caused by a deficiency of the two substances that control intracellular glutathione levels. Those two substances are Selenium and L-Cysteine or its more bioavailable form – N-Acetyl Cysteine (NAC). The following studies show that selenium is a key nutrient in the control of Candida

Albicans. Here are some excerpts:

"The effects of selenium deficiency on the responses to Candida albicans infection were examined in mice. When selenium-deficient mice and selenium-supplemented mice were given i.v. injections of 0.1 ml suspensions of 1X10(5) or 5X10(4) C. albicans in 0.9% sterile saline, deaths in the selenium-deficient animals started after 2.5 to 3.5 days compared with 7 to 8.5 days in the selenium-supplemented animals. Further studies demonstrated that 3 days after an i.v. injection of 1X10(5) C. albicans, significantly more of the microorganisms were found in the kidneys (P less than 0.001,) livers (P less than 0.025) and spleens (P less than 0.01) of the selenium-deficient mice, compared with the same organs of the selenium-supplemented animals. Selenium deficiency was also demonstrated to impair the ability of mouse neutrophils to kill C. albicans in in-vitro tests." (1) This excerpt was from the Journal of Nutrition.

In an experiment in rats, Boyne, Arthur and Wilson found that "Selenium deficiency in rats impairs the ability of neutrophils and peritoneal macrophages to kill Candida albicans organisms in vitro." (2)

In India, Kukreja and Khan reported that "The role of selenium in the diet of rats has been examined with respect to the Neutrophil function. Feeding of Se-deficient diet for 75 days resulted in reduction in candidcidal activity, superoxide production, oxygen consumption, glucose utilization and glutathione peroxidase activity. Supplementing the diet with Selenium for 30 days resulted in partial restoration of all the activities. (3)

Consider the millions of people, who have been, and are today, suffering from the overgrowth of candida albicans and other yeast and fungal infections. Very few of these people know, or have been told, that selenium supplementation is absolutely crucial for their recovery. Last week a reader, who started taking selenium supplementation reported on our Message Board that it has cleared up the coating on his tongue. The coating may be due to yeast overgrowth and lymphatic congestion. Several people who have started on higher doses of selenium (800 to 1200 mcg daily of high-selenium yeast or high-selenium mustard greens) have reported the candidiasis is rapidly going away, and that many food allergies and intolerances are being reduced each day. They also report that the whites of their eyes are now a bright white, instead of being gray or yellow in color.

A gray tinge is often seen in elderly people due to overall buildup of toxins in the blood and the yellow tinge in the whites of the eyes is often due to elevated liver enzymes. The white part of the eyes is a very bright white as seen in young healthy growing children. Is it not rewarding to see tangible results when using selenium – tongue clearer, eyes that sparkle and the whites that are bright?

Glucose (sugar) has been found to suppress the anti-candida activity of neutrophils. Supplementation with Cysteine and Methionine in rats reversed the suppression of Neutrophil activity against the Candida Albicans (1). Cysteine binds with selenium to help produce glutathione peroxidase, which increases the functional activity of neutrophils, free macrophages and the Natural Killer (NK) cells. Here is what Tancho found from testing various groups of amino acids for their effect in promoting the anti-candida activity of neutrophils.

"In all groups tested, amino acids containing cysteine and methionine clearly neutralized the suppression, especially cysteine, at the concentration of more than 20 mcg/ml significantly recovered the anti-Candida activity of neutrophils, which were suppressed in the presence of 1% glucose. Correspondingly, cysteine augmented production of lactoferrin by stimulated neutrophils; which functions as a major effector molecule in growth inhibition of Candida by neutrophils. These results suggest that cysteine in alimentation solution augments anti-Candida defense mechanisms through recovery of Neutrophil function." (4).

As we can see the beneficial effects of methionine, cysteine and selenium in promoting the anti-Candida activity of neutrophils, it makes sense to consume foods naturally high in these substances.

References:
1. The Response of selenium-deficient mice to Candida albicans infection – by Boyne and Arthur. J Nutr 1986 May;116(5):816-22
2. An in vivo and in vitro study of elenite deficiency and infection in rats – by Boyne, Arthur and Wilson. J Comp Pathol 1986 Jul;96(4):379-86
3. Effect of experimental selenium deficiency and its supplementation on the candidcidal activity of neutrophils in albino rats, by Kukreja and Khan. Indian J Biochem Biophys 1994 Oct; 31(5):427-9
4. Reverting effect of cysteine on the suppression by glucose...of anti-Candida activity of human neutrophils, by Tansho. Kansenshogaku Zasshi. 1998 Jul;72(7):727-37

Lack of L-glutathione induces TH2 responses

The value of restoring intracellular Glutathione levels on antigen processing and presentation and activating CD8 CTL's was reported in Positive Health News, Report No 16. Glutathione has a very important role as an anti-oxidant and removes many toxins from inside the cells. New research indicates that a lack of intracellular glutathione leads antigen-presenting cells to shift from a Th1 to a Th2 cytokine profile, in response to infections.

Peterson JD et al reports: "By using three different methods to deplete glutathione from T cell transgenic and conventional mice, and studying in vivo and/or in vitro responses to three distinct antigens, we show that glutathione levels in antigen-presenting cells determine whether Th1 or Th2 response patterns predominate." (1)

Substances that increase intracellular glutathione levels include alpha lipoic acid, N-Acetyl Cysteine (NAC), organic Selenium (from food sources) and L-glutamine. Alpha Lipoic Acid is found in raw potatoes.

Note: Jerome Deutsch CNC reports from his experience that the most effective form of NAC is time-released. He reports that regular NAC has a half-life of about one hour, and that the timed-release form provides benefits throughout the day, whereas the regular NAC is short-lived. He uses one of two brands. They are "NAC Sustain" by Jarrow Formulas or "Resbid" from Ecological Formulas.

1. Proc Natl Acad Sci USA 1998 Mar 17;95(6):3071-6

The "Cure" for Candidiasis are immune-based therapies that restore immune function

Selenium from plant sources – Use Phytosel (Nucycle – 200 mcg per capsule).. For therapeutic purposes, use 100 to 200 mcg per 20 pounds of body weight each day. Example. If the person weighs 160 lbs, divide by 20 which equals 8. 8 times 100 =800 mcg daily. That would be 2 capsules twice daily and up to 4 capsules twice daily if needed. The high selenium mustard greens contain mostly L-selenocysteine and a lesser amount is bound to methionine.

SelenoMax (high-selenium yeast). Yeast grown in a medium that converts inorganic selenium into mostly natural L-selenomethionine, although there is still some selenium bound to cysteine. Source Naturals and some other companies distribute this brand called SelenoMax. It is a high quality product that also comes in 200 mcg tablets. Note: if you have an allergy to yeast then use the Bio-Active Selenium. Eating 3 or 4 Brazil Nuts daily can add another 300 to 400 mcg of selenium to your daily diet. Each Brazil Nut contains on average about 100 mcg organic selenium.

Suggestion: If you are not allergic to yeast, you can use both products. Take one of each two or three times each day.

NAC Sustain (by Jarrow Formulas or Resbid by Ecological Formulas. Both products are a timed-release form of NAC that produces very good results. Jerry Deutsch CNC, who has compared regular NAC to the time released forms, as in Resbid or NAC Sustain, and states; "the time-released forms are 4 to 6 times more effective than the regular forms of NAC." According to Jerry Deutsch, L-Cysteine and NAC have a half life of about one hour. He has tested both types of NAC (regular and time released) in persons with low glutathione levels and chronic fatigue and found that patients reported a sustained benefit all day with the time-released formulas. In persons under chronic immune challenge, he uses only the time-released N, Acetyl Cysteine or NAC, the most bio-active form of Cysteine. Take one tablet once a day or one tablet twice daily, spaced about 8 hours apart. I would advise against using more than 1000 to 1200 mg of NAC daily (about 2 tablets) for long term use.

Alternative sources of Cysteine: Aged Kyolic Garlic extract, Formula 100. Use 8 capsules twice a day. This is a great product that a controlled study found restored Natural Killer cell function in about 6 weeks. Ion exchange membrane filtered whey products like Immunocal and ImmunePro – use as directed.

Other supplements that help increase Glutathione levels include Silymarin (200 to 400 mg daily), IP6 (4 to 6 grams daily), L-Glutamine and Alpha Lipoic Acid – food source – raw potatoes or (consider an ALA dissolved in oil as in thiogel www.thiogel.com).

Beta 1 3 D glucan helps improve macrophage funciton and has helped a number of people control candidiasis. Dose 100 to 500 mg daily.

The importance of avoiding synthetic selenium compounds

These include any dietary supplements simply called "Selenium" and containing any of the following substances: sodium selenite, sodium elenite, L-selenomethionine or selenium aspartate. Sodium selenite and elenite are beneficial and effectively assimilated, but have adverse effects at doses over 500 mcg daily. At 1000 mcg daily, your hair may start to fall out, so avoid these supplements in the h igher dosage range. L-selenomethionine and selenium aspartate are made in a laboratory and in 14 cases I have followed, failed to provide any benefits. Two out of 14 persons using L-selenomethionine developed numbness on the right side of their bodies, and had to discontinue using the product. The symptoms cleared in a few days.

Five other persons also reported side effects from using synthetic L-selenomethionine, that included feeling ill, nausea and skin eruptions. The problem is that dietary supplements called "L-selenomethioine are not that. They are simply a mixture of inorganic selenium with L-methionine and water and spray dried. The reason these kinds of selenium compounds are sold by many discount houses is that they are cheaply made and the public buys them, not knowing that they don't work and may even have harmful side effects. Unfortunately, there is no present law against manufacturers selling dietary supplements that are neither safe nor effective. The immune system cure for Candidiasis also requires the restoration of normal thyroid function. See related chapter in this book.

Other helpful treatments for Candidiasis

Fiber/Pectin/probiotic blend. Be sure that the probiotics include L Salivarius, which may also be added to water and used as a douche for vaginitis or yeast in the colon.

The most effective herbs for Candidiasis are Oregamax (wild crafted oregano), Lomatium Dissectum (LDM-100), Venus Fly-trap extract and raw garlic, caprylic acid (Kaprystatin and Caprycidin from Ecological Formulas). Caprylic acid is found in coconut oil.

Oregamax – use 2 or 3 capsules 3 times a day. Lomatium Dissectum or Venus fly-trap extract – 40 drops in water 3 times daily. Raw garlic – eat 1 clove sliced on rye crisp 3 to 4 times daily. Eat parsley with it to deodorize the effects of the garlic.

The following 3 herbs, taken together, are also beneficial – White Oak Bark, Mathake and Pure Purple Lapacho. Use one teaspoon of each or one tea bag of each. Drink 3 cups times a day. Diflucan, available from your physician, is used for thrush and yeast infections, as is Nystatin. Bee Propolis also kills yeast infections.

No treatment for yeast overgrowth, including ozone therapy, will last very long, if you have depleted glutathione levels. White sugar or corn syrup found in processed pastry, candy bars, soda depresses neutrophil and macrophage function, needed to control fungal infections. The diet plan in this book is helpful for long-term relief. To reduce sugar cravings, take Chromium Picolinate – 100 mcg twice a day or Hypo-Ade, by Enzymatic Therapy – 1 tablet twice a day. If you bite the sides of your cheeks, this could be due to facial swelling, caused by candida overgrowth in the head. The spice "Thyme" will kill candida in the head. "Fenu-Thyme" by Nature's Way is highly recommended. Dosage: 3 capsules three times a day.

In most cases, taking 800 to 1200 mcg daily of organic food based selenium will eliminate candidiasis within a few weeks, and then you can enjoy carbohydrates again.

Colon Cleansing – Colonic – weekly, then drink cultured cabbage juice daily. Give yourself enemas with garlic, vinegar and chlorophyll added on a daily basis or as needed.

Mouth rinse – gargle with 3% hydrogen peroxide. Rinse mouth with clear water. This may be repeated 3 to 5 times a day as needed. Colloidal silver also kills most yeast infections. Grapefruit seed extract also kills candida but is very acidifying to the system and should not be used continuously.

Probiotics: Use L-Plantarum, B Longum, L Salivarius and Acidophilus. Raw shiitake mushrooms – 2 or 3 daily eaten raw or use shiitake capsules.

The role of HHV-6 in AIDS, CFIDS and Candidiasis

Robert Gallo discovers HHV-6

In 1986, Robert Gallo, while doing research at the National Institute of Health, discovered a new virus, shortly after his meetings with John Beldekas, on the possible role of the African Swine Fever Virus (ASFV) in HIV/AIDS. Gallo and the NIH dismissed Beldekas's research on ASFV, while never attempting to explain why antibodies to ASFV showed up in 9 AIDS patients.

A few months after Beldekas's presentation, Gallo discovered a new virus that he called Human B cell Lymphotropic Virus or HBLV. The name means that HBLV likes to infect B cells, a factor that it has in common with other herpes viruses and even ASFV. A few months later he named it "Human Herpes Virus 6" or HHV-6, the name that survives to this day.

As for Beldekas's research, the positive antibody test in the 9 AIDS patients for ASFV may have resulted from a cross reaction with HHV-6 co-infection in these same AIDS patients, giving a false reading for ASFV. Another example of cross-reactivity is when a person is inoculated for Rabies and then gives a false antibody positive test result for HIV although never exposed to the HIV virus. This happened in one Florida case that led to a lawsuit.

Texas physician finds HHV-6 in 98% of her AIDS patients

Dr. Patricia Salvato MD (Houston, TX) found that 98% of her patients, who had full-blown AIDS, also had HHV-6 by PCR amplification. This does not mean the other 2% were not also infected with HHV-6, as the blood sample may not have had the presence of the virus that was elsewhere in the patient (i.e. lymph system). Antibody tests for HHV-6A are not 100% accurate. It is well known that some persons testing negative for the HIV antibody that are actually infected with HIV. In July 1997, I asked Konstance Knox and Donald Carrigan if they had found HHV-6A in all of the AIDS patients, in which they had done lymph node biopsies. They told that they found the variant A strain of HHV-6 in 23 out of 23 cases. As of 1999, this number has grown to 28 out of 28 cases. They also told me that in examining tissues of deceased AIDS patients, they found that HHV-6A was widely disseminated and had done all of the cellular destruction in the lymph nodes.

AIDS patient has flare-up in KS lesions after eating pork

In Dec.1995, I had a discussion with a PWA from Rio Rancho, NM, who has Kaposi

Sarcoma. At the time, he told me that on three occasions, when he ate pork, he had a flare-up and growth in his KS lesions. He did not get this effect from beef, turkey or chicken. He said: "when I eat pork, the KS goes wild." He was not aware that research by Gallo and others has shown the presence of HHV-6A in KS lesions, although since then, HHV-8 has been implicated in KS. This virus likes pork. HHV-8, widely reported in KS lesions, may be a variant strain of HHV-6A.

Chocolate may increase herpes and HHV-6 replication

A client of Dr. Patricia Salvato MD has reported that she has advised all her AIDS and CFS patients not to eat chocolate, as it will increase HHV-6 viral activity. Herpes Zoster virus and Epstein Barr Virus (EBV) as well as HHV-6 that live in the B cells. The free form amino acid - L-Arginine can stimulate herpes viruses into activity when other conditions like elevated interleukin-6 levels are also present. Chocolate contains high concentrations of this free form amino acid. Several persons who have AIDS or Chronic Fatigue Syndrome (CFS) have reported extreme fatigue associated when eating chocolate candy bars although the sugar in the candy bars may also be a contributing factor. Whether Carob is an effective substitute is unknown at this time.

Note: In support of chocolate, when the herpes virus is not active, the L-Arginine in chocolate can actually improve thymus function and the anti-oxidants in chocolate can protect cells from free radicals. Also chocolate added to milk neutralizes the adverse effects of lactose. When Herpes type viruses including CMV, EBV or HHV-6 are dormant or inactive, chocolate does have to be avoided.

Gallo and Carrigan on HHV-6

Dr. Robert Gallo, in his article on "Disseminated Human Herpes Virus 6 Infection in AIDS," stated "this concept, which has gained additional ground, is primarily based on the frequent isolation of HHV-6 from AIDS patients and its ability to infect and kill CD4 T cells, and on the demonstration of several unique interactions between HHV-6 and HIV."

A growing body of scientific research by Robert Gallo, Donald Carrigan and others indicate that HHV-6 (A) can infect and disrupt the function of B cells and at least one weaker subset of NK cells. According to Carrigan, HHV-6A stops B cells from maturing into plasma cells. Plasma cells produce antibodies.

Gallo found a subset of NK cells that was immune from attack by HHV-6A. This subset of NK cells was capable of destroying other immune cells infected with HHV-6A.

HHV-6A activates HIV infection of CD8 cells and B cells

In Dec 1995, I ran a computer search for HHV-6 on AIDSLINE at the National Library of Medicine and retrieved several articles. One abstract by P Lusso et al (Int. AIDS Conf, Jun 1991) showed why HIV is more dangerous in the presence of HHV-6A. HHV-6A causes many more immune cells, besides the CD4 cell, to present the CD4 receptor on their membrane, that makes the other immune cells also subject to infection by HIV. Like HIV,

HHV-6A also uses the same CD4 receptor to invade immune cells. The immune cells with the CD4 receptor may be invaded by both HIV and HHV-6A at the same time, using different CD4 receptors.

Of HIV in the presence of HHV-6A, Lusso wrote: "Since CD4 is the receptor for HIV-1, HHV-6 may thus broaden the cellular host-range of HIV-1, favoring its spread in co-infected patients." What Lusso is saying is that HIV, in the presence of HHV-6, is invasive of many more immune cells than without HHV-6.

Several authors, including Gallo, have published scientific reports that did not specify if the HHV-6 virus they were referring to was strain variant A or B. This has caused some confusion in the scientific community. However, several scientific journals, where articles were published, have identified HHV-6 (A) as being either of the following isolates: U1102 or GS. One Abstract cited U1102 as a HHV-6, variant A, isolate from a Ugandan AIDS patient. References to U1102 as being a strain of HHV-6A have been published in the following medical journals:

1. J. Virol. 1995, Aug; by Araujo JC et al
2. Virology, 1995, May; by UA Gompels et al
3. J. Virol Methods., 1995, Feb.; by L Foa-Tomasi et al
4. J. Immunology, 1994, Jun.; by M Furukawa et al
5. Virology, 1994, May; by F Kashanchi et al
6. Oncogene, 1994, Apr; by J. Thompson et al
7. J. Virol. 1993, Aug; by B Pfeffer at al
8. J. Med. Virol, 1992, Aug; by B Chandran et al
9. Int. AIDS Conf, 1994. by K Yamanishi et al.

HHV-6A may be a co-factor in AIDS progression

In the Journal of Acquir Immune Defic Syndr Hum Retroviral, 1996, Apr 1:11(4):370-8, Konstance Knox and Donald Carrigan, of the Medical College of Wisconsin, published the following findings:

"Studies published previously by this laboratory have demonstrated that patients with AIDS have widely disseminated, active infections with HHV-6 at the time of their death (Lancet, March 5, 1994). However, it remains unclear when, in the course of the human immunodeficiency virus (HIV) infection, the active HHV-6 infection first appears. To address this question, lymph node biopsies from 10 HIV-infected persons were analyzed for active human herpesvirus 6 (HHV-6) infections by immunohistochemical staining....In total, 10 of 10 (100%) of the lymph nodes studied contained cells productively infected with HHV-6; in contrast, three lymph nodes with follicular hyperplasia and four normal lymph nodes from patients not infected with HIV were negative for HHV-6 infection...The variant A strain of HHV-6 was found to be the predominant form of the virus present in the lymph nodes biopsies from all of these HIV-infected patients,... Of special note, the absolute CD4+ lymphocyte counts of 75% of the HIV-infected individuals in the study were > (greater than) 200/mm3, at the time of their lymph node biopsy."

This study by Knox and Carrigan is very significant, as it shows that HHV-6A infection occurs early in AIDS and in persons with CD4 Helper cells above 200, and is not just another opportunistic infection. At least one of the biopsies came from an HIV+ person with over 700 CD4 cells. Jim P. (Milw, WI) told me that in 1990, Dr. Patricia Salvato MD found HHV-6 by PCR when Jim was experiencing hyper-CD4 activation; that is, his CD4 count was over 1400. Equally significant, Knox and Carrigan told me late in July, 1997, that HHV-6A was found in 100% of the lymph node biopsies taken in studies of AIDS patients living as well as those deceased. If it was not found in 100% of the lymph node biopsies examined, then it could be reasonably argued that it was an opportunistic infection, and not the primary AIDS virus. In an earlier article (Lancet, 1994, Mar 5), Knox and Carrigan found "Human herpesvirus 6 (HHV-6) infected cells were detected in all lung, lymph-node, spleen, liver and kidney tissues, obtained at necropsy (death) from an unselected series of nine patients with AIDS."

Knox and Carrigan (Medical College of Wisconsin) have concluded from their probes of the lymph nodes of PWAs, for both HHV-6A and HIV that it is the HHV-6, variant A strain that is destroying the cells, not the HIV. They have observed that HIV gathers outside the follicular dendritic cells in the lymph nodes while HHV-6A eats out and destroys the germinal centers of the lymph nodes. These observations have been also observed in examining lung, brain, liver and kidney tissues. It is the HHV-6A that is causing the cellular destruction, not the HIV. Their findings in this area are also strengthened by studying the two viruses in cell cultures. Robert Gallo reported earlier (ABC News, Dec. 7, 1995): "When you compare the two viruses (HIV and HHV-6) in a laboratory, the most destructive by far is HHV-6."

Where can I learn more about HHV-6?

Anyone with a computer and modem can access AIDSLINE or MEDLINE at the National Library of Medicine at http://igm.nlm.nih.gov/. There, you can find ample published research on the role of HHV-6 in several disease conditions. When you are connected to the National Library of Medicine, run a computer search for "HHV-6," and prepare to receive over 200 abstracts from articles published in medical journals.

Knox and Carrigan have a website with links to over a dozen other websites on the human herpes virus 6 (HHV-6) at www.viracor.com, or you can write to them at Viracor, 1210 NE Windsor Dr, Lees's Summit, MO 64086. Fax 816-347-0143

HHV-6A may be a cause of CFIDS

What does HHV-6A do without HIV? You can look at over one-half million people, sick and debilitated with Chronic Fatigue Immune Dysfunction Syndrome (CFIDS), and infected with HHV-6, variant A and the answer is obvious. While published reports indicate that 70% of CFIDS patients are infected with HHV-6, these numbers are low, because antibody tests for HHV-6 in the blood are only about 50% accurate, and PCR for HHV-6 in the blood are not 100% accurate. This is because HHV-6A infection spreads primarily cell-to-cell. Staining of lymph node biopsies for HHV-6A is a 100% accurate test for the presence for HHV-6, variant A. Unfortunately, this test is not available in many areas.

A CFIDS case report

Ginny Kloth suffered from CFIDS since 1976, when she believes she was infected with HHV-6A from a vaccination for the Swine Flu. Since Oct 1995, after discovering the Keep Hope Alive web page on the INTERNET, she has found benefits from the daily use of the whole lemon/olive oil drink. She started on Naltrexone, a prescription drug that triples Natural Killer cell activity (Dr. Bihari MD., NYC) about March 13, 1996. At the time, her CD4s were 1100; her CD8s were 220 and a CD4/CD8 ratio of 5.0, not a normal 1.8. Ginny had hyper CD4 activation, that is very common in CFIDS patients who also have multiple allergies, chemical sensitivities, and digestive problems. After just 5 weeks on Naltrexone, her CD4/CD8 ratio reversed and her symptoms subsided. On April 26th, 1996, she reported her CD4's were 237 and her CD8s were 1270, a ratio of .19, similar to an AIDS profile. She sent an e-mail message that said her last swollen lymph node was gone. She wrote; "I had to share the good news! I have been calling all my family members. Praise the Lord! I spent all day working...am feeling so good!" (Positive Health News, Report No 11).

Update, Jan 26, 1997: In phone call to Ginny Kloth today, she reported that she has seen over 12 lab reports of CFIDS patients, of which all had a CD4/CD8 ratio in the range of 3.0 to 6.0. CD4's are above normal, and CD8s are way below normal. All these patients are reporting multiple allergies, chemical sensitivities and digestive disorders. Three had wasting syndrome and were continuing to lose weight. Ginny also found in all these cases elevated CD26+ several times above normal. Her research found that elevated levels of CD26+ are related to a type of lymphoma called mycosis fungoides.

Several CFIDS patients have contacted Keep Hope Alive within the past and reported symptomatic relief, using Naltrexone, the lemon/olive oil drink, low-dose hydrocortisone, the immune enhancement diet from my book and Beta 1, 3 glucan supplements. John Dettling is a CFIDS patient of Dr. Patricia Salvato (Houston, TX). In a phone call to me, John said Dr. Salvato is giving him injections of L-Glutathione with ATP (adenosine triphosphate) and said she claims an 80% success rate in treating CFIDS. John is currently 36 lbs underweight - has wasting syndrome and is HIV negative.

Recently, John Dettling added immune based and nutritional protocols to his daily regimen. He reports weight gain and other areas of improvement in his health and well-being. He can be reached by e-mail at dettling@tenet.edu

HHV-6A impairs antigen presentation and NK cell function

The Dendritic Antigen Presenting cells (APCs) present antigen (a foreign invader or substance) to the CD4 cells that either signal the B cells to produce antibodies (A TH2 CD4 type response) or signals the CD8 CTLs to kill the infected cells (A TH1 CD4 type response). As Donald Carrigan pointed out, "Without the dendritic antigen presenting cells, the CD4s don't know what to do." Monocytes and Macrophages also present antigen, but both of these subsets of white blood cells are also infected by HHV-6A, and their ability to present antigen is also impaired.

An antigen presented to a CD4 cell could be a particular foreign protein that is part of a virus, such as P24, a key viral protein for HIV or a viral protein on HHV-6. The CD4 cells look at the antigen and decide if it is friend or foe (self or non-self). Antigen presentation is

done by Antigen Presenting Cells (APCs). These include dendritic cells primarily and also monocytes and macrophages. If the CD4 recognizes the antigen is from a friend (self) it signals the APC to let it go. If it is an alien (non-self), it signals a cell-mediated immune (C.M.I.) response (to kill the infected cell), or a humoral (antibody) response. These conferences between CD4s and APCs are usually done in the lymph nodes (the Courthouse). Antigen Presenting Cells are like Policemen picking up prisoners (viruses etc) and the CD4s are like the judges. CD4s either signal the APCs to let their prisoners go or execute them and other look-a-like viruses. However, Dendritic cells are infected with both HHV-6A and HIV. This raises a question whether HHV-6A contains genes that suppress the cell-mediated immune response (antigen presentation).
1. Canals A et al; Arch Virol 1995;140(6):1075-85
2. Gregg DA et al; J Vet Diagn Invest 1995 Jan;7(1):44-51 and 23-30.

HHV-6A retinitis - eye "floaters" in CFIDS

An article was published in Invest. Ophthalmol. Vis. Science, …36:2040, 1995 by Qavi, Hamida, Green, Lewis, Hollinger, Pearson and Ablashi on " HIV-1 and HHV-6 Antigens and Transcripts in Retinas of Patients with AIDS in the absence of Cytomegalovirus." The article was reviewed by Neenyah Ostrom in the New York Native, in Oct 1995. Ostrom writes: "Powerful evidence has just been published suggesting that Human Herpes Virus 6 (HHV-6) may be a frequent cause of vision loss, suffered by more than half of all AIDS patients. Although most eye disease has been attributed to cytomegalovirus (CMV) infection, it now appears that, along with the identification of HHV-6 as the most common infection found in AIDS patients, HHV-6 may in addition be causing a significant percentage of the AIDS retinitis, formerly blamed solely on CMV."

In CFIDS, several persons have told me of having a significant amount of "eye floaters." Whether the eye floaters are directly related to active HHV-6A, CMV or to oxidative stress, or both, remains to be determined. Some persons with AIDS or CFIDS have reported a twitching eyelid syndrome and/or the feeling like something is poking them in the eye (HHV6-A activity?)

HHV-6 infection in chronic candidiasis

Where chronic yeast infections continue to reoccur, when carbohydrates are consumed, an underlying infection with HHV-6A should be suspected, and tests for the virus and its activity should be undertaken. While many cases of chronic yeast infection can be traced to over use of antibiotics or steroids, or over consumption of simple sugars (white sugar, corn syrup etc), when the consumption of complex carbohydrates, such as beans and whole grains cause illness, HHV-6 may have an underlying role.

The treatment of HHV-6 infection and candidiasis

The immune-based treatment for HHV-6 is the same as the treatment for Candidiasis: Selenium (organic from plant sources only). For activation of Neutrophils, macrophages and

Natural Killer cells, organic selenium activates these immune cells by increasing intracellular Glutathione levels. Diet: Pork needs to be avoided, and chocolate and sugar can activate herpes infections.

The natural plant based sources of selenium (from mustard greens or yeast) can be used in higher doses, 800 to 1200 mcg daily, without any known adverse effects. Usually, about 800 mcg of the plant based selenium used daily is sufficient to restore Neutrophil function and resolve Candida Albican and fungal infections in a few weeks. Body temperature increases and sweating resumes. Low body temperature and lack of ability to sweat are common factors in persons with CFIDS, HHV-6 infection, Candidiasis and Cancer.

Interleukin-6 inhibitors – low-dose hydrocortisone, fish oil, Royal Jelly, cayenne and others

Naltrexone – 3- to 4.5 mg daily to enhance Natural Killer cell function.

Selenium – natural (Phytosel) – 400 mcg 2 or 3 tjmes daily. (i.e. Brazil nuts)

L Cysteine (raw and undenatured). Try undenatured whey protein, like Immunocal, ImmunoPro, or aged garlic extract (Kyolic Formula 100), raw onions, raw garlic, sprouted seeds and nuts.

Lomatium Dissectum or Oregamax – use as directed to kill herpes viruses.

Whole Lemon/olive oil drink, once a day, OR Mango/Lemon drink (see chapter on free radicals).

BHT - 250 mg daily – an antioxidant to inactivate herpes

Prescription Drugs to treat herpes viruses: Valtrex? Consult with your physician.

5
The immune response in AIDS and CFIDS

The "AIDS Research Alliance" bombshell

In the winter 98/99 edition of Searchlight, the official publication of AIDS Research Alliance of West Hollywood, CA, there is an article by Andrew Korotzer, Ph.D. titled "The Gut Reaction to HIV." Korotzer cites research in 3 major scientific publications (1,2,3), including "Nature's Medicine," "AIDS" and the "Proceedings of the National Academy of Sciences," that indicates about 14% of HIV replication occurs in the blood, while 86% occurs the mucosal membranes of the intestinal tract and in the lymph nodes. IN OTHER WORDS, AIDS IS NOT PRIMARILY A DISEASE OF THE BLOOD, BUT RATHER OF THE GUT AND THE LYMPH NODES! These findings have profound implications in designing future treatments for HIV, by focusing anti-viral therapy on the areas where the highest concentrations of HIV is found - the intestinal tract and the lymphatic system.

1. Dianzani F et al. Nature Medicine (1996) 2:832
2. Fackler O.T. et al. AIDS (1998) 12:139-146
3. Pantaleo G. et al. Nature (1993) 362:355-358
4. Wong J.K. et al. Proc. Natl. Acad Sci USA (1997) 94:12574-12579.

Korotzer states: "Mucosal membranes in the rectum and the urogenital tracts serve as entry points for sexually transmitted HIV; therefore, viral dynamics in these tissues are particularly relevant to the etiology of HIV/IDS. This holds true even for lymphoid tissue in mucosal membranes, when the initial infection occurs elsewhere. SIV, a virus related to HIV that infects monkeys, will become established in GALT (Gut-Associated Lymphoid Tissue) within days of infection - even when the virus was inoculated intravenously. This highlights the special vulnerability of GALT to infection with HIV."

Korotzer cites 3 factors that make the mucosal membranes of the gut vulnerable to HIV infection. They are (1). the presence of a large population of activated CD4 helper cells (2). mucosal membranes in the gut transporting digested food material into the body for evaluation by immune cells and 3. surface molecules that HIV uses as a point to gain entry into the cells (i.e. CD4s) that are highly expressed in the gut making them vulnerable to infection.

Interferon-gamma blocks HIV-1 infection in colon epithelial cells

France: Tantini, Yahi and de Micco reported that human cells from the mucus membranes of the colon (large intestines), called HT29 cells, pretreated with gamma interferon at 100 U/ml, was sufficient to block their infection with HIV-1 and HIV-2 isolates. They concluded that "IFN-gamma, at a concentration compatible with clinical use, has a potent anti-HIV effect on human colon epithelial cells. Therefore, this cytokine should be tested for the prevention and treatment of gastrointestinal disorders with HIV-1 or HIV-2 infection." (1)

1. Int AIDS conf. 1993 Jun 6-11;9(1):171 (abstract no PO-A13-0221)

Stress and the immune response in digestion

CD4 and many other types of white blood cells are in the intestines to inspect and determine the safety of the byproducts of digestion. Proteins and other nutrients, that are not properly digested, are attacked by the immune system, when they get past the mucus membranes. Hence, the importance of eating foods in a way to assist in their complete digestion, that is, eating slowly and mixing a lot of saliva with each mouthful. The use of cultured, fermented, raw or living foods high in natural digestive enzymes, or the taking of supplemental enzymes, will assist in the digestion process. When you combine poor digestion with leaky gut syndrome caused by Candida Albican overgrowth, you have a combination that causes serious stress on the immune system and weakens the capacity of the immune system to deal effectively with infectious organisms elsewhere in the body.

This stress is further exacerbated when the mucus membranes are weak and there is a failure of mucosal immunity (i.e.. lack of IgA and CD8 cytotoxic lymphocytes in the mucosal membranes). These factors, that can stress the immune response, occur not only in HIV infection, but also in HHV-6A, CFIDS, Candidiasis, Hepatitis, GWS, cancer and in persons with allergies and multiple chemical sensitivities.

Lower CD4s in the blood linked to HIV infection of the gut

While it is well known that HIV preferentially infects activated CD4 cells, Korotzer reports, that because CD4 cells in the lamina propria of the gut are highly activated, they present surface molecules that make them very susceptible to infection by HIV. The lamina propria are under a single layer of mucus membrane called epithelial cells. Korotzer reports that HIV clings to a type of cell in the mucus membranes called "M" cells and the M cells are thought to present antigen to the CD4 helper cells in the lamina propria. He states:

"M cells are the cell type within the epithelium thought to be responsible for the transport and presentation of antigen to lymphoid cells within. Lymphocytes migrate towards the M cells to become educated about the material the gut is being exposed to. Many of these lymphocytes are the activated helper T cells that are particularly vulnerable to infection with HIV. HIV can adhere to the surface of M cells, and it is possible that T cells inside the gut mucosa become infected when they migrate out to meet M cells."

Korotzer continues:

"there is a selective loss of CD4+ helper T cells within the lamina propria, and there are indications that helper T cells are depleted in the lamina propria before there is loss detected in the blood."

Korotzer raises two questions in conclusion to his article on "Whole-body viral burden.' They are (1). Does HIV viral replication in the gut have an impact on the course of HIV disease? and (2). Does the high rate of HIV replication in the gut contribute to drug resistant strains of HIV?

1. Searchlight, 621A North San Vicente Blvd, West Hollywood, CA 90069 Winter 98/99 issue. Ph No 310-358-2423. Subscriptions available with a $35 donation.

Scientific research on HIV in the gut & lymphoid tissues

1. "HIV-1 p24, but not proviral load, is increased in the intestinal mucosa compared with the peripheral blood in HIV-infected patients." Fackler OT et al. AIDS. 1998 Jan 22;12(2):139-46.

Fackler states: "The high viral antigen load in the intestine therefore indicates that mucosal HIV production is upregulated at the transcriptional and/or translational level. The intestinal mucosa is a major reservoir for HIV in HIV-infected patients."

2. "Tumor necrosis factor-alpha (TNF-alpha) stimulates bi-directional production of HIV-1 in polarized human colon epithelial cells," Yahi N et al, Int Conf AIDS. 1993 abstract no PO-A13-0220)

Yahi states: "TNF-alpha is a potent stimulator of HIV-1 replication in chronically infected differentiated HT29 (gastrointestinal epithelial) cells…"

3. "Perturbations of glucose metabolism associated with HIV infection in human intestinal epithelial cells." Lutz et al, AIDS. Feb; 11(2):147-55

Lutz states: "HIV-1 infection results in a disturbance of glycolytic and oxidative activities in human intestinal epithelial cells."

4. "Intracellular calcium release, induced by HIV-1 surface envelope glycoprotein, in human intestinal epithelial cells: a putative mechanism for HIV-1 enteropathy," by Dayanithi G et al Cell Calcium. 1995 Jul.18(1):9-18

Dayanithi states: "HIV-1 may directly alter ion secretion in the intestine, and thus be the causative agent of the watery diarrhea associated with HIV-1 infection."

5. "Physical contact with lymphocytes is required for reactivation of dormant HIV-1 in colonic epithelial cells," Faure E et al, Virus Res. 1994 Oct; 34(1):1-13

Faure et al state: "observations provide a putative molecular mechanism for transmission of HIV-1 from mucosal epithelial cells to lymphocytes."

6. "Replication and apical budding of HIV-1 in mucus-secreting colonic epithelial cells," Yahi N et al. J. Acquir Immune Defic Syndr. 1992 Oct 2(10):993-1000.

Yahi et al state: "data suggest that HIV-infected goblet cells in the colonic mucosa may produce the virus in the colorectal lumen; this could explain the route of transmission of HIV in the case of anal intercourse."

7. "Selected HIV replicates preferentially through the basolateral surface of differentiated human colon epithelial cells," Fantini J et al. Virology. 1991 Dec; 185(2):904-7

Fantini et al state: "data suggests that epithelial cells of the colon, productively infected with HIV, are able to produce the virus through both sides of the epithelium, but mainly through the serosal side."

CD8 cytotoxic lymphocytes kill cells infected with HHV-6

In my discussion with Donald Carrigan (12/18/95), he said that CD8 Cytotoxic T cells (CTL's) could kill cells infected with HHV-6A, if there are a sufficient number of CD4 cells and Antigen Presenting Cells available. The Antigen Presenting Dendritic cells, also known as CD35, are produced in the lymph nodes. However, if the CD4s and Antigen Presenting cells are insufficient, or serious damage has been done to the lymph nodes, then the Killer T cells do not know what to do and would not be effective in lowering the HIV and HHV-

6A viral load.

The subsets of CD8s and NK cells

The subsets that are effective against the two AIDS viruses are the CD8/CD57+ and the Natural Killer (NK) cells.

One subset of CD8 CTL's is CD57+. Usually, they will appear on a lab test form as (CD8 CD57+). Physicians can order a test to measure the quantity or percentage of CD8 CTLs (Cytotoxic Lymphocytes) including the other CTL subsets.

There are three subsets of Natural Killer cells, CD3-, CD16+ and CD56+. All three are added together as a total when testing for the "Total Absolute NK Cell Count." Of the three types, the CD16+ and CD56+ are thought to be the most important. There are two types of tests - Quantative and Function. A test that counts the number of subsets of immune cells is a quantitative test. A second test is known as a "Natural Killer Cell Function" test, and the function is measured in "Lytic Units," which is sometimes abbreviated on Lab tests as "LU." A NK Function Test measures how active and effective the NK cells are in killing cancer cells in a lab. A function test is not to be confused with a quantitative test.

To further understand the difference, if a subset of immune cells were Mexican Jumping Beans, the total number would be a "quantitative " test while the total number of beans that "jumped" would be a function test. If you had 1000 Mexican Jumping Beans and found that only 500 jumped, then your beans are only 50% functional. The same would apply to your immune cells.

6
Diagnostics: Monitoring immune health
Laboratory Tests for Measuring Immune Function

Anyone who has any of the following chronic illnesses (e.g. CFIDS, MS, Lupus, Cancer, AIDS, Hepatitis, Candidiasis, Heart disease or Alzheimer's etc), that their doctor cannot cure in 30 days, should have their physician proceed with tests to measure and determine immune function and whether the immune system is in or out of balance. (TH2 dominant or TH1 domnant or balanced).

1. Interleuken-6 levels as a key indicator of TH2 activity. With IL-6, you want normal or low levels. Specialty Labs (Santa Monica, CA) . Test code 3828 measures IL-6.
2. Blood serum levels for Selenium.
3. Delayed Cutaneous Hypersensitivity (DCH) - a skin Anergy test.
4. Natural Killer Cell Function.
5. Th1 cytokine profile - measures Interleukin 2 levels. With IL-2, you want high normal levels. If you can obtain a test for IL-12 and gamma interferon, this will enhance your Th1 profile test results.
6. T cell and B cell function (Lymphocyte Mitogen Proliferation Analysis).

The bottom line is that, if have nearly normal values in all six tests and maintain those values, it is unlikely that you will break with an onset of infections, whether you have AIDS or CFIDS. The Th1 and Th2 cytokine profile tests are important as they will indicate if the cytokine profile of the immune system is in the TH2 direction or the more effective TH1.

1. Interleukin-6 – elevated when HIV is progressing to AIDS, Cancer growth, CFIDS, Candiasis, Adrenal insufficiency (low cortisol, low DHEA and other hormones), low body Temperature. Specialty Labs, Santa Monica, CA 310-828-6543 Test code 3828 for IL-6.

2. Blood serum test for selenium

Selenium is a key trace mineral in maintaining and supporting cell-mediated immunity. Researchers have found 30 seleno-proteins in humans. Selenium is an essential and necessary component of Glutathione, the principal cellular antioxidant. Deficiencies of selenium prevents the immune system from mounting an effective response against cancer, HIV, HHV-6, EBV, CMV, Candidiasis and many other types of fungal, viral and bacterial infections. Selenium primarily and N-Acetyl Cysteine secondarily are the two main factors controlling glutathione levels. Each testing lab has its own reference range for selenium and other nutrients. A typical reference range is from 60 to 160 mcg/l. However, from our research and experience, these numbers are too low. We find that 135 to 270 mcg/l is a good range for normal healthy people not immune challenged. When chronic immune challenges exist, a target therapeutic ra.ge is from 250 to 500 mcg/l. Researchers in China found that when selenium is derived from natural food sources, blood serum levels must exceed 1000 mcg/l before side effects occur. Usually when blood serum levels of selenium reach 250 mcg/l or higher, symptoms of candidiasis will disappear and the individual's tolerance for carbohydrates is restored. Specialty Labs in Santa Monica, California will test for selenium in either blood serum or whole blood. www.specialtylabs.com. (310-828-6543)

3. Skin test for DCH or anergy.

The immune system can be challenged with a skin test, when inactivated antigens are injected just under the surface of the skin. A strong response (i.e. large welt) is indicative of a strong immune response where no welt indicates anergy - a condition that occurs when an immune system does not react to a challenge.

One skin test for anergy or DCH includes at least 3 of the following antigens: tetanus, candida, diphtheria, tuberculin, Streptococcus, proteus, trichophyton plus glycerin, which is added as a control (neutral). The tester pricks the surface of the skin and inserts a small amount of inactivated antigens. The test is read 48 to 72 hours later. If the patient was previously exposed to an antigen (i.e. tetanus) there should be a strong reaction in the form of a welt, an area that becomes red and sometimes itchy.

The strength of your immune response is determined by the size of the welts that form. The average size welt is 2 mm or larger. The size of the welt is measured in millimeters. The larger the welt, the greater is your immune response. The formation of the welts is direct proof that antigen presentation is taking place.. No immune response is called Anergy. Skin tests for Anergy measure CMI (Cell Mediated Immunity), also called DTH (Delayed Type Hypersensitivity- Type IV) or Delayed Cutaneous Hypersensitivity or (DCH) and is a direct indicator of antigen presentation and immune response. As a surrogate marker, skin tests for Anergy and other immune function tests are unsurpassed as a marker to determine the efficacy of any immune-based treatment protocol.

Key points: Persons with Anergy (little or no DCH or DTH response) is a condition associated with a selenium deficiency, low glutathione levels, heavy metal toxicity, low body temperature, metabolic defects in adrenal and thyroid metabolism, toxic liver and colon. Other factors - chronic infections that promote TH2 cytokine responses, IL-6, histamine and excessive antibody production.

4. Natural Killer cell function.

NK function is measured in "lytic units" (LU). LU measures, in a lab, the ability of NK cells to lyse or kill cancer cells. The normal reference range for NK lytic units is from 20 to 250. Anyone with less than 20 lytic units has little or no NK function and almost no natural immunity against cancer.

What makes Natural Killer Cells so important in chronic conditions of immune dysfunction is that, unlike other immune cells that must hold conferences with the CD4 Helper cells, the Natural Killer (NK) cell is policeman, judge, jury and executioner, all in one. NK cells target infections both outside and inside the cells. NK cells target and kill cancer cells, viruses and bacteria. Unlike Memory T and B cells that have to acquire the knowledge of which foreign invaders to target, the NK cells have an innate knowledge of what to do.

NK function can be impaired only by a failure of antigen presentation from infected cells. Infected cells present antigen on their cell surface to signal NK and other white blood cells that they are infected. If this event fails to happen, the NK cells cannot see the infected cells and fail to clear the infection by destroying the infected cell. This is what makes skin test for DCH and the tests for selenium so valuable, when used in combination with an NK Function Test. If you have selenium levels of 200 mcg/l or higher, and a good DCH response to a skin test as well as a test score in "lytic" units (at least 50 or higher, preferably 100 or higher), then the NK cells can "see" the infected cells aa well as have the energy to destroy them.

NK Function tests are available from ImmunoSciences Labs (800-950-4686 or 310-657-1077) or Specialty Labs (800-421-7110 - test code 5420)

5. Th1 cytokine profile - measuring Interleukin 2 levels (IL-2).

IL-2 is an important Th1 cytokine that increases T cell counts and improves NK function, when used in small doses. It is an indicator or surrogate marker of other Th1 cytokines like Interleukin 12 and gamma interferon. Test code 86318 from Immunosciences Labs measures IL-2 levels. When IL-2 levels increase and reach normal or high normal, it indicates stronger cell-mediated immunity (CMI). (Immunosciences – Beverly Hills, CA)

6. T and B cell function (ImmunoSciences Labs) or (Lymphocyte Mitogen Proliferation Analysis - Specialty Labs - test code 1060).

This test uses 3 different mitogens for stimulating the B cells, CD4 and CD8 cells in lab cultures. The proliferative response is necessary for the immune system to clone the troops and mount an attack against the invaders. If the proliferative response fails, then anergy exists in one or more of the subsets. B cells that are anergic will not produce antibodies. CD4s and CD8s both produce various cytokines. Without the cytokines (chemical messengers), no effective immune response will occur. Individually or together, these tests are important diagnostic tests for measuring immune function.

Note: A poor man's self-test for antigen presentation is a topical skin test for Delayed-Type Hypersensitivity using a topical solution of DNCB (DiNitroChloroBenzene). More on DNCB in the next chapter that covers treatment options. Remember, antigen presentation is absolutely the first event that must take place before the immune system can mount a successful attack against a virus.

Testing for HHV-6A
"Rapid Culture Assay" or "Lymph Node Biopsies"

Constance Knox Kiehl and Donald Carrigan have two types of tests for determining the presence of HHV-6A and B. They are Lymph Node biopsies and Rapid Culture Assay. Only lymph node biopsies will determine the condition of your lymph nodes and requires a surgeon. Rapid Culture Assay only requires a blood draw. Staining is used to determine the presence of HHV-6 and their subsets, Variant A and/or B. Any anti-viral and/or immune-based protocol that reduces HHV-6 to non-detectable levels is an effective treatment for AIDS and HHV-6 related CFIDS. For example, Dr. Jesse Stoff MD used a transfer factor that activates Natural Killer Cell function in a CFIDS patient; as the NK function improved, the HHV-6 titers in the patient dropped to non-detectable levels and her symptoms of severe fatigue, myalgias, dyplagia and insomnia completely disappeared. This demonstrates the importance and effectiveness of increasing NK function in CFIDS

patients with HHV-6 infection.
To order Rapid Culture Assays for HHV-6, contact Knox and Carrigan at
VIRACOR, 1210 NE WINDSOR DR.,
LEE'S SUMMIT, MO 64086
800-305-5198 FAX 816-347-0143 www.viracor.com

Note: www.viracor.com contains links to more than a dozen websites for persons with CFS or MS and more information on HHV-6.

In March, 1998, I received an announcement that Medical Diagnostic Labs now offers testing for the subsets of HHV-6, variant A and B.

Address: Med Diagnostic Labs, 133 Gaither Dr, Suite C, Mt. Laurel, NJ 08054 Phone 877-269-0090. Contact person - Dr. Eli Mardechai. www.mdlab.com

Body temperature and pH tests

In addition to all the above, two other very critical tests that can be self-administered and cost pennies are body temperature and saliva pH.

1. Low Body Temperature is a condition widely reported in persons with AIDS, CFIDS, Epstein Barr Virus (EBV), Candidiasis and Cancer. Body temperature should be a normal 98.6_ Fahrenheit. Temperatures even 1 degree below normal indicate impaired energy production and anergy in the white blood cell response to infections. No treatment for any chronic infection will ever be completely satisfactory until body temperature returns to normal. When body temperature returns to normal, most symptoms disappear. A thermometer is all you need to take this very important test. Low body temperature correlates directly to increased HIV, HHV-6A viral loads, increases thrush and fungal infections and growth of cancer cells. See the chapter on low body temperature for suggestions on how to restore it to normal.

2. Saliva pH. Low saliva pH, below 6.4, measures acidosis in the body and directly correlates to increased viral replication, impaired enzyme function and malabsorption of nutrients that directly impacts white blood cell counts and immune function. See the chapter on Balance your pH for more information.

Beta 2 micro-globulin level test

Beta 2 micro-globulin levels measure an antibody that indicates the rate of cell destruction going on in a person. In AIDS, levels of 2.0 or less correlate with non-progression and low HHV-6A activity. The same is true in CFIDS. Levels above 2.0 correlate with a higher rate of cell destruction and increased HHV-6A infection, or other lytic viruses such as hepatitis in the cells. It is important to ask your physician to give you a Beta 2 micro-globulin test at the same time testing is being done for HIV viral load, using either PCR or dDNA. If the viral load is low and the beta 2 levels are high, it indicates another possible active virus or oxidative stress (low Glutathione levels) may be contributing factors. This will necessitate further testing for other active viruses or a blood test to measure intracellular levels of L-Glutathione. Medical research has correlated low glutathione levels with a failure of antigen processing. Cells infected with viruses must be able to process and present antigen on the cell surface before a CD8 cytotoxic lymphocyte response is activated. Another factor that impairs antigen presentation is low Adenosine Tri-phosphate (ATP) production in the mitochondria of the cells.

Find an immunologist and a nutritionist

Never ask an I.D. (infectious disease) physician for advice in areas in which he is not trained - immunology and nutrition. I.D. physicians spend too much time listening to the pharmaceutical salesmen, and not enough time reading scientific journals. Find an Immunologist and consider him or her your primary physician. Look in your local Yellow Pages phone directory under "Immunology" to find a medical doctor who has training in the arena of immune function and nutrition. In other words, interview the doctor, before you let him examine you. What training or education have you had in immunology and nutrition?

We have a list of physicians who have purchased this book and will provide anyone who writes to us with a list of local names and addresses on request.

6.4: Balance your pH
What is pH?

pH is a measure of "hydrogen potential." It is a measure, on a scale of 0 to 14, of the concentration of hydrogen ions in a solution. 0 means a substance is saturated with hydrogen ions and cannot absorb more, such as sulfuric acid. 0 is the most acid you can get. 14 means there are no hydrogen ions in the solution and it is the most alkaline you can get, such as calcium. A neutral Ph is around 7. Solutions below a pH of 7 are generally considered acid and those with a pH of 7 or higher are considered alkaline.

Why is pH important? pH is a controlling factor for hundreds of enzymes in the body involving digestion and assimilation of nutrients and the production of energy in the cells. Normal saliva pH is 6.4 in a resting state and is the ideal pH number to indicate balance and homeostasis within the body. After eating food, normal saliva pH increases to 7.2 to help digest carbohydrates, then later returns to a lower level. Low saliva pH (below 6.2) is linked to poor absorption of nutrients in the gastro-intestinal tract and is indicative of liver toxicity. Accordingly, restoring normal saliva pH is a prerequisite to increase nutrient absorption and to a healthier functioning liver. Saliva pH parallels the pH value of the blood and lymph system. An acid blood and lymph, as indicated by an acid saliva pH, creates a favorable condition for the growth of viruses. Low saliva pH is linked to acid blood that may also indicate a deficiency of potassium, magnesium, calcium and trace minerals. Low saliva pH is also linked to a high pulse rate (over 80 beats per minute at rest). Restoring normal saliva pH values is necessary for restoring normal metabolism, digestion and assimilation, and is indicative of a pH value in the blood and lymph unfavorable for the growth of viruses. The more the pH value moves away from 6.4 in either direction, the more serious the imbalance is within the body.

How to test for pH values.

pH is measured with pH tape or testing strips that are sold in drug stores and some health food stores. To test saliva pH, place saliva in a spoon, dip pH paper in it and read it immediately by comparing it to a color chart. To test urine pH, place a small amount of urine in a glass, dip pH paper in it and read it immediately. Saliva pH tends to be more stable than urine pH and is the more important value of the two. The most important urine pH reading is the first urine pH value in the morning that should read 5.5 to 5.8. Urine pH readings during the day will fluctuate considerably. In normal healthy people, they will average 6.4. It is mainly the first urine pH reading in the morning with which we are concerned. To test for saliva pH in the morning, first drink a glass of water and wait 3 minutes, then place some saliva in a spoon and test the saliva pH value. It should read 6.2 to 6.6 (normal value is 6.4). Saliva pH values are closely linked to blood and lymph pH values.

pH – the big picture

The big picture on pH is that it is likely the single most basic and broad control of every aspect of body chemistry, so taught Arthur G Guyton, M.D. author of MEDICAL PHYSIOLOGY.

The major mechanisms, by which pH controls work, are chemical, hormonal and electrical. The bio-chemical control is mediated through enzymes, which are catalysts for all bio-chemical activity. Enzymes are very pH sensitive. Hormones are very pH sensitive and electricity is pH sensitive. Together, enzymes, hormones and electricity affect many body functions. The late Carey Reams made pH values, and how to interpret them, part of what is now known as "the Reams Formula." Dr. Gary Martin, DN, of Phoenix, AZ carried the Reams Formula a step further and made it incredibly complicated. Both men apparently overlooked the importance of restoring normal body temperature and adding it to their equation of normal metabolism.

Normal saliva pH values before eating or when taken 2 hours after eating, should be 6.4. Immediately after eating food, normal saliva pH is 7.2. pH testing is used as a tool to measure how far out of balance your blood chemistry is and is used as an instrument to measure your progress toward a normal metabolism. However, when fighting an infection, it is best for urine pH to fall in a range of 5.5 to 6.0 and saliva pH should be slightly above 6.4. If urine pH is constantly higher than 6.4 and saliva pH is constantly lower than 6.0, it is a set of numbers associated with many health problems such as chronic infections, fatigue, adrenal exhaustion or even cancer. The further these numbers are out of balance, the more it is associated with extreme blood and liver toxicity. Saliva is the more stable of the two pH numbers and should be kept in a range of 6.0 to 6.8. If saliva pH falls below 6.0, vital nutrients, (amino acids and many minerals), are not being absorbed and the liver and blood becomes toxic. Saliva acidity may be caused by a diet high in refined white sugar and refined grains (white flour products). Other contributing factors are heavy metal poisoning, prescription or street drugs. Excess smoking of tobacco may also depress saliva pH. Saliva pH of 6.8 to 7.0 (on the alkaline side) is certainly better than being acid, but indicates a slow digestion, which could be indicative of a deficiency of amino acids and hormones like Thyroxin. The ideal pH for blood is 7.4. Buffering systems including amino acids and bicarbonate ions control the pH of the blood.

Carbon dioxide in the blood is a source of acidity. As the blood goes acid, the brain tells the lungs to breathe faster to expel the CO_2. This increases the pulse rate, a condition associated with blue and in extreme cases, even black blood, which is due to excess levels of CO_2 and lack of oxygen. Oxygen, and its more reactive forms like Ozone and H_2O_2, has an immediate alkalizing effect on the blood. Kidneys excrete many kinds of metabolic acids. Lack of heat in the kidneys may impair removal of CO_2 from the blood, hence the relation to low body temperature. Drinking more water helps dilute acids and makes the blood more alkaline and helps the kidneys excrete acids. Drinking warm ginger root and cayenne tea together can have a warming effect on the body as well as increasing your intake of liquids high in potassium, which will help the cells release toxins into the blood and expel them via the kidneys and lungs. Liquid vegetable juices are one of the richest sources of potassium, and drinking them will quickly alkalize the blood and help expel excess CO_2, thereby causing the blood to become more red and less acid. A glass of low sodium V8 juice spiked with Tabasco sauce has the same effect. It is even more effective, when you add a spoonful of Barley or Wheat grass juice powder. Blood buffers are amino acids that can switch polarity and move blood in either an acid or in an alkaline direction. Potassium, sodium, calcium and magnesium all have an alkalizing effect on the blood. Saliva acidity is related to upper body respiratory problems.

PWA's have told us that taking a Tbsp of blackstrap molasses up to three times a day moves saliva from an acid condition closer to the normal value of 6.4. More recently, we discovered that a drink made from whole lemons and olive oil quickly moves saliva pH to normal values within a few days and in some cases, in a matter of hours.

pH – the first reading in the morning

First, measure both urine and saliva pH at the same time. Like body temperature, pH values can fluctuate considerably during the day. The best time to take both pH readings is in the morning before eating any food. In the morning, drink one glass of water and wait a few minutes. Then take both your saliva pH and your urine pH. The first reading of urine pH in the morning should read between 5.5 and 6.0 and saliva should be 6.2 to 6.4. If the first urine pH is alkaline (over 6.2), it means the cleaning out phase or catabolic cycle of sleep is not working and too many waste products are building up in your blood. With this pattern, the person is likely to wake up feeling tired. These are important numbers, especially if weight loss, cancer or KS is involved. After your first urine test, your second reading should be 6.4 for both saliva and urine pH values. After you eat food, these numbers will naturally change again. It is the first set of numbers in the morning that are the most important. You do not want your first urine pH reading to be alkaline, over 6.0 while your saliva pH is under 6.0. This set of numbers is associated with a congested and toxic liver, adrenal exhaustion, digestive disorders, acid blood and lymph. Alkaline urine pH and acid saliva pH also indicates an inability to assimilate essential fatty acids. While I would advise anyone against spending all day testing their saliva pH, keeping a record of daily pH changes will help you monitor your progress in normalizing pH values.

Most dangerout pH tendencies

The most dangerous pH levels are reached when the saliva pH goes acid, below 6.0, or urine pH goes very alkaline, over 6.8.

Normal pH patterns

Early morning: Saliva - 6.2 to 6.4; urine - 5.5 to 6.0.

pH and cancer

Note: The St. Jude's Cancer Clinic in Mexico reports that the first morning urine pH reading of cancer patients is alkaline when they arrive at the clinic. As their bodies began to heal, the first urine pH reading in the morning becomes acid. I have found the same pattern in AIDS patients with wasting syndrome or rapid loss of body fluids.

pH and AIDS

When HIV first infects a person, saliva pH tendencies should tend to be alkaline. In advanced HIV infection, saliva pH goes acid and urine pH goes alkaline. The whole Lemon/Olive oil drink or Rapid Recovery Procedures and the ACD diet will reverse and normalize these profiles.

Supplements and diet to correct pH deviations

A: Normal: Saliva pH is 6.4 and urine pH is 6.4 most of the time (when measured during the day between meals.)

Note: It is normal for urine pH to deviate during the day but saliva pH should be stable. When the pH of urine and saliva are taken at the same time and then added together and then divided by 2, it should equal 6.4. This is your overall systemic acidity or alkalinity number. Example: Saliva pH 6.8 Urine pH 6.0. Add 6.8 and 6.0 = 12.8 divided by 2 = 6.4 If you are overall too acid, you need to drink more water, stop eating foods with salt added and increase your intake of absorbable calcium, magnesium and potassium rich foods, juices or supplements. If you are too alkaline, reduce supplements that are causing the alkalinity problem (also reduce fruit and vegetable intake) and increase your intake of whole grains, quality proteins with very little fat. Consider fasting on whole grain bread and water for a meal or two or a whole day once or twice a week.

B: Saliva pH is above 6.4 and urine pH is below 6.4: (closest to normal)

Take supplements to increase body temperature and strengthen the kidneys if the pH deviation is more than .6 off (i.e. saliva-7.0 and urine-5.8). Eat more whole grains, gluten-free.

C: Both saliva and urine pH are alkaline (above 6.4): (third from the worst)

When both saliva and urine pH are alkaline, over 6.4, take large doses of regular Vitamin C and Liquid Amino Fuel and increase your intake of proteins to bring both numbers down. This profile is often found in persons on strictly vegetarian diets that are low in protein. However, this is not a bad set of numbers. Alkaline urine means that the kidneys are working to remove the substances that are causing excess alkalinity in the saliva and blood.

D: Advanced illness - both saliva and urine pH run acid: (second from the worst profile)

Drink more water. Use Whole Lemon/Olive drink daily. Increase your intake of vegetables and fruits. Eliminate your intake of white sugar, white flour products, salt , salt flavored foods (lunchmeat, ham etc) and canned soda.

E: The Worst Profile:

Urine pH is alkaline (over 6.4) and Saliva pH is acid (below 6.4): commonly seen in advanced HIV associated with weight loss, cancer or KS.

When urine pH tends to be alkaline and saliva pH is acid, it indicates the worst pH profile of all four that are listed here. It indicates that your blood is very toxic, probably blue or black along with serious absorption problems and nutrient deficiencies. We recommend that drinking the whole lemon/olive oil formula for a few days. If you need more help to restore a normal pH profile, add Rapid Recovery Procedures or the immune enhancement diet until your pH values are normal. Dark green vegetables are high in magnesium, calcium and potassium, all of which help reverse serious blood and saliva acidity. Red beets will help in digestion, as they are a natural source of betaine hydrochloride. Other beneficial foods: blackstrap molasses, flax oil, evening primrose oil and cod liver oil. Avoid eating just before going to bed. Eat your evening meal about 3 hours before bedtime.

Supplements: You will need supplements to restore normal body temperature and you should take warm baths twice a day. You will need to take 1 betaine hydrochloride tablet and 1 digestive enzyme tablet with each meal. (Use lemon juice and olive oil with each meal if saliva pH is below 6.0). Use lemon juice before bedtime and if you feel you still have a full stomach, take one betaine HCL and 1 vegetarian enzyme tablet. This will help you digest your food, sleep better and will give you a better set of pH numbers in the morning. Coral Calcium powder – 1/2 teaspoon in water in the evening once a day. Co-enzymated B vitamin complex (Source Naturals), the most bio-available form of B Vitamins. Dissolve one tablet twice daily about 8 hours apart.

Zinc is the nucleus of an enzyme called "carbonic anhydrase" which converts carbon dioxide to carbonic acid in the blood. Zinc sulfate (220 mg ea) – one every other day. As zinc lowers copper levels, you may need some blackstrap molasses as a source of copper. Use magnesium chloride (Alta Health Products) – 4 to 6 tablets daily, or magnesium sulfate (Epson Salt) 1/2 tsp daily to help the body retain potassium, which helps increase saliva pH and to produce ATP (energy) in the cells.

Foods that move urine and saliva pH in an alkaline direction

All fruits and vegetables. The most alkaline fruit is figs, followed by apricots, grapes and citrus fruits. Almonds are the only protein food that always promotes an alkaline reaction. All vegetables, especially parsley, spinach and other dark green vegetables, promote alkalinity. Other factors that promote alkalinity are drinking large amounts of water and juices. Herb's: peppermint tea and watermelon seed tea. Cayenne and blackstrap molasses also promote alkalinity. Any other foods high in potassium, magnesium and calcium. Coral Calcium will help overcome severe acid saliva conditions. Almonds are naturally rich in protein and calcium. Amino acids can switch polarity in the bloodstream and cause your pH to go from acid to alkaline or vice-versa. When your saliva pH is constantly acid, it could mean that your blood levels of amino acids are low; also, it most likely means your blood levels of calcium, magnesium and potassium are low. Green juice (made from wheat grass, barley grass, spinach, carrot tops, beet tops, endive and parsley etc.), are rich in amino acids, calcium, magnesium and potassium and are a perfect food for the person whose saliva pH is too acid. Start off with one cup a day and increase to 4 cups a day until saliva pH returns to normal.

Foods that usually more both urine and saliva pH in an acid direction – in normal health people

All proteins (except for almonds) and most starches. legumes (beans), grains (corn, brown rice, millet, quinoa, rye etc.), fish and meats are all acid forming. Acid forming herb's: hyssop, juniper berry and desert herb. Acid forming supplements: Apple cider vinegar and Vitamin C. Any foods high in phosphorus or sulfur. EXCEPTIONS: When Cancer or AIDS patients have low blood amino acid levels, amino acid supplementation may move saliva pH in an alkaline direction, because amino acids can switch polarity and act as a blood buffering system.

Mixed reaction foods to move saliva pH up and urine pH down

All foods high in fresh oils - Flax oil, olive oil, butter, cod liver oil, evening primrose oil, most nuts and seeds. Pectin, found in citrus rinds and in applesauce, helps assimilate fatty acids. The whole lemon/olive oil drink produces rapid results in moving saliva pH up and urine pH down.

Mixed reaction foods to move saliva pH down and urine pH up

All grains (corn, brown rice, millet, rye etc.) wheat germ and bran, and, to a lesser extent other starches, like potatoes, rutabagas and turnips.

In **THE NUTRITION AND DIETARY CONSULTANT,** Feb., 1990, Sal D'Onofrio, M.S., C.N.C., writes in an article on "The Digestive pH Factor" about the effects of saliva pH ranges. Here is some of what he says on the effects of various saliva pH values.

"6.4 to 6.6. Ideal range if all other numbers are perfect.

6.0 to 6.3. Bile is weakening. Loss of soluble Vitamins A, D, E, K. Too much alcohol, coffee, cigarettes or drugs may be the cause.

5.7 to 5.9. Digestion is too fast and nutrients are bypassed. Suspect heavy metal poisoning. Vital organs not being nourished.

5.2 to 5.6. Same conditions of acid urine stress. Bile is no longer working and liver is extremely toxic and weak.

0.0 to 5.1. Jaundice can set in, death near. "

pH tape

pH tape is sold in drug stores and in some health food stores. A tape with pH values in a range from 5.5 (acid) to 8.0 (alkaline) in .2 increments will give you a reasonably accurate reading.

How to use pH tape

Tear off a one-inch piece of pH paper from the roll. Place some saliva in a spoon and dip the pH paper in the saliva and then immediately compare the change in color to match a reading on the color chart that comes with the pH tape. For urine, or any other solution, dip the pH paper in the solution and then immediately read the color chart to determine the pH value. For accuracy, the reading should be done about 4 to 6 seconds after dipping the pH tape in the solution.

Use limewater (calcium hydroxide) to move saliva pH in an alkaline direction when all else fails. Also consider Coral Calcium

Limewater, not the fruit, is high in calcium hydroxide. Originally, limewater was derived from "limestone." When diet alone and the whole lemon/olive oil drink will not move saliva pH in an alkaline direction, limewater has always worked. Add 1 tablespon to a quart of water. Drink 1 or 2 glasses daily. If after 3 days, saliva pH has not returned to a normal 6.4, then increase to 4 glasses daily. When saliva pH returns to a normal 6.4, adjust the dosage downwards to maintain that level. When pH is continuously on the acid side, it may indicate a deficiency of ionic calcium in the blood.

Coral calcium that comes from coral reefs near Japan is highly alkalizing as well. The coral calcium is high in trace minerals and is one of the cleanest mineral supplements on the planet. Take Coral calcium capsules with a glass of water in the evening.

Note: Because of the risk of Mad Cow Disease, bone meal should be avoided although the riskiest part of a cow to transfer this disease continues to be the pituitary gland. See Positive Health News, Report No 22 for a detailed report on Mad Cow Disease or Progressive Health News for March 2001 on the internet at www.keephopealive.org.

8

Adrenal Cortisol lowers IL-6 and helps restore balanced immunity

The benefits of low-dose cortisol

There are several components to any successful program to balance the immune system including a hypoallergenic diet and anti-inflammatory supplements including low-dose cortisol that have a supportive role by reducing an overactive TH2 arm of the immune system and balancing the TH1 and TH2 branches.

By helping to normalize IL-6 levels (a TH2 cytokine active in cancer and AIDS), low-dose cortisol along with low dose thyroid therapy has many benefits to offer. Besides restoring immune function to prevent nad help remit malignancies including various forms of cancer, there are also reduced food allergies and chemical sensitivities. These benefits include reduced replication of HIV, candidiasis, CMV, HHV-6, CMV, EBV, herpes, less fatigue during the day and more restful sleep at night along with improvements in Natural Killer cell function and macrophage function.

Cortisol deficiency and Chronic Fatigue Syndrome

In an article on the Adrenalcortex Stress profile at Great Smokey Diagnostic Laboratory website www.gsdl.com, they state that chronic fatigue syndrome (CFS) is actually a disease of the hypothalamic-pituitary-adrenal axis and add, "Unlike ordinary fatigue, however, CFS is typically characterized by low free cortisol levels and adrenal insufficiency. Raising cortisol levels by even small amounts has been found to improve unexplained fatigue in many CFS patients." Plechner is not alone in his view and experience, that small physiological doses of cortisone relieves numerous symptoms, including fatigue, and promotes the ability of the immune system to control infectious disease. (1)

Researchers have found that melatonin increases cortisol levels in aged, but not young, women (2). Taking melatonin before bedtime may help resolve fatigue related to cortisol deficiency in some persons.

1. Jeffries WM, Mild adrenocorticol deficiency, chronic allergies, autoimmune disorders and the chronic fatigue syndrome: a continuation of the cortisone story. Med Hypotheses 1994;42(3):183-9
2. Cagnacci A et al, Melatonin enhances cortisol levels in aged but not young women. Eur J Endocrinol 1995;133:691-5

IL-6 and Tumor Necrosis Factor (TNF) - fatigue-inducing cytokines

Chronic fatigue syndrome most likely is associated with defects in the hypothalamus, pituitary and adrenal glands or HPA axis. This could involve overactive B cells that produce cytokines (TH2 types – IL-4, 5 6 and 10) and antibodies that are not effective against infections and inflammatory conditions. The cytokines may contribute to daytime fatigue.

Vgontzas An et al report in the journal of "Metabolism" (1) "Interleukin-6 and tumor necrosis factor are fatigue-inducing cytokines, and the daytime secretion of IL-6 is negatively influenced by the quantity and quality of the previous night's sleep."

The researchers hypothesized that fatigue during the day is caused by increased secretion of IL-6 and tumor necrosis factor (TNF) during the daytime hours.

Eleven insomniacs and 11 healthy controls were matched for this study. Patients were tested for 4 days in a sleep laboratory and on the 4th day, plasma levels of IL-6 and TNF were taken during the 24-hour period.

The authors concluded "that chronic insomnia is associated with a shift of IL-6 and TNF secretion from nighttime to daytime, which may explain daytime fatigue."

At the same time, the pituitary continues to pump out ACTH that stimulates the adrenals to produce more cortisol until the adrenals become exhausted and are unable to keep up with demand.

Ref:
1. Chronic insomnia is associated with a shift of inteulukin-6 and tumor necrosis factor secretion from nighttime to daytime. Vgontzas An et al, Metabolism, 2002 Jul;51(7):887-92

HPA Axis in HIV disease

Freda PU (*) et al report that "Abnormalities of the endocrine system, and of the hypothalamus-pituitary adrenal (HPA) axis in particular, are associated with HIV infection. Opportunistic pathogens, neoplasms, and drugs used to treat infections may all contribute to the reported abnormalities, which range from subtle subclinical disturbances of HPA axis regulation to frank adrenal insufficiency. Patients with AIDS should be considered to be at high risk for primary or secondary adrenal insufficiency, and those with symptoms should be evaluated. Subclinical abnormalities may progress to clinically significant adrenal insufficiency as therapies improve and patients with AIDS live longer."

* The hypothalamus pituitary adrenal axis in HIV, Freda PU et al, AIDS READ 1999 Jan-Feb;9(1):43-50

Adrenal insufficiency in HIV: A review and recommendations.

Eledrise MS (1) et al in 2001 report from the Univ. of Texas, Galveston that "Adrenal insufficiency is known to be a complication of HIV infection, although estimates of its prevalence and severity vary. Adrenal insufficiency is the most serious complication that occurs in persons with HIV infection. Patients with AIDS are considered to be at high risk for primary and secondary adrenal insufficiency. We describe 3 patients with AIDS who had clinical features suggestive of adrenal insufficiency, but their Corticotrophin (ACTH) stimulation tests were normal. Repeat testing confirmed the diagnosis in one patient, and further testing with the overnight Metyrapone test revealed evidence of secondary adrenal insufficiency in the other patients. Persistent clinical improvement was evident on subsequent glucocorticoid therapy. A normal response to the ACTH stimulation test can be dangerously misleading. Patients with AIDS and suspected adrenal insufficiency who have normal screening by the (high dose) ACTH stimulation test should undergo further testing for secondary adrenal disease."

1. Adrenal insufficiency in HIV infection, Eledris MS et al, Am J Med Sci. 2001 Feb;321(2):137-44

Researchers find glucocorticoids (cortisol) reduces Interleukin 6 levels

Geneva, Italy. J. Rheumatology.

Cutolo M et al from the University of Genoa in Italy report in the J Rheumatology April 29, 2002 on a 12 month study involving 41 patients recently diagnosed with polymyalgia rheumatica (PMR). Basically this is a form of rheumatism associated with muscle pain. Patients were monitored for serum cortisol levels, DHEA, androstenedione and IL-6 concentrations at baseline and after 1, 3, 6, 9 and 12 months of glucocorticoid treatment.

They report that "serum concentrations of IL-6 at baseline were significantly higher in PMR patients than in controls. During 12 months of glucocorticoid treatment IL-6 levels dropped significantly at one month; thereafter they remained stable and did not increase again despite tapering of the glucocorticoid dose."

They concluded: "This study found reduced production of adrenal hormones (cortisol, DHEAS) at baseline in patients with active and untreated PMR. The defect seems mainly related to altered adrenal responsiveness to the ACTH stimulation (i.e. increased 17-OHP), at least in untreated patients. The 12 month glucocorticoid treatment of patients reduced the production of inflammatory mediators (i.e. IL-6) in a stable manner that persisted after glucocorticoids were tapered off."

This study validates the use of low-dose anti-inflammatory steroids (cortisol etc) long-term to down regulate an over active TH2 cytokine (i.e. IL-6). Researchers have also found that in humans, injections of IL-6 increases ACTH secretion, but more so in males than in females (1) Since ACTH stimulates the adrenals to produce more cortisol, the use of low-dose cortisol to reduce IL-6 ultimately reduces ACTH that in turn reduces the signals to the Adrenals to produce more cortisol. Thus the HPA axis comes back into balance and helps to restore a normal 24-hour hormonal and cytokine cycle.

1. Differential male and female adrenal.... cortisol responses to interleuken-6 in humans. Silva C et al.; ANN NY Acad Sci 2002 Jun;966:68-72

German study finds inadequate adrenal steroid hormones in patients with rheumatoid arthritis

Straub RH et al report in March 2002 (1)

Straub et al reported that the number of swollen joints correlated inversely with the ratio of serum cortisol to serum IL-6 in rheumatoid arthritis patients. In rheumatoid arthritis and reactive arthritis patients, they found lower levels of ACTH, cortisol, ASD, DHEAS, and 17-OH-progesterone in relation to levels of IL-6 and TNF (tumor necrosis factor). They concluded that the level of cortisol and ACTH are relatively low in relation to levels of IL-6 and TNF in untreated patients with early rheumatoid arthritis and reactive arthritis.
1. Arthritis Rheum, 2002 Mar;46(3): 654-62

Low levels of cortisol and elevated IL-6 in persons with PTSD

Post Traumatic Stress Disorder or PTSD was first brought to my attention after the Vietnam War although media reports state it was first diagnosed after World War II. Interrupted sleep, fatigue, nightmares and uncontrolled nervous reactions to loud noises that bring back reactions to the trauma of past combat experiences are some of the symptoms.

According to an article published in "Neuroimmunomodulation" in 2001 by Baker SDG et al, at the University of Cincinnati College of Medicine, Baker et al report that "Interleukin-6 (IL-6) secretion is suppressed by glucocorticoids and stimulated by catecholamines. Patients with PTSD have decreased cortisol and increased catecholamine secretion."

In a study that measured the IL-6 and norepinephrine levels in the Cerebrospinal fluid of PTSD patients vs. healthy controls, the researchers found that "PTSD patients had increased concentrations of IL-6 in their Cerebrospinal fluid." They report that low cortisol secretion in patients with PTSD may account for the elevated IL-6 secretion.

Adrenal hormones including cortisol start with cholesterol

Cholesterol is the raw material from which hormones in the body are produced. When cholesterol levels are too low, 125 or less, it will reduce the production of all the body's hormones, and the immune function will suffer. For a strong immune system, total cholesterol levels should be 160 or higher, and HDL, the "good" cholesterol should be above 39. Treatments that detoxify the liver and foods high in cholesterol, like soft-boiled organic eggs, will raise both the HDL and the total cholesterol levels.

In the late 1980's, egg yolk lecithin containing all the natural cholesterol components, was widely used in the treatment of HIV infection, with some noticeable decrease in symptoms. Liquid egg yolk would have increased the output of adrenal hormones like cortisol and DHEA; however, egg yolk that is hard-boiled or completely cooked would have a damaged lecithin component but still retain the cholesterol. Dietary lecithin (derived from soybeans), as a supplement, should be considered and used with meals that contain cooked foods that are high in cholesterol (eggs, red meat, shrimp, oysters, liver, cheese, lobster, butter), so that the cholesterol can be utilized in a positive way, and not cause damage by clogging up the arteries.

From cholesterol, the mother of all hormones is produced called pregnenolone. From pregnenolone are produced cortisol, adrenaline, DHEA, testosterone, estrogen and other hormones in the estrogen family, like estrone and estradiol. DHEA can be a pathway for the production of androgens, testosterone, cortisol, estrone and estradiol. DHEA is involved in mitochondrial respiration and thyroid hormone function. Both of these functions are critical for maintaining normal body temperature. A decrease in DHEA has been found in persons with hypothyroidism. Low DHEA levels have been associated with aging, cancer, alzheimers, insulin resistance, obesity, high blood pressure and lower sex drive.

It is increasingly apparent that millions of people who suffer from low body temperature and immune dysfunction have exhausted adrenals and impaired detoxification pathways. These are events that are not isolated, but are all interconnected in some way. Plechner has found that low dose cortisol turns off the feedback back loop through the Hypothalamus and Pituitary that results in lower ACTH levels. Lower ACTH reduces demands on the adrenals resulting in reduced adrenal estrogen output. Plechner maintains that the excess adrenal estrogen binds to the thyroid hormones and depresses the immune response. Thyroid hormone is also given, and this increases the energy output and ATP production in the cells, thus improving the detoxification pathways, antigen production and cellular immune responses. Thyroid hormone helps the liver process toxins and bound hormones.

The Great Smokies Diagnostic Laboratory (www.gsdl.com) states in their Adrenal Cortex Stress Profile "Researchers have proposed that CFS is actually a disease of the hypothalamic-pituitary-adrenal axis. Unlike ordinary fatigue, however, CFS is typically characterized by low free cortisol levels and adrenal insufficiency. Raising cortisol levels by even small amounts has been found to improve unexplained fatigue symptoms in many CFS patients."

In Depression and Schizophrenia, researchers have found an abnormal circadian rhythm in cortisol levels. Normally, the highest level of cortisol is at 8am in the morning. In Depression, high levels are also found at midnight. The Great Smokies Report states that Cortisol is a major steroid produced by the adrenal gland. High or low levels, along with disrupted amounts in the circadian rhythm, can play a role in many conditions including depression, insomnia, AIDS, aneroxia nervosa, stress, obesity and chronic fatigue. To this may I add food allergies.

Researchers recommend combination therapy of DHEA and corticosteroids. DHEA inhibits IL-6

Straub RH et al report from Germany that "In chronic inflammatory diseases, such as rheumatoid arthritis, an alteration of the HPA stress response results in inappropriately low cortisol secretion in relation to adrenocorticotropic hormone (ACTH) secretion. Furthermore, it has recently been shown that the levels of another adrenal hormone, DHEA, were significantly lower after ACTH stimulation in patients with rheumatoid arthritis without prior corticosteroids than in healthy controls…We recently confirmed that DHEA is a potent inhibitor of IL-6, which confirmed an earlier study in mice."

Straub also reports that DHEA inhibits NF-Kappa B and that DHEA deficiency is linked to osteoporosis. Thus the authors concluded that a combined therapy of hydrocortisone or other corticosteroids be used along with DHEA in chronic inflammatory diseases.

Brownstein in his book recommends the natural hydrocortisone over Prednisone and other synthetic steroids and he suggests a maximum of 30 mg daily of hydrocortisone (but more preferably 10 to 20 mg daily). For DHEA use in women, Brownstein recommends 10 mg daily and slightly higher in men. Several other soruces recommend up to 25 mg DHEA daily in men, but levels need to occasionally monitored by your physician.

Reports on the use of hydrocortisone

Sept 2004: One of our readers from Miami who has HIV/ AIDS and osteoporosis is trying 20 mg hydrocortisone daily along with 25mg of DHEA plus two Red clover capsules twice a day and 1/2 to 1 grain of natural thyroid daily. So far, he has tolerated this 4 part combination well and reports feeling much better even though he has taken a vacation from his anti-HIV meds. Since he has just started he has no lab results to share with us at this time. He also takes coral calcium and a number of other nutritional supplements.

He also uses hydrocortisone cream on his leg and the bone pain is nearly gone. This is just after a few days. He has added red clover capsules and low dose DHEA to help increase his bone density. He also plans on adding 1/2 grain of thyroid daily to his regime. He is currently on his new regimen while taking a drug holiday from his HIV meds.

Oct, 2004: One person with chronic fatigue and symptoms of Lupus told me that he took 20 mg of hydrocortisone last year for several months and all his symptoms disappeared. When he stopped using the hydrocortisone, his symptoms have re-emerged.

In Nov, 2004 two other persons with long term chronic conditions of ill health whom physicians have been unable to diagnose or treat have reported improvement in how they feel with low dose-hydrocortisone - one taking 5 mg daily and aother taking 10 mg daily. They say they are very encouraged by the results.

Sign of adrenal exhaustion

If you are lying down and quickly stand up and feel disoriented or a little dizzy, it indicates a possible drop in blood pressure and weak adrenals. Test blood pressure while lying down and again immediately after standing up. If it drops, it indicates weak adrenals.

Signs of overactive adrenals – high blood pressure, anxiety, mood swings, mental instability.

Indications of low adrenal cortisol

1. Candidiasis and other chronic infections
2. Hypoglycemia/insulin resistance
3. Low blood sugar (hypoglycemia)
4. Strong cravings for salty foods, sweets or alcohol
5. Autoimmune disorders
6. Feeling like taking a nap during the day or mid afternoon.
7. Asthma or a tendency toward asthma (wheezing)
8. Fatigue that comes on easily after physical or mental exertion.
9. Food allergies and sensitivities (lactose/gluten intolerance)

10. Aching joints
11. Depression
12. Insomnia – interrupted sleep
13. Low IgA
14. Fluid retention
15. Weight gain/obesity for both men and women
16. In men, growth of tits on the upper chest
17. Weak sex drive (low DHEA and Testosterone)
18. Digestive disorders
19. Low Natural Killer cell function
20. Elevated Il-6 and Anergy/loss of DTH

Factors in adrenal exhaustion/imbalance

1. **Toxemia - kidneys are sluggish** (from toxins in the food, water, air). Protein intake is either too high or too low. Water intake is insufficient to flush out toxins.
2. **Heavy metal toxins, especially mercury,** in the air and food supply.
3. Stress – significant fluctuations in blood sugar caused by eating refined sugar and sweets, toxins in the liver. Other - excess noise, worry, fear, anxiety etc. Anti-stress treatment – talk a long walk every day – listen to soft classical music, sing a song, play a musical instrument, meditate or pray.
4. Excess estrogen from processed food, meats, and beverages and from the adrenals
5. Pesticides in food that have an estrogenic effect that are toxic inside the cells.
6. Hormones (estrogen) given to beef for weight gain prior to marketing them. Milk from cows fed bovine growth hormone contains higher levels of IGF-1.
7. Nutritional factors –
    a. Excess consumption of sugar, candy, soda, sweets, bakery and refined carbohydrates including alcohol.
    b. Excess salt intake and lack of high potassium foods; foods with MSG added, foods deep fried or cooked at high temperatures, foods containing hydrogenated fats, trans-fatty acids or cooked with polyunsaturated fatty acids.
    c. Deficiency of vitamin B5 (pantothenic acid) and natural vitamin A, C, E, chromium and B vitamins.
    d. Diet lacks fresh fruits and vegetables, whole grains, legumes and seafood.
1. Environmental factors
    a. Microwave ovens, exposure to computers without screen filters to block ELF and VLF radiation, living near TV and radio stations, high power lines, within 1000 ft of cellular phone towers.
1. Chronic infections – HIV, HHV-6, Hepatitis viral
2. Protease inhibitors, used to treat HIV, can inhibit thyroid function. Check the Physicians Desk Reference.
3. Intestinal dysbiosis – unfriendly flora predominate.

Natural & prescription remedies for adrenal function

1. **Natural**: a. Herbs with adrenal hormones precursors are **Black Cohosh, Wild Yam, Yucca and Ginseng**. Try one capsule of each herb twice daily - early morning and mid or late PM but not before bedtime. Licorice root can be used in small doses to boost cortisol levels when blood pressure is low or normal. However, licorice root can increase blood pressure so this must be monitored. **Note: Black cohosh also lowers blood pressure**.

    b. **Plant Sterols/Sterinols** (Steroids) precursors to adrenal hormones: Chestnuts, **Rice bran** or unrefined oil, unrefined (black) **Sesame seeds** or oil. Rice bran - 1/4 cup daily.

2. **Prescription: Hydrocortisone** - available by prescription. Comes in 5 mg, 10 mg and 20 mg tablets. Low dose for adults weighing from 140 to 180 20 mg once a day in the AM for adults or 10 mg twice daily (8 am and 2 pm). Over the Counter remedy: Hydrocortisone Cream 1% - 1/2 teaspoon massaged into the skin daily contains about 20 mg of hydrocortisone. However, it is thought that the tablets may have a stronger systemic effect.

3. **Diet – Food allergies promote inflammatoryresponses and increased need for adrenal cortisol.** Thus food allergies promote both adrenal exhaustion and obesity and the storage of cortisone in abdominal fat. A **hypoallergenic low calorie diet** - eat snacks (small meals) 5 times a day and use **grapefruit** and small amounts of **licorice root** to reverse these effects and lose weight while increasng free cortisol levels (reduces abdominal cortisone).

    Hypoallergenic – Give up any food to which you are allergic or sensitive, such as corn, wheat and other grains with gluten, lactose (milk, ice cream), but usually not yogurt, naturally cultured cottage cheese or whey protein, that are better tolerated. Consider the immune enhancement diet in this book. Eliminate commercial beef, pork and poultry that are contaminated with antibiotics and steroids. Avoid all soy products including soymilk as it will depress thyroid hormones and body temperature. The exception to this caveat is Miso, a fermented soy product that does not seem to cause any problems.

    a. Aged Kyolic Garlic Extract – Kyolic Formula 100. Four to 8 capsules twice daily. Reduces stress and both estrogen and cortisol levels. Japanese researchers have found 80% less corticoids in mice under stress and given Kyolic garlic preparations than the control group that was not given the aged garlic. In his book, "Garlic for Health," Dr. Benjamin Lau MD cited 3 studies (on animals and humans) on the benefits of Kyolic garlic in reducing the effects of stress. In his own patients, Dr. Lau has found that Kyolic Garlic reduces fatigue, depression and anxiety. In chemotherapy patients', side effects were reduced by 67%. In mice, Kyolic garlic reduced the size of tumors, starting in the 3rd week.

    b. Manganese – eat 1/2 cup oat bran daily and 2 cups of pineapple (juice or fruit). Both foods are very high in manganese. (Avoid amino acid chelates, proteinates or complexes). Serve Oat Bran cereal or whole oatmeal with diluted coconut milk. Coconut oil and milk are thermogenic and increase body temperature and promote weight loss in persons who are obese.

    c. Chromium – wheat germ and whole grains.

4. Two soft boiled organic or free range eggs daily, if total cholesterol levels are below 160. (increases adrenal hormone output).

    a. Watercress, parsley*, slippery elm, yucca, hydrangea*, kelp and bayberry - all help

improve adrenal output and function. *improves kidney function.
   b. Coconut oil and coconut milk - increases metabolic rate, burns fat and helps normalize body temperature. Use 3 tablespoons of coconut oil daily. Use coconut milk on breakfast cereal.
   c. Except for supplemental freshly ground flaxseed, eliminate soybean, corn, canola and other oils high in poly-unsaturated fatty acids (suppresses thyroid function) and of course margarine (except for Smart Balance) and all partially hydrogenated vegetable oils/ shortening. Use olive oil mainly – high in monounsaturated fats. It is OK to use some sesame or peanut oil in moderation as these also contain substantial amounts of monounsaturated fats (40% to 47%).

5. Supplements: Niacin and Pantothenic acid. Consider "Coenzymated B Vitamins" by Source Naturals. This product is taken sublingually and contains a full range of B vitamins in their most bioavailable form. Dissolve one tablet in mouth twice daily. B vitamins not coenzymated may not be bioavailable. Natural B vitamin sources - liver, brewers yeast and royal jelly.
   a. Royal Jelly – 500 mg freeze dried once or twice a day. (Do not use if you are allergic to it) High in Pantothenic acid and contains a full spectrum of all vitamins, minerals, amino acids and some special compounds found nowhere else.
   a. D'Glucarate – 400 mg 2X – binds estrogen receptors – major detox pathway. (Found in health food stores)
   b. Vitamin A – Cod Liver oil capsules (fresher than the liquid) Take about 6 a day.
   c. Vitamin C – Rose hips or Acerola cherries – 5 grams of whole dried fruit powder contain 500 mg of natural C plus bioflavinoids and trace minerals and co-factors. Amla (gooseberries) are also very high in vitamin C. Oranges – about 70 mg per whole fresh orange, also very high in glucaric acid, a powerful anticancer detox substance.
   d. Magnesium – 500 mg daily of magnesium oxide, magnesium citrate or magnesium chloride. (Avoid the amino acid chelates)
   e. Herbs containing the good natural phytoestrogens that block the bad estrogens from getting into the cells are - Red clover (estrogen blocker – studies show increases in T3, bone density and the good HDL cholesterol), Tumeric (Curcumin) and Yucca - act as estrogen blockers to stop their entry into the cells. In-Vitro studies found that the combination of Curcumin and Red Clover is powerful against breast cancer. Red clover caps- 3 2X plus Curcumin – 2 – 2X. At the same time, plant phytoestrogens support cell functions in persons that are low in natural estrogen.
   f. Fresh flaxseed ground daily – one tablespoon. Flaxseed is high in lignans and this binds estrogen receptors on the cells surface, blocking excess estrogen and chemicals with estrogenic effects in the environment (pesticides etc). Pesticides, unlike natural phytoestrogens that support cellular functions, poison the mitochondria inside the cells.
   g. Stress Reduction – avoid loud noises – listen to soft classical music.
   h. Avoid Soy products (except Miso and Tempeh)
   i. Use Resveratrol (an antioxidant and phytoestrogen from the skin of red grapes - antioxidant (binds estrogen receptors – inhibits breast cancer).

Use white button mushrooms raw – species Agaricus bisporus (reduces estrogen production, inhibits breast cancer cell .proliferation) *J. Nutr. 2001 Dec;131(12):3288-

Plechner on cortisol, estrogen and immune dysfunction

Alfred J. Plechner D.V.M. a graduate of the University of California-Davis School of Veterinary Medicine, has practiced in West Los Angeles for more than 35 years. Early in his career, he developed an interest in nutrition, allergy, and the relationship of hormone-immune imbalances to small animal diseases. His research and clinical experiences have been published in veterinary journals as well as popular animal magazines. In the mid-1980's, he co-developed the first successful commercial lamb and rice diet, a new hypoallergenic pet food diet that has been widely copied. He later served as a consultant for Natures Recipe in developing a new generation of hypoallergenic foods for pets. Plechner is co-author, with Martin Zucker, of a 1986 book "Pet Allergies: Remedies for an Epidemic." (Very Healthy Enterprises), and a new book, "Time bomb Pets" to be published in 2003 by New Sage Press.

Martin Zucker, a mutual friend and medical writer, first brought my attention to this work by sharing a fascinating scientific paper he wrote with Plechner that is based on the veterinarians more than thirty years of clinical experience. The paper, published in a medical journal, is entitled "An effective veterinary model may offer therapeutic promise for human conditions: cortisol and thyroid hormones." The article sparked my immediate interest. According to Zucker, Plechner has treated numerous cats with serious FIV infections. The treatment restored normal immune function.

In 2003, I interviewed Alfred Plechner DVM on his theories and protocols for normalizing endocrine (hypothalamus, pituitary and adrenal) [HPA] and thyroid hormones to normalize immune function in animals with chronic immune dysfunction such as cats with FIV (feline immune deficiency) and pets with allergies, cancer, fatigue and other chronic conditions. Most of this interview is published in two chapters in the "Immune Restoration Handbook."

To recap Plechner's theories, a defect in the Adrenal Cortex limits the amount of cortisol it can produce. Under stimulation from ACTH produced by the Pituitary, Plechner theorized that this causes the Adrenal glands to produce estrogen from the middle adrenal cortex when the adrenals are unable to produce more cortisol. Plechner states that the excess estrogen levels then impairs immune function.

[On this point I now disagree with Alfred Plechner. I don't find collaborative research that supports the theory that low cortisol levels causes an immune shift from TH1 to TH2 because of estrogen dominance. What I have found in the published literature is that low cortisol levels is linked very strongly with elevated Interleukin 6 (IL-6) and IL-6 is the TH2 cytokine that is a major factor in a wide range of illnesses from Cancer to AIDS to Arthritis to Chronic Fatigue syndrome to Candidiasis. What is really significant is newly discovered research that supplementation with hydrocortisone and even synthetic look-a-like drugs such as Prednisone and Prednisolone lower IL-6 levels dramatically.]

Since the 1980's, Plechner reports he has successfully treated over 35,000 pets by using a low-dose of thyroid in combination with low-dose cortisol or prescribed equivalents. He has observed improvements in the health and conditions of these animals and frequent remissions of their illnesses. Many aspects of Plechner's work are corroborated by other researchers but the link of immune dysfunction to elevated estrogen levels is not conclusive and has inconsistencies.

For example, I have talked to many persons who have chronic fatigue syndrome and/or multiple food allergies that actually have low rather than high estrogen levels. A search of the scientific literature fails to link elevated estrogen to immune dysregulation such as a predominance of TH2 cytokines (Interleukin 4, 5, 6, 8 and 10) with IL6 being the most problematic of the TH2 cytokines. In cancer and AIDS, there is substantial research linking high levels of IL-6 and tumor necrosis factor (TNF) to wasting syndrome and HIV progression to AIDS.

In candidiasis, chronic insomnia and CFIDS, elevated plasma levels of IL6 have been widely and consistently reported for several years. Elevated IL-6 is linked to increased replication of HIV, HHV-6, CMV, EBV, herpes and other viruses.

Cortisol has a reputation for being immunosuppressive. Why would anyone with Candidiasis, Cancer, HIV/AIDS, allergies, rheumatism and CFIDS want to use low-dose hydrocortisone.? Why?

The answer is that like a teeter-totter, the TH1 arm of the immune system is on one side and the TH2 is on the other. When the TH2 arm is over-active, it depresses the TH1 arm. Lowering the TH2 arm of the immune system raises the TH1 arm. In the middle is, in theory, the TH3 balance point with TH3 being the digestive tract. When food allergies and sensitivities develop and a person develops leaky gut syndrome, these conditions will lead to inflammatory reactions by increasing IL-6 and antibody production.

IL-6 is an essential TH2 cytokine needed to support the function of humoral immunity – particularly antibody production, although researchers have reported neuroprotective effects as well. The problem of imbalance occurs when levels of IL-6 do not return to normal and as a result depresses TH1 cytokine function. Several factors appear to contribute to elevated interleukin-6. They are:

1. Chronic infections
2. Chronic oxidative stress and free radicals
3. Insomnia
4. Toxins in food, water, air and environment
5. Stress from multiple causes – noise, strenuous exercise as in weight lifting, emotional and electromagnetic pollution (microwave, cell phone relay towers, violence on television and movies, rapid scene changes on TVs and computers without EMF blocker screens etc).

Researchers have found that in acute stress, both cortisol and IL-6 levels increase. With lower levels of stress, cortisol and other glucocorticoids reduce IL-6 secretion. **IL-6 has been found to stimulate the pituitary to release ACTH, the hormone that then stimulates the adrenals to produce more cortisol.** Over time, the body has evolved a unique set of checks and balances to control the effects of stress and immune challenges. It is now very evident that proinflammatory cytokines like TNF and IL-6 influence the functioning of the HPA (Hypothalamus, Pituitary and Adrenal) axis.

Revising Plechner's theories

While Plechner believes that elevated estrogen levels causes immune dyfunction when adrenal cortisol is insufficient, I propose that it is elevated IL-6 and other inflammatory cytokines, not estrogen, that were the primary cause of immune dysfunction in Plechner's 35,000 pets that he successfully treated with low-dose cortisol along with thyroid. The correct use of low dose cortisol may also help restore normal circadian cycles of cortisol (high in the morning and low at night) essential to restore normal sleep patterns.

The use of low-dose cortisol would probably not be needed if we learned how to get the liver to convert cortisone (the inactive form) to the active form of cortisol. In immune-compromised patients, levels of bound cortisol (called cortisone) will sometimes be high while levels of free cortisol - the active form - will be low. In persons under the stress of chronic infections, the need for free cortisol will be higher than in the normal population. In lab tests on persons with cancer, AIDS or chronic fatigue sysdrome, normal or lower cortisol levels should not be considered good news for this group while elevated cortisol levels should not be considered bad news. This is because of the increased needs for cortisol in persons under the stress of chronic illness. Being at or slightly above the normal reference range for cortisol would be desireable in these conditions.

Plechner uses Cortisol to treat Cancer in Pets

Plechner reports that cancer not only kills humans but dogs as well and states that it "accounts for almost half of canine deaths over the age of ten years."

Plechner states that *"Cortisol is an essential adrenal hormone with a paramount regulatory influence over immune and inflammatory activity in the body...that a defect triggers a domino effect of problems, among them a profound destabilization of the immune system."* He goes on to list several forms of cancer that are a result of cortisol deficiency including skin cancer, mammary cancer, lymphoma, fibrous sarcoma and leukemia and states: *"I have successfully treated many cases by addressing this cortisol defect, in my opinion, a major causal factor."*

Excerpts from an article by Alfred Plechner:

In June, 2003, I treated a dying Siberian Husky. The dog had been diagnosed two months before by another veterinarian with multiple metastasis tumors of the lungs. The site of the primary cancer had not been identified. The patient was eating poorly, breathing with difficulty, and coughing persistently. The animal had lost 12 pounds since the original diagnosis.

I suggested doing an endocrine-immune test and proceeding directly with steroid injections before the results came back. The owners agreed.

I injected the dog with 5 mg Vetalog (long acting hydrocortisone) and 60 mg of Depomedrol (methylprednisilone). Test results showed the animal had endocrine-immune imbalances including 52 mg/dl IgA suggesting probable malabsorption.

Two weeks later, the owners returned with a healthier dog. He had regained four pounds and was breathing easier. I rechecked the blood levels. The key estrogen and antibody levels had improved significantly. I now switched the dog to 6 mg of oral Medrol daily.

After another two weeks, I retested. The levels had normalized even further. Thoracic X-rays revealed that the lung lesions had disappeared. There was no evidence of tumors. The dog now weighed 78 pounds and had regained his appetite. Breathing was normal.

Although the dog has been on the therapy program for only a short period of time, the initial response has been excellent — and not unusual. The potential exists for normal health as long as the dog is *maintained on the program.*

For humans, Plechner writes: "The testing and therapy program I have described here has produced outstanding results for many years in the treatment of many different types of cancer. Can cortisol deficiency increase the risk of cancer? Do my findings in animals with cancer apply to humans?"

Editor's note: The successful Gerson Treatment for cancer, developed over 50 years ago includes thyroid supplementation and adrenal support. Coincidence?

The above case with a dog is one of several reported by Plechner who states he has successfully treated over 35,000 pets with these methods since 1978 including cats with FIV (Feline immunodeficiency virus), the cat equivalent to HIV.

For a thyroid medication for dogs, he has used Soloxine. Interestingly, he finds that cats often do not need thyroid supplementation although they still respond to the steroid (cortisol) treatments the same as the dogs do.

Why Plechner sometimes uses injectables in treating cancer

IgA is critical to mucosal immunity, digestion and absorption. **Plechner reports that malabsorption occurs when IgA levels are below 60 mg/dl.** This is why it is critical to test for IgA levels. When the levels are low (below 60), not only will oral hydrocortisone or synthetic substitutes like prednisone and prednisolone fail to be absorbed but also dietary nutrients and Chemotherapy will fail to be absorbed as well and the patients condition can be expected to worsen. When IgA levels are low, injectable hormones/steroids and other injectable drugs are used to bypass the intestines. Thyroid supplements are given to increase and restore normal IgA levels as well as improve other thyroid functions. When IgA levels return to the normal reference ranges, injectables can be discontinued and the oral supplements will be absorbable and provide effective treatment.

Interleukin-6 Test

An important test is to measure for plasma levels of IL-6. Specialty Labs (Santa Monica, CA **www.specialtylabs.com**) tests for IL-6. **The test code for IL-6 is 3828.** You can also ask your physician for a "TH2 cytokine panel test." This test will measure IL-6 and other TH2 type cytokines.

Cortisol supplementation can be given and then adjusted up or down to bring IL-6 levels back to the normal reference range which is a desirable goal and will have wide range benefits and symptomatic relief for many chronic conditions of inflammation. There are also several other supplements (i.e. fish oil, some anti-oxidants etc) and other dietary factors that can increase free cortisol levels and help return IL-6 to normal reference ranges.

Where to get a prescription for natural hormones?

Cortef has been discontinued. Generic alternatives to the brand name "Cortef" are available and usually come in 5, 10 or 20 mg tablets. Ask for the generic version of **"hydrocortisone"** tablets. Your physician may also know where to obtain it. For anyone with AIDS or Cancer, 5 mg per 40 lbs of body weight would be the minimum to consider. A 160 lb person (160 divided by 40 = 4 x 5 = 20 mg hydrocortisone). However, if IgA levels are below 60, you will not absorb the oral form and will need an injectable alternative.

Hydrocortisone and other natural hormones are made available in any strength through a compounding pharmacy. To locate a compounding Pharmacist, contact

Int'l Academy of Compounding Pharmacists (IACP), PO Box 1365, sugarland, TX 77487 800-927-4227 or Fax 281-495-0602. Their web site is http://www.iacprx.org and they can provide you with a list of local compounding pharmacists. Natural hormones are also available through www.womensinternational.com. 800-279-5708

If you cannot afford the you can obtain some benefits from a **1% hydrocortisone cream** that is available as an over-the-counter item at your local durgstore. There are about 20 mg of hydrocortisone in 1/2 teaspoon of the cream. Massage about 1/2 teaspoon daily in the morning on your skin or joints. It may be debatable as to how much is actually absorbed systemically, but some is.and enough to give noticeable results.

Natural Hormone sources or precursors

Urine, herbs and plant steroids. **Morning urine contains free cortisol.** Some alternative physicians have successfully treated cancer by injecting the patients own urine back into their body. Some persons drink a glass of their own urine daily for its health benefits. For those who cannot get past the thought or the taste, a urine retention enema has benefited persons. Urine can be applied topically to absorb its properties.

Cortisol precursors can be found in **Wild Yam** (cortisol/progesterone), **Black Cohosh** (cortisol/DHEA), **Yucca** (cortisol) and **Ginseng** for testosterone. Licorice root elevates cortisol, also blood pressure so must be used in small doses or not at all. Note: Black Cohosh supports Adrenal steroid production and also lowers blood pressure.

Plant Steroids (Sterols): Soy should be avoided due to presence of estradiol. **Plant sterols are precursors to Pregnenolone and DHEA**. Best sources are **Brown Rice bran** and **unrefined (black) Sesame seeds** or oil, **Avocados** and most other raw unprocessed seeds and nuts especially **sunflower seeds**, peanuts and **pumpkin seeds**. Other sources are **seafood**, **buckwheat** and **barley**.

Fish Oil reduces IL-6 - cancer patients gain weight

Barber MD et al reporting in Nutr Cancer. 2001;40(2):118-24 from Edinburgh, UK that nutritional supplements with fish oil given to pancreatic cancer patients who were losing weight resulted in weight gain. In this study, 20 patients who were wasting away were asked to consume daily a 600-calorie nutritional supplement that contained 2 grams of EPA (eicosapentaenoic acid) derived from fish oil. After 3 weeks of consumption of the fish oil-enriched supplement, they reported "a significant fall in production of IL-6, a rise in serum insulin concentration and a fall in the proportion of patients excreting proteolysis inducing factor." These blood parameter changes were associated with a median weight gain of 1 kg per patient. They stated, "Various mediators of catabolism in cachexia are modulated by administration of a fish oil-enriched nutritional supplement in pancreatic cancer patients.

This may account for the reversal of weight loss in patients consuming this supplement."

Note: If using "EPActive" by Jarrow Formulas, it would take 10 capsules daily to reach the level of 2000 mg of EPA (eicosapentaenoic acid).

Anti-cancer benefits of fish oil

In an article titled "The Traditional Diet of Greece and Cancer" Simopoulos AP (1) writes that the diet on the island of Crete represents the traditional "Mediterranean diet" prior to 1960. Analysis of the diet shows a number of protective substances including selenium, glutathione, high fiber and antioxidants and Resveratrol from red wine and polyphenols from olive oil and a balanced ratio of omega 6 and omega 3 fatty acids. The Omega 3 (DHA and EPA) fatty acids from fish "exert protective effects against some common cancers, especially cancer of the breast, colon and prostate." The Omega 3 fatty acids suppress "Cox-2, IL-1 and IL-6 gene expression." Other Cox-2 inhibitors (Pharmaceutical or botanical) may also inhibit IL-6.

Note: Cox 2 inhibitors are widely marketed for treatment of arthritis. Recently Vioxx, a pharmaceutical cox-2 inhibitor was pulled form the market after causing heart disease in several thousand users.

Treble T et al (2) reports that tumor necrosis factor and Il-6 decreased with dietary fish oil supplementation in healthy men in a dose dependent manner.

1. The Traditional diet of Greece and Cancer, Simopoupos AP Eur J Cancer Pre 2004; Jun;13 (3):219-230
2. Inhibition of tumor necrosis factor and Interleukin 6 by mononuclear cells following dietary fish oil supplementation….. Treble T et al Br J Nutr. 2003 Aug;90(2):405-12

Fish oil – How much is needed to reduce IL-6 in a healthy vs immune-challenged group?

In an article published in the Br J Nutr by Wallace FA. Miles and Calder titled "Comparison of the effects of linseed oil and different doses of fish oil on mononuclear cell function in healthy human subjects" the authors report on 3 types of Omega 3 fatty acids and their effects. In Linseed oil also known as flaxseed oil that is high in alpha-linolenic acid, they reported an increase in EPA but not DHA in plasma phospholipids. With fish oil (DHA and EPA) they reported a decrease in IL-6 in a daily dose between .44 and .94 grams daily. That would be 440 to 940 mg daily in healthy adults. It is important to remember that this dose was in a population of healthy adults, not a group of seriously immune compromised patients.

In the study with patients with pancreatic cancer, 2000 mg of EPA was used daily. However, I have read research that both DHA and EPA have similar anti-inflammatory effects and reduce IL-6, (Note: The "Max DHA" product from Jarrow Formulas will provide 2088 mg of DHA/EPA at about 6 capsules daily or 3 twice a day).

It takes about 3600 mg of sardine oil to yield around 2088 mg of a mixture of DHA/EPA and other Omega 3 fatty acids. Six capsules of Jarrow Formula DHA/EPA will yield that exact amount. Based on published research, that level of supplementation should reduce IL-6 plasma concentrations within a few weeks and bring a noticeable improvement in symptoms.

Note: Avoid taking rancid fish oil or rancid flaxseed oil as these can have the opposite effect of actually increasing IL-6 levels. Buying the lowest priced fish oil supplements on the market from mass merchandisers could be detrimental to your health. Fish oil should always be sealed in a dark capsule that prevents entrance of light or sealed in a can (canned sardines are good choice). Also avoid cod liver oil that is bottled in a clear bottle that allows light in and sits on a store shelf. Avoid all fish oil capsules that are "clear." The capsules must be brown or black in color to prevent the entrance of light and prevent rancidity from forming while on the shelf.

Never use flax oil or fish oil that has been long exposed to either light or oxygen (example – a nutritional bar that sits on a store shelf with either flax oil or deodorized sardine oil added should be considered rancid and avoided).

You can tell rancidity by the taste. If it has a fresh taste it is not rancid. If it tastes bitter, sour or flat, it may be rancid or going in that direction. Freezing or refrigeration helps prolong the shelf life of all oils.

Royal Jelly inhibits IL-6 and TNF

Okayama, Japan. Kohno K et al report (1) that when supernatants of Royal Jelly, the food of the Queen Bee, were added to a culture of mouse peritoneal macrophages that were stimulated with lipopolysaccharide, the production of proinflammatory cytokines such as TNF-alpha and IL-6 were efficiently inhibited in a dose-dependent manner without having cytotoxic effects on the macrophages. Macrophages are a type of white blood cell that fight infections in the body. The factors that had this effect in Royal Jelly were not identified and the dose was not mentioned in the abstract. Based on other research, a dose of 1000 to 2000 mg daily should be a good starting point.

My own opinion is that the least processed Royal Jelly is likely to have the most benefits (i.e. fresh Royal Jelly rather than freeze dried). Royal Jelly should to be kept under refrigeration or sealed in opaque (light resistant) capsules.
1. Royal Jelly inhibits the production of proinflammatory cytokines by activated Macrophages, Kohno K et al; Biosci Biotechnol Biochem. 2004 Jan;68(1):138-45

Vegetable Oils increase inflammatory cytokines (IL-6, TNF)

Chiba Univ. Hayashi N et al in Japan measured the effects of intravenous Omega 3 from fish oil (DHA/EPA) versus Omega 6 (poly unsaturated fatty acids) or PUFAs from vegetable oils on delayed-type hypersensitivity reactions in burned rats. They concluded that the Omega 6 from vegetable oils increased proinflammatory cytokine levels (IL-6, TNF etc) while the Omega 3's from fish oil prevented immunosuppression in burned rats receiving TPN.

The pro cancer effects of high fat diets are widely reported and the fats themselves are almost universally the wrong kind of fats (processed vegetable oils, margarine, hydrogenated fats etc). Compare the high cancer and heart disease rate of the western use of "vegetable oils" to the "Mediterranean diet" that uses olive oil and the Eskimos who eat high fat diets from fish that have little or no heart disease or cancer. The results speak for themselves.

Note: It is evident that under stress conditions, the consumption of these vegetable oils (canola, soybean corn, sunflower, safflower etc) promote inflammatory cytokines (IL-6, TNF etc) and would weaken the immune response against cancer, HIV, HHV-6 etc). The safe oils to use would be palm oil and olive oil, the latter containing 90% monounsaturated fatty acids.

Note on Flaxseed oil: The research I have read thus far suggests that the Omega 3 fatty acids from fish oil are more effective than the alpha linolenic acid from flax seed oil for their suppression of inflammatory cytokines. This does not mean that there are fewer benefits from using fresh flaxseed oil, except that there are more documented benefits from using high quality fish oils. The quality of these oils is critical for obtaining their benefits. If either is rancid, (oxidized), the effects will be the opposite of what is expected.

Vitamin E inhibits IL-6

Copenhagen. Fischer CP et al report (1) that 400 i.u of vitamin E daily inhibited the release of interleuken-6 from contracting human skeletal muscle after 3 hours of knee-extensor exercise. Lipid peroxidation levels did not increase in the group treated with the vitamin E. This was a small controlled study involving 7 volunteers.

Godbout JP et al report in experiments in mice that vitamin E inhibits peroxide formation and interleuken-6 secretion. (2)
1. Vitamin C and E supplementation inhibits the release of interleukin-6 from contracting human skeletal muscle. Fischer CP et al, J Physiol. 2004 May 28 Univ of Copenhagen.

Note: Other researchers report that vitamin C when used in doses above 500 mg daily can increase oxidative stress.
2. Alpha-Tocopherol reduces lipopolysaccharide-induced peroxide radical formation and interleukin-6 secretion..." Godbout JP et al. J Neuroimmunol. 2004 apr;149(1-2):101-9

Glucose and other sugars increase IL-6 from macrophages

Researchers Yu WK et al (1) in China found that increases in glucose levels in the blood raised macrophage production of IL-6, TNF and insulin. These conditions are more pronounced in persons with impaired glucose tolerance or have type 1 or 2 diabetes, sepsis or hyperglycemia. What does this say about the stress effects of consuming corn syrup and white sugar found in soda and thousands of processed foods? These simple sugars clearly promote IL-6, TH2 dominance and immune imbalance.
1. World J Gastrolenterol, 2003 Aug;9(8):1824-7

Specialty Labs on using IL-6 inhibitors to treat Breast Cancer

Speciality Labs web site at www.specialtylabs.com has an article on "Interleukin-6." IL-6 is an important cytokine to stimulate the B cells and thus antibody production and it is produced in the body by many types of cells including B cells, T cells, monocytes and hepatocytes. However, IL-6 is also produced by carcinomas, kaposi sarcoma cells, other sarcomas and melanomas and is elevated in Hodgkins disease. Specialty labs states that "neutralizing the effect of IL-6 may result in tumor regression. In recurrent breast cancer, IL-6 and IL-8 at the beginning of treatment are predictive indicators of response to therapy and prognosis; continuous elevation of IL-6 levels indicates poor prognosis in heavily pretreated patients. Combination therapy including agents that reduce IL-6 will become a new strategy for aggressively treating recurrent breast cancer."

IL-6 elevated in Heart Disease/mycocardial infarction

Specialty labs also reports that "IL-6 was significantly elevated in 28 persons with acute myocardial infarction compared with 15 normal controls, a recent study suggests that IL-6 with its proinflammatory role, plays a key role in the pathogenesis of coronary artery disease. The amount of IL-6 produced is closely related to the severity of myocardial dysfunction." Specialty Labs also reports that persons with the high plasma levels of IL-6 also have the highest mortality rates.

Summary on normalizing Interleukin-6 and TNF

1. **Use herbs for steroid precursors and plant sterols or low-dose hydrocortisone** (prescription may be required) – 5 to 10 mg taken early 8 or 9am and at 1 or 2 pm only, not in the evening. Also consider using low-dose thyroid – 1/2 grain once or twice daily as prescribed – helps the liver process cortisone into cortisol and detoxify the body. Avoid using cortisol long term without also using thyroid at the same time.
2. Low-dose DHEA – 25 mg daily for men and 10 mg daily for women.
3. Fish oil – DHA and EPA – Sardine and/or Salmon oil. Max DHA from Jarrow Formulas and/or EPActive. Three capsules twice daily should lower IL-6 based on the scientific literature. Fish oil lowers tumor necrosis factor as well as IL-6. Critically needed for all cancer, CFIDS and HIV patients.
4. Avoid vegetable oils high in Omega 6 PUFAS that stimulate the secretion of inflammatory TH2 cytokines. These oils include canola, soybean, corn oil, sunflower and safflower oil primarily. Peanut oil that has 50% monounsaturated fatty acids and is less problematic but the best choices are the oils very high in monounsaturated fatty acids like olive oil – all types even the ultra light have 90% monounsaturated fatty acids. Special strains of safflower oil are also very high in monounsaturated fatty acids and are so labeled. Avoid eating in restaurants where fats of unknown origin are used.
5. A Hypoallergenic diet reduces stress on the digestive tract and thus IL-6 levels. (Avoid milk, ice cream, soy flour, and gluten from wheat if you are gluten intolerant etc). Note: You can try using cultured milk products (yogurt, kefir) and cultured soy products (Tofu, Miso). Soy milk is usually well tolerated while soy flour causes digestive problems. Consider using fiber and probiotics together daily.
6. Complex carbohydrates (with no added fat or protein) normalize IL-6 and other inflammatory cytokines. For an anti-inflammatory breakfast, consider plain whole grain toast with natural applesauce and tea (green/licorice). Whole grains, fruits and vegetables with little or no oils added and some fish are the ultimate diet for balanced immunity and health.

7. Cox-2 inhibitors, NF-Kappa B inhibitors and anti-oxidants [Tumeric, Holy Basil, Skullcap, Green tea, Hu Zhang aka Solomon's Seal (high in Resveratrol), Rosemary, Ginger, Red grapes, Oregano, Hops, raw potatoes - high in catalase – breaks down H_2O_2 into O_2 and H_2O]

8. Licorice root and Grapefruit. Both grapefruit and licorice interfere with an enzyme (11-beta-OHSD) that oxidizes cortisol into cortisone, thus elevating cortisol levels. Grapefruit and licorice should be used in the morning and afternoon and not late evening. Too much licorice will raise blood pressure. Suggestion: Find an herbal tea with licorice root as the 2nd, 3rd or 4th ingredient mentioned on the label. (e.g. Red Zinger" by Celestial Seasonings").

9. Vitamin E – use "mixed tocopherols" only for best results– for adults 400 i.u daily.

10. Royal Jelly – fresh only 1000 mg to 2000 mg daily.

About lab tests results for cortisol levels

Researchers have found that Metyrapone and low dose (LD-ACTH) test are far more accurate than the standard high dose ACTH test.

The second problem with lab test results whether it is selenium, DHEA, cortisol or something else is that lab reference numbers are based on what is average for normal healthy people. Unfortunately, many people who get these tests are not normal healthy people but suffer from various conditions from HIV/AIDS to CFIDS to MS to cancer to candidiasis to intestinal dysbiosis and much more. People with these conditions most likely will have a need for higher plasma levels of cortisol and many other nutrients including selenium. What would be high levels in a normal person would be low levels in someone with chronic inflammation and immune dysfunction.

It is my opinion that the need for cortisol in someone with cancer or AIDS may be up to twice as high as what is found in healthy persons. It is my opinion that it is more important to get interleuken-6 (IL-6) levels back to its normal reference range than to worry about getting cortisol down to its normal reference range. Researchers have found that as free cortisol levels go up IL-6 goes down.

The most important test is to measures IL-6 levels. By tracking the effects of various doses of hydrocortisone from 10 mg to 20 mg to 30 mg daily and adjusting the dose up or down until IL-6 reaches the normal reference ranges, you can determine the effectiveness of the treatment. In HIV, I would expect the CD4 counts to rise and viral load to fall as IL-6 returns to a normal level. In CFIDS, fatigue should go away and energy should return to normal. In cancer, tumors should stop growing and start receding. The IL-6 test can also measure the effects of other IL-6 inhibitors and normalizers like fish oil, royal jelly, turmeric, holy basil and others.

Plechners Protocol for Pets

2003: In a phone call to Alfred Plechner, I asked him to describe his treatment protocol for pets and small animals. Here was his reply.

Plechner: The treatment consists of giving low dose thyroid hormones along with low-dose cortisol..

Konlee: Do you mean low-dose thyroid hormones like "Armour Thyroid" that provides the natural thyroid hormones "Thyroxin" (T4, T3, T2 and T1) and hydrocortisone that the body uses to make cortisol, the natural adrenal hormone?

Plechner: Yes, the equivalent of these drugs for use in humans is available by prescription for household pets and other animals. The amount given varies according to the weight of the animal and the results of diagnostic tests. If I were treating an animal that weighed 150 pounds, I would start off with 1/2 grain of thyroid (about 32 mg) and 5 mg of cortisone twice a day. You will need to monitor blood pressure when giving thyroid as too much could cause it to rise as well as increase the pulse rate. The process of increasing thyroid use has to be gradual. Usually the amount of cortisol used is maintained at a low level.

Konlee: I can understand the role of the thyroid hormone, as it controls cellular metabolism throughout the body, the production of ATP and will help in normalizing body temperature that is critical for restoring cell-mediated immune responses, but cortisol, is it not immunosuppressive?

Plechner: Absolutely, if you take too much of it. The same is true for zinc. Research has shown that too little zinc or too much is immunosuppressive and this has been shown for other nutrients as well. You absolutely need zinc for your thymus gland to function properly and mature T cells, but you don't want too much or too little.

Now for cortisol, it is a natural anti-inflammatory hormone, and the normal healthy human body produces about 40 mg daily. It is well established that most of the pharmaceutical versions of "cortisone" like Prednisone are synthetic steroids, powerful anti-inflammatory agents, but also immunosuppressive at high doses. In fact, at doses over 5 mg daily (the equivalent of 30 mg pf hydrocortisone), Prednisone will completely shut down your adrenal gland production of cortisol. When going off Prednisone, which is over 6 times stronger than hydrocortisone, it has to be tapered off gradually over a period of several days or weeks. At high doses, all kinds of adverse effects can develop with the synthetic steroids, and this has given them a bad reputation.

Low-dose natural free cortisol or hydrocortisone reduces levels of interleuken-6, a TH2 cytokine, that is overactive in HIV/AIDS, Candidiasis, CFIDS cancer and many other conditons.

The amount of cortisol produced by the adrenals is controlled by ACTH from the Pituitary gland and controlled through a feedback loop with the Hypothalamus gland that produces Corticotropic-Releasing Factor (CRF). When the adrenals are exhausted and not producing enough free cortisol, the Hypothalamus continues to pump out CRF that, in turn, stimulates the Pituitary to produce more ACTH. The elevated ACTH signals the Adrenals to produce more Cortisol that the exhausted adrenals are unable to do. However, the adrenal glands respond to the ACTH stimulation by continuing to produce estrogen. In other words, ACTH can stimulate the adrenal glands to produce either cortisol or estrogen. (In some instances, total adrenal exhaustion causes the adrenals to fail to produce either enough cortisol or estrogen).

What turns-off the CRF/ACTH feedback loop is sufficient free cortisol levels in the blood. At a certain level, cortisol turns off the CRF that regulates the ACTH output from the Pituitary. In a normal 24-hour period (circadian cycle), cortisol levels are highest at 8 A.M. in the morning and lowest in the evening (8pm to midnight). Cortisol supplements, given before bedtime, can interfere with sleep. Cortisol supplements should only be given between 8am and 2pm (early afternoon).

There are many people treated with thyroid hormones that get their body temperature back to normal and many who do not. One reason is that part of the Adrenal glands are exhausted and are not producing enough cortisol, while another part of the Adrenal glands are producing too much estrogen that binds to thyroxin. The production of cortisol and adrenal estrogen is controlled through the Hypothalamus/Pituitary feedback loop.

Konlee: IgA is a TH1 Immunoglobulin needed for mucosal immunity. Bifidobacteria Longum has been found to increase the levels of IgA as does vitamin A. What are some of the benefits of supplementing with low-dose thyroid and cortisol that you have observed in your clinical practice?

Plechner: After a trial and error period, I have developed a testing and treatment strategy that has proved to be safe and highly effective. The central modality is replacement with physiological doses of hydrocortisone preparations to address the root issue of cortisol deficiency. The low-dose cortisol preparations normalize ACTH levels, stop the overproduction of adrenal estrogen and the accompanying estrogen blockade of the thyroid hormones and reregulates the immune system. The use of low-dose cortisol long-term has also been reported by Jefferies for treating allergies, autoimmune disorders and chronic fatigue syndrome (1).

The second important modality is the simultaneous use of thyroid hormone. The thyroid hormone is needed, because the excess adrenal estrogen has bound some of the thyroid hormone. The low dose thyroid hormone helps increase the metabolic rate and the liver to detoxify, as well as process cortisone. By giving cortisol and thyroid replacement simultaneously, the body is able to effectively utilize and process cortisone (the inactive form) without developing side effects.

Once the testing and low-dose hormone therapy is underway, *it is very important to follow a hypoallergenic diet and remove foods to which the animal or person is sensitive*. After a few weeks, the sensitive foods may be reintroduced one at a time.

Konlee: Have you written and published other articles on this subject?

Plechner: In the late 1970's, I wrote four articles (2, 3, 4 and 5) on my experiences and theories but found no germane research in veterinary journals to provide guidance.

Konlee: I understand you have worked a lot with animals that have the FIV virus, the equivalent of HIV in humans. Can you tell us more about your experience?

Plechner: FIV is one of several retroviruses that affect cats. Like terrorists, they infiltrate into the body of cats, live in a dormant state for periods of time, even years, replicate as conditions allow, and then attack, causing serious damage and even death. From my perspective, the ability of a cat to combat viruses like these hinges on its endocrine-immune resources. The presence of the abnormal endocrine-immune mechanism I have described to you renders an animal less able to fight. The immune cells are deregulated, unable to establish a strong unified defense. As the underlying hormone and immune irregularities intensify with time, errant defenses run amok. When cats die, people say the virus killed them. To me it's more a case of a dysfunctional immune system that has not only failed to deter the viruses, but also turned on the cat and helped to kill it. Cats with clinical signs of the disease are regarded as incurable. They are often euthanized.

Many cats have no symptoms, but are nevertheless positive for this or perhaps other retroviruses (such as feline leukemia or feline infectious peritonitis). The blood test I have developed shows whether an animal has the endocrine-immune imbalance. When I do the test, and the results indicate no imbalance, it is highly unlikely an animal will break with the disease. If the results indicate imbalance, the situation has to be corrected otherwise an animal will become sick or sicker.

After the hormone replacement program is started, a cat often will test negative for the (FIV) virus. This is true, whether the cat previously was merely positive for the virus or actually symptomatic. The underlying defect has been corrected. The immune cells are back in business. They fight back and vanquish the viruses. This is my experience in numerous cases. Multiple felines under one roof might be positive for a particular virus but the huge majority of them live long and healthy lives, if they are put back into hormonal balance and their owners keep them on the program. If the program is stopped, the imbalance will return and the animal become at risk again.

You test for the defect. If you find it, you correct it, and stay the course. The imbalance is there. You are correcting it with the therapy, and putting an animal's derailed immune system back on the tracks, enabling it to fight off any virus. The cat will respond by testing antibody negative. I have seen this reversal so many times that it doesn't surprise me anymore, even though the veterinary textbooks say it doesn't happen. Supposedly, once you have the virus, you always have it. But that's not my clinical experience. I have been able to turn around approximately 70 percent of sick animals with FIV. Obviously, the earlier you correct the imbalance the better the chance for recovery. You want to intervene before severe damaged is inflicted to organs and vital parts. Remember what I said about elevated estrogen in the system. If the level is high enough it can suppress bone marrow and red blood cell production. The animal will develop anemia, and blood transfusions may be needed.

Konlee: How might this relate to HIV?

Plechner: If my experience with animals is any indication, perhaps when a human is exposed to the HIV virus, whether or not he or she breaks with symptoms of AIDS may depend on the health of that person's endocrine-immune integrity. If an imbalance is found through testing, correction with appropriate hormone replacement could be a significant strategy for both prevention and therapy.

I have suggested to interested physicians that they test for the same range of hormonal-immune relationships as I do for animals. That means a blood test measuring cortisol, total estrogen, thyroid (T3/T4), and Immunoglobulin. Other factors could be added, such as T cells and perhaps other hormones, in order to develop a more precise picture of the defect's total range of impact. Testosterone and other androgens, also produced in the adrenal cortex, might be included and measured against immune cell levels. I have not done this in my clinical practice because of increased testing costs. However, researchers have begun looking at the immune and inflammatory modulating effects of androgen/estrogen ratios and concentrations. Patients can be retested after biweekly or monthly intervals to monitor changing relationships. The bottom line is that hormonal replacement must be measured against B and T cell levels.

Note: The active form of thyroxine, T3, is a strong inducer of IgA, a TH1 cytokine needed for intestinal and mucosal health.

Ref:
1. Jefferies, w. McK.Mild Adrencortical deficiency, chronic allergies, autoimmune disorders and the chronic fatigue syndrome: a continuation of the cortisone story. Medical Hypothesis, 1994; 42;183-189

2. Plechner A. J., Shannon M., Canine Immune Complex diseases. Modern Veterinary Practice, November 1976; 917
3. Plechner A. J., Shannon M., Epstein A, Goldstein E., Howard E. B., Endocrine-immune surveillance. Pulse. June-July, 1978
4. Plechner A.J., Theory of endocrine-immune surveillance. California Veterinarian, Jan 1979; 12.
5. Plechner A.J. Preliminary observations on endocrine-associated immunodeficiencies in dogs? A clinician explores the relationship of immunodeficiencies to endocrinopathy. Modern Veterinary Practice, 1979; 811

Diagnostic tests for humans – available from Specialty Labs in Santa Monica, CA www.specialtylabs.com 310-828-6543

Tests for both males and females
A. Blood (Serum or Plasma) Tests
   1. Interleukin-6 (IL-6) code 3828
   2. Thyroid Panel Hypothyroidism- Code 3074
   3. Cortisol – Code 3128 or Low Dose ACTH Test
   4. Testosterone – total and free – Code 3248
   5. IgA, IgG and IgM -Code 1045
   6. TNF-a (CFIDS, cancer, KS or wasting syndrome is present) Code 3294
      Note: if IL-6 is high, then test for C-Reactive Protein as it may also be high. C-Reactive Protein is a marker for heart disease. IL-6 inhibitors and some Cox-2 inhibitors may also lower C-Reactive protein (www.specialtylabs.com article on cytokine inhibitors.)

A. **Urine tests for both males and females**
   1. Active /Free Cortisol – Code 3128U
   2. Free T3 and T4

C. **Basal metabolic temperature (using a digital thermometer)**

Traditional method: Shake down thermometer and place on bed stand the night before. Upon awakening in the morning, while still in bed, place thermometer in armpit for 10 minutes before getting up. Normal basal temperature should be between 97.8 and 98.2_F. Note: Mercury thermometers are no longer being sold due to the hazards of mercury, should a thermometer break.

A convenient digital thermometer called a "Talking Thermometer" is available from Walgreens for about $10. Just click the button and wait for 3 beeps then it is ready to use. The thermometer will talk to you and tell you your temperature when it stabilizes. Upon awakening, the basal temperature may be taken under the tongue. Manufacturers of thermometers state that the basal temperature taken under the tongue can be done faster and with the same accuracy as under the armpit.

Note: Because of its fast readout, the Talking Thermometer and other digital thermometers will not give you an accurate reading under the armpit and should be taken under the tongue instead. The normal basal temperature range under the tongue upon awakening in the morning is from 97.6 to 98_F or .2 degrees less than the armpit reference range. A basal temperature of 1/2 degree below normal indicates mild hypothyroidism, whereas 2 degrees or more below normal is quite serious hypothyroidism.

Note: Basal test is only accurate in a menstruating women from 2nd to 4th day.

In addition to the above, the following tests are also recommended for Females:
- a. Progesterone (lack of this hormone can cause osteoporosis)
- b. Ferritin

Summary of Plechners findings

1. Low immunoglobulins, especially IgA, will indicate to the clinician that the cortisol is at least partially inactive, and active thyroxine (T3) is deficient. This is true, even when T4 and blood cortisone levels are normal or high.
2. Binding of thyroid hormone by estrogen can be indicated, when both T3 and T4 test normal and the patient has these symptoms – excessive sleeping, sluggishness, hyperkeratosis of the nose and pads of the feet; excess pigmentation in skin of ventral abdomen; high cholesterol; high triglycerides, underweight or overweight.
3. Suppression of IgA, IgM and IgG.

Plechner states that the role of cortisol as an immune regulatory agent has been grossly neglected. An unknown, but probably very large percentage of cats and dogs, produce inadequate or bound cortisol, as a result of contemporary breeding practices primarily, and, to a lesser degree, stress, aging, poor diet, and other environmental inputs. The cortisol defect triggers a deregulation of major immune system cells.

Health care professionals may and others who want a copy of Plechner's 14 page report can write to Keep Hope Alive, PO Box 270041, West Allis, WI 53227. Include $2 and a stamped self addressed envelope.
Alfred J Plechner, D.V.M. email: drplechner@hotmail.com.Phone 208-765-0456
Testing for Pets: National Veterinary Diagnostic Services, Lake Forest, CA 949-859-3648)

Note: There are several reports on the internet that agree natural thyroid works better and with fewer side effects than their manufactured alternatives, like Synthyroid. If you decide to try a natural formula, avoid any with "pituitary" gland extract, as this is the gland that can spread "mad cow disease" from infected cows. Pituitary of bovine origin is one glandular to avoid in all supplements. Pituitary of porcine origin (pigs) is not known to contain any risk factors.

Melatonin linked to deep sleep and increases in DHEA

When darkness comes to the eyes at night, the body begins to produce melatonin. Melatonin promotes deeper and more restful sleep. When light strikes the optic nerve in the morning, melatonin production stops. Sometimes, people have a hard time waking up in the morning because of melatonin spillover – that is, a small amount of melatonin continues to be produced after a person wakes up. This lowers the metabolic rate and the person goes through the day feeling half awake. To solve this problem, expose the eyes to a bright light for a few minutes or go outside and take off the sunglasses and take brisk walk for about 15 minutes. This will stop melatonin spillover. More information on melatonin spillover can be found at www.drdebe.com/barriers.htm in an article written by Dr Joseph Debe.

Melatonin is also important, as it stimulates the adrenal glands to produce DHEA. DHEA is itself a precursor of other hormones. Melatonin supplements are available over-the-counter (OTC). Start off with a small amount like 1 mg and gradually increase its use, until sleep is optimal. Exposing part of a persons body to the north-pole seeking side of a magnet for 30 to 60 minutes before bedtime also increases melatonin production. However, I would advise against exposing a person to a magnet, or a magnetic pad or mattress, all night long, as this may interrupt sleep.

Tart cherries found to contain melatonin

Cherries have been used to lower uric acid crystals in the body to prevent and treat gout. Cherries have also been found to have other anti-inflammatory properties, including Cox 1 and Cox 2 inhibitors for relieving arthritis pain. Sour cherries also contain Melatonin, a hormone produced by the pineal gland. (1) "Consuming cherries could be an important source of melatonin," according to Texas scientists. Drinking a glass of sour cherry juice, or eating about 20 red tart cherries before retiring at night, may assist in inducing a deeper state of sleep and supporting adrenal glandular function. Without actually measuring melatonin levels, I found that the tart red cherries, the kind used to make pie, were more effective than the red, sweet, eating cherries, in promoting a deeper and more restful sleep. Red tart cherries can be found in many areas year round in the frozen food section. Just thaw out about 1/2 a cup of frozen cherries and eat 20 or 25 as a late evening snack.

ImmunePro: You can also help yourself to a night of deep restful sleep by taking 10 grams of a cold processed whey protein, like Immunepro, before bedtime, or eating 1/2 cup of cottage cheese or Ricotta cheese on rye bread, as a source of Glutamine and calcium lactate, and, when used with cherries, may induce a deep sleep. I believe these choices that are natural and gentle may be better than a sleeping pill or a melatonin pill, both of which have "manufactured" ingredients. When it comes to synthesizing pharmaceutical compounds, I have found that plants usually "get it right" more often than laboratory technicians. If cherries and whey protein or cottage cheese used at the same time don't help you fall into a deep restful sleep, there is always "Ambien," a pharmaceutical sleeping aid with a reasonably good reputation. Sources: Tart cherry juice concentrate – Sunrise Dried Fruit Co, 6530 NW Bayshore Dr., Northport, MI 49670. 800-488-5762 or www.sunrisedriedfruit.com/concentrate.htm. For ImmunePro, 800-735-1047 or www.wellwisdom.com

Note 1/19/03: Last week two local persons here in West Allis, who had chronic interrupted sleep (insomnia) for over one year, used ten grams of ImmunePro plus 4 ounces of tart cherry juice before bedtime and had instant success – 7 hrs in one case and 9 hours in another of deep continuous restful sleep. Both persons now report that the combination of the cherries and the whey protein, together, works better than either used alone. One of the two persons, who had used sleeping pills every night, finds he no longer needs them. The other no longer wakes up in the middle of the night to urinate.

1. Ralph Moss newsletter No. 13 www.cancerdecisions.com

9

Thyroid hormone activity, body temperature and immunity

The thyroid gland is located in front of the throat below the Adam's apple and above the breastbone. It regulates metabolism in the cells and the rate at which the body utilizes oxygen. The thyroid functions like a kind of biological thermostat. Broda Barnes MD who wrote the famous book on "Hypothyroidism" in 1976 stated that 40% of the American people were hypothyroid, that is, had underactive thyroid glands. This sluggish activity, Barnes reports, is linked to a weakened immune response to infections, fatigue, to low body tempaerature and a long list of chronic health conditions including obesity, skin problems and even heart disease. Barnes cites significant clinical data from his life long experiences to back up his statements. (1)

Dr. Regan Golob has an article on "How's Your Thyroid" on his website at http://www.docgolob.com/thryoid.htm. He states: "the thyroid a lot of times reaches burnout due to over-stimulation of the adrenals, which become exhausted. This over-stimulation can be from coffee or pop, excess protein, stress etc. The thyroid picks things up for a while, until it becomes exhausted and then a persons experiences fatigue, intolerance to cold, weight gain, muscle weakness, depression, dry and scaly skin."

Thyroid and adrenal insufficiency go hand in hand. The major glands are linked so closely that when one does not function properly it can throw the others off. The key to normalcy is to detoxify and nourish and return all the organs to homeostasis or balance. This is easier said than done. Sometimes the fastest and easiest path to recovery is to supplement daily with low-dose natural hormones. Too often, under the influence of pharmaceutical salesmen, synthetic look-a-like drugs are used that are not in the patients best long-term interest.

1. Hypo-thyroidism – the unsuspected illness, by Broda Barnes, 1976. Fitzhenry and Whiteside Ltd, Toronto.

A self-test for iodine deficiency

Dr. Golob recommends a skin test for iodine deficiency, as iodine is the most important mineral for thyroid function. He suggests getting a bottle of tincture of iodine, the kind that stains your skin yellowish brown (not the colorless kind). You paint a 1-inch square area on your arm. The stain should stay for 24 hours. If it goes away in a few hours, or before the 24-hour period has elapsed, it means your thyroid gland is looking for and needs more iodine. Keep up the daily skin treatments until the stain is present after 24 hours, then try the test every other day, or until it is not needed.

The basal temperature test under the armpit needs to be taken in the morning. As your iodine level increases, there should be a corresponding increase in body temperature.

General signs of thyroid deficiency

1. Low Body Temperature (LBT) (not always conclusive as LBT can coexist with normal T4 and T3 values for thyroxin.) www.wilsonssyndrome.com
2. Susceptible to all kinds of infections
3. Low white blood cell counts
4. Anergy – lack of DCH response to a skin test to challenge immune system
5. Fatigue
6. unrefreshing sleep – can't completely wake up
7. Headaches
8. Chronic sinusitis
9. Dry scaly skin (eczema, psoriasis, acne etc)
10. Rheumatic pain in joints
11. Depression
12. Menstrual problems for women

Dr Brownstein's list of factors that impair thyroid function (1)

1. Aging linked to a gradual decline of both thyroid and adrenal hormones.
2. Alpha Lipoic Acid (does not affect everyone)
3. Alcohol
4. Chronic illness
5. Cigarette smoking
6. Diet factors. Soy products and cruciferous vegetables – dose dependent (avoid large quantities). Studies in animals show soy impairs T4 to T3 conversion.
7. Drugs (Birth control pills, Lithium, Estrogens, Propranolol, Beta blockers, Dexamethasone, Methimazole and Propylthiouracil)
8. External radiation
9. Growth hormone deficiency
10. Heavy metal toxicity including mercury and lead, pesticides, sodium chloride as well as sodium fluoride in city water.
11. Hemochromatosis
12. High Stress
13. Low adrenal states
14. Malnutrition (mineral deficiencies) consumption of trans fats and hydrogenated fats and a lack of good fats – monounsaturated – avocados, olive oil, palm, omega 3.
15. Mineral and vitamin deficiencies (selenium, Vitamin A, B6 and B12)
16. Postoperative state
17. Physical trauma.

Besides the above list, Brownstein cites research that in a state of hypothyroidism, hydrocortisone production and metabolism is usually low. Hypothyroidism can be established by chronic low basal body temperature as measured by the Barnes method upon rising. Thus a direct link has been established between subnormal thyroid and inadequate adrenal production of hormones.

Toxemia or the buildup of toxins in the body and an impairment of the detoxification pathways can be a major cause of impaired thyroid function. Link by link, the health of one organ affects the health of another. The liver, the organ through which most detoxification occurs, has the greatest burden of all.

Today, I reasonably estimate that due to toxins in the diet, air pollution and contaminants in the water we drink and electromagnetic pollution, that the combined effect contributes to overworked adrenal and subnormal thyroid activity in at least a third or more of the population in the United States.

1. Overcoming Thyroid Disorders, David Brownstein MD; published by Medical Alternatives Press, 4173 Fieldbrook Rd, West bloomfield, MI 48323 www.drbrownstein.com 888-647-5616

Remedies to support the thyroid and mitochondria

1. Armour Natural Thyroid – derived from pigs – prescription required - use as directed by a health care professional. OTC – desiccated thyroid sold in some health food stores. Start off with 16mg (1/4 grain) or 32 mg (1/2 grain) twice daily after consulting with a health care professional - monitor blood pressure. Reduce amount if too much stimulation occurs. Not recommended for persons with congestive heart failure. The following are alternatives to Armour Thyroid or synthetic prescribed drugs like Synthroid that may be sufficient for some peoples' metabolic needs.

    a. Thyrophin PMG – by Standard Process Labs. Made from bovine thyroid, with the thyroxine removed. Standard Process introduced this product 50 years ago. Several persons report it has helped restore normal body temperature in 2 to 6 weeks. 1 to 3 tablets daily are used with meals. Cost about $10 a month. Sold through health care professionals. To locate a health care professional in your area, contact Standard Process Labs at 800-848-5061 or 262-495-2122 (PO Box 904, Palmyra, WI 53256 www.standardprocess.com). Thyrophin is recommended when body temperature is more than 1 degree below normal.

    b. Homeopathic Thyroid and Adrenal preparations (tablets or liquid are available) are manufactured by Natra Bio and found in health food stores. This product may be sufficient for some persons if body temperature is less than 1 degree below normal. Otherwise, go for the Armour Thyroid or use Thyrophin PMG. Use as directed.

2. Iodine – Tincture of iodine used as a daily or every other day skin test for a few weeks then monitor weekly. Kelp – 2 capsules 1 to 3 times daily or as directed. Seafood - fish, Seaweed – Dulse, Wakame, Kombu, Nori, Arame, Dulse, Hijiki, Purple Laver, Agar-agar, Sea-cabbage, Mekabu and Sea palm. Miso soup made with Wakame is a good choice for a daily meal. Note: Seaweed sources - Gold Mine - 800-475-3663 or Mountain Ark - 800-643-8909

3. Cayenne, African Bird Pepper, Chili, other hot peppers, Curry, ginger root. Hot Salsa. Vitalerbs (Dr Christopher's Original Formula) is the only true whole food based vitamin/mineral/enzyme formula I know of in the United States that is not fortified with synthetic vitamins.

4. Selenium - 400 mcg to 800 daily of Phytosel (high-selenium mustard greens) or high-selenium yeast - helps convert T4 to T3. Selenium is found in Brazil nuts, fish, seaweed and brewers yeast.

5. Exercise in the morning raises metabolic rate and body temperature. After sunrise, upon awakening, drink a glass of water and go for a 30 to 45 minute brisk walk (about 1.5 to 2 miles) before you eat. Do not run or jog, just walk at a moderate pace or take a ride on your bicycle. Do not wear sunglasses. The diffused sunlight hitting the retina of the eye stops the melatonin spillover effect and, combined with the exercise, will raise the body temperature from 1/2 to 1 full degree, a benefit that will last most of the day. You can measure the increase in body temperature by taking your temperature before you walk and then again about 20 to 30 minutes after you return to your home or after having breakfast. The results are truly amazing.

6. Whey protein – (5 to 7 grams per 100 pounds of body weight) before bedtime or as a late evening snack, will promote deep restful sleep with REM and raise basal temperature. Raises glutathione levels and builds muscle while you sleep. One scoop of ImmunePro, Immunocal or other quality cold processed whey protein in the evening with a glass of tart cherry juice is a very good choice. Lack of certain amino acids, particularly tyrosine and taurine, impairs thyroid function and immune function. Whey is a good source of tyrosine, taurine and glutamine. Glutamine increases human growth hormone (HGH) while you sleep).

If for any reason you are intolerant to whey protein, try predigested rice protein powder or fresh almond/pineapple shake once a day in the evening. Add a glass of tart cherry juice or pineapple juice to a blender and add 1/4 cup of raw almonds and one tsp. raw grated ginger root or one whole kiwi fruit. Blend and drink. Natural calcium and trace mineral supplements, like ground marine Coral, may also be used at the same time.

7. Oolong tea – a black tea from China with a natural sweet taste that raises the metabolic rate and body temperature. Helps burn fat in overweight persons.

8. Venus flytrap extract – 20 drops 2 times daily. Severl persons have reported normal body temperature after u sing VFT daily for about 3 months. Sources: Vital Health Products (vhp4.com) or Generation II

9. Two raw apples and 2 oranges daily – both are very high in Glucaric acid. D'Glucarate (Solaray or another brand) – binds estrogen – major detox pathway. Therapeutic dose: Two 400 mg capsule every 8 hours each day or eat apples and oranges.

10. Manganese – Best sources: pineapple and oat bran. Suggestion – 1/2 cup of oat bran daily along with 2 glasses or servings of pineapple. Other sources are barley, brown rice, buckwheat and blackberries, beans and other legumes.

11. Coconut Oil, Coconut milk and fresh coconuts - richest natural source of medium chain triglycerides (MCTs). 3 Tablespoons of coconut oil daily or 1/2 cup of coconut milk or 1/2 a fresh coconut will enhance metabolic function and increase body temperature. Highly recommended to help burn off fat calories in persons who are overweight. If you are not using coconut milk or fresh coconuts, I highly recommend Virgin Coconut Oil imported from rural villages in the Philippines from Tropical Traditions 1-866-311-2626. They have the freshest and most aromatic coconut oil on the planet.

12. Royal Jelly – 1000 to 2000 mg daily; A rich source of pantothenic acid needed for adrenal function and RNA/DNA to support the mitochondria.

13. Chlorella or Spirulina – 5 grams daily to support Mitochondria function inside the cells (converting T4 to T3). (Note: Vitalerbs contain alfalfa, barley and kamut extract that also support mitochondrial function).

14. Transfer Factor Plus (4-Life Products) Case reports on the Internet indicate improved

thyroid function using transfer factor products. Two to 4 capsules daily.

15. Fat and Sodium. Diets high in vegetable oils high in polyunsaturated fats (canola, corn, soy etc) increase estrogen levels, lower body temperature, contribute to obesity and loss of lean muscle mass and promote cancer. Foods high in salt decrease potassium reserves needed as electron donors to produce energy in the mitochondria of the cells.

16. Ojibwa tea - readers report normalization of body temperature after several months of use.

17. Detoxification - Critical to recovery.
 a. Whole lemon/olive oil drink has increased body temperature in many persons.
 b. Bitter Melon extract – 2 to 4 capsules daily to help balance blood sugar levels.
 c. Red clover tea- Drink 1 to 3 cups daily with the last one before bedtime - one tea bag per cup or take 3 capsules twice daily. In animal experiments, increased total and free T3, the most active form of thyroxine. Stimulates the P450 liver enzyme detoxification system. Other herbs: Tumeric (Curcumin), Black cohosh, Thyme and/or Hops.
 d. Exercise directly increases ATP production and moves toxins out of the body
 e. Water - clean – oxygen or ozone added with ionic trace minerals or coral - drink one large glass every hour. Water is just as critical to move toxins out of the body and clean your inner self as water is needed to wash your hands and outer self.

18. Raw Foods – raw vegetables, fruits and sprouts, Chlorella, Spirulina all enhance the production of energy in the cells, whereas foods cooked at high temperatures stress the white blood cells and can contribute to fatigue. Always include some raw foods with any meal of cooked foods, to avoid a stress response. Unless recently harvested, avoid buying room temperature rancid seeds or nuts that are not frozen or refrigerated.

Which thyroid supplement is best – natural or synthetic?

Among prescription drugs for the thyroid, there are several choices of brand names, but actually only two groups – natural or synthetic. Laboratory made synthetic brands like Synthroid or Levothroid only contain the T4 hormone whereas natural Armour Thyroid, that is derived from pigs (porcine), contains all 4 types of thyroid hormone, T1, T2, T3 and T4. The problem with the synthetic brands of thyroid is that many patients cannot convert T4 to the active form T3. This is often due to deficiencies of selenium, that is required to convert T4 to T3 but could be due to deficiencies of other nutrients like L-tyrosine, iodine, manganese, glutathione levels, Vitamin A, certain B vitamins, C and E.

Most doctors will prescribe a synthetic pharmaceutical thyroid like Synthroid, instead of the natural Armour Thyroid, that is actually desiccated thyroid glandular of porcine origin. Several case reports on the Internet indicate that hypothyroid persons do better on Natural Thyroid than Synthroid. For those of you who surf the Internet, the source on Thyroid under Holistic Health Topics has a 24-page article on hypothyroidism, with 102 scientific references, located at www.holistichealtopics.com/HMG/thyroid.html.

The Broda Barnes Foundation continues to educate doctors on the proper use of hormones and can provide references to physicians in your area.

Broda Barnes MD Res. Fdn
PO box 98
Trumbull, CT 06611

1. Web Site: www.brodabarnes.org.

Another list of local physicians trained in using natural hormones can be founds at www.wilsonssyndrome.com.

Recommended readings:

1. **Hypothyroidism** by Broda Barnes and Lawrence Galton, Harper and Row, NY
2. **The Miracle of Natural Hormones,** by David Brownstein MD Medical Alternatives Press 888-647-5616 www.drbrownstein.com. In his book, Dr. Brownstein has found that when the adrenal output of cortisol is very low, thyroid supplementation may make symptoms worse, unless small amounts of cortisol (10 to 20 mg daily) are first administered. Brownstein states that normal cortisol levels are needed to help T4 convert to the active form T3.

Ojibwa tea restores thyroid function

Dec 5, 2002.
To Michelle at Ojibwa Tea of Life.

It's time to let you know what has happened to me since I started taking Ojibwa Tea a little over two months ago. My annual physical was about a week after I started using the tea. Three days after my appointment, the doctor called to say my thyroid medication had to be reduced (I've been taking medication for hypothyroidism for over 30 years). He decreased it, and I went back 30 days later for another test. Three days later, I got another call saying it had to be reduced even more. The third test was a week ago. Yep! It has been dropped again. I figure it will take him about 6 months to get me off the medication altogether.

I am not sure you wanted all this info, but I really wanted to let you know what good results I'm getting in areas that I didn't even think about. Had my one year after surgery mammogram last week and everything is clear. I think what I'm trying to say is a great big Thanks for providing the means of getting myself healthier than I've ever been.

Happy, Healthy Gale

Note: Michelle Kalevik (Denver, CO), who sent me a copy of Gale's letter, can be reached at 303-322-7930 or www.ojibwatea.com. Ojibwa tea is premixed for home brewing and contains sheep sorrel, turkey rhubarb, burdock and slippery elm. The formula is based on a recipe discovered by the Ojibwa Indians in Canada early in the last century. The tea has been used to enhance immunity against Cancer, helps reduce symptoms of **Autism** in children and is used to heal the intestines.

Energy at the cellular level linked to cell-mediated immunity

The great scientist, "Albert Szent-Gyorgi," called ATP molecules "the energy currency of the cell." The sequence of events can start with exciting thoughts or when the Pituitary gland releases a hormone called "Thyroid Stimulating Factor." TSF then stimulates the Thyroid to produce a hormone called "Thyroxin." There are two kinds of Thyroxin - "T4" and "T3". T3 is the active form and T4 is the stored form. When cells remove one of the iodine ions from T4, it readily becomes usable T3, that is a major factor in producing ATP

(Adenosine Tri-Phosphate). ATP is produced in the mitochondria of the cells. Electrons give ATP their energy. The transport of electrons into the cells is carried out by two enzymes produced by Vitamin B-2 (Riboflavin). An enzyme called ATPase carries electrons into the mitochondria, in exchange for ATP molecules. The production of ATP is not a fragmented process and also involves the amino acid, L-Tyrosine, glycogen from the liver and DHEA, a hormone from the adrenal glands. There is a pump at the cell membrane that removes sodium from the cells and brings potassium in, along with electrons. Both potassium and magnesium are important minerals and carriers of electrons involved in the production of ATP - the energy currency of the cell.

Foods high in white sugar (sweets and pastry) will reduce levels of key minerals in the blood, like potassium, magnesium and calcium, leading to a depletion of electrons in the body and reduced production of ATP at the cellular level, causing fatigue and exhaustion.

The person with active infections and low body temperature will have a sluggish and ineffective immune system, and is likely to have long term chronic infections that do not respond well to any medication. The person with a fever may also be fatigued, but has a better chance for rapid recovery, as his bone marrow will produce more white blood cells, which produce all of the subsets of T-cells to actively fight the infection. The person with a fever will respond quickly to the proper medication.

Body heat increases red blood cells absorption of B-12

In a discussion on "Anemia," in his book, HYPO-THYROIDISM - THE UNSUSPECTED ILLNESS (Harper and Row, NY), Dr. Broda O. Barnes M.D. writes: "Red blood cells are manufactured in the bone marrow...A study has been done on the effect of temperature on the formation of red cells." In the study done on a white rat, they found that in the tail of the rat, where the body temperature was cool, the bone marrow was white, indicating no ongoing production of red blood cells. Where the body temperature is higher, the bone marrow is red and red blood cells are being formed. In the experiment, they warmed the tip of the rat's tail and saw the color of the bone marrow change from white to red, indicating that red blood cells were being formed.

Dr. Barnes then discusses anecdotal cases, where anemia that did not respond to iron supplements, because of low body temperature, did respond, when thyroid medication was given. Higher body temperatures increase red blood cell production.

Dr. Langer M.D. writes: "Unless we feed the Thyroid gland properly, we can't efficiently absorb another critical vitamin, (B12). In laboratory tests, rats without thyroid glands could not absorb vitamin B-12 at all...supplying subjects in starvation experiments with missing B-complex vitamins, with accent on B1 and B12, brought about enhanced thinking and remembering, among other positive results."

What causes low body temperature?

Normal body temperature is 98.6 degrees Fahrenheit. In a random survey of 25 people at stages of HIV ranging from 0 to 700 T4 cells, I found that everyone with normal body temperature had good energy levels and rarely got sick. I also found that everyone with low body temperature had chronic infections ranging from CMV to KS. I found that the lower the body temperature, the more severe were the infections and the more difficult were they to treat. Low body temperature is directly related to the low production of ATP (Adenosine Tri-Phosphate) that, in turn, is linked to low hormone levels, low output of hormones from the Pituitary, Thyroid and Adrenal Glands, low output of enzymes from the Liver and Pancreas and poor Kidney function to remove toxins from the blood.

In an interview with Dr. Frank Shallenberger M.D. of Minden, NV on Jan 5th, 1994, we discussed the low body temperature theory. Dr. Shallenberger says that as the body becomes more loaded with toxins and heavy metals, it further depresses body temperature. He was fascinated by the low body temperature theory and was amazed that kelp and cayenne produced such fast results. He said the usual reaction to an infection is that the body will produce a fever that speeds up metabolism throughout the body. The body cannot sustain this indefinitely, as it will burn out and exhaust nutrient reserves.

Low amino acid levels, copper and manganese

In persons with low vitality and low energy levels, low amino acid levels in the blood may lower body temperature. This is suspected when blood tests show low albumin levels, when there is weight loss associated with loss of muscle mass or when the person is underweight or has wasting syndrome.

In his book, Dr. Langer M.D. says that low copper levels are linked to Adrenal and Thyroid malfunction. Manganese is needed to help the thyroid produce thyroxin, as well as make the antioxidant - SOD. Seafood, nuts and Blackstrap Molasses are good sources of copper and all trace minerals. Whole foods and whole supplements are far less likely to create imbalances in the body than man-made concentrates of one or the other individual nutrients. The latter is a fragmented approach to nutrition, while the former is whole-nutrient approach. Dr. Langer also says that Vitamin E deficiency has been linked to both Pituitary and Thyroid malfunction.

Mercury, lead & other toxic metals

A letter from one reader told of a friend who had an increase in body temperature after having her dentist remove Mercury (Amalgam) fillings from her teeth and replacing them with a plastic composite material. Millions of Americans have high levels of lead, mercury and other toxic metals in their body. Having your doctor take blood and/or hair analysis tests for lead and other toxic metals might be a good start. Foods that are reported by various sources to remove heavy metals are garlic and pectin. Pectin is found in apples, applesauce and in the rinds of lemons, oranges and grapefruit. Citrus pectin and apple pectin are sold in powdered form in health food stores. Formaldehyde, found in new carpeting and new furniture, is a poison that can also depress your immune system. Several readers have reported increases in body temperature with the whole lemon/olive oil drink, indicating that detoxifying the liver and lymph system helps remove a roadblock to increased ATP production. Citrus pectin, the rind of lemons, also helps reduce heavy metals.

Fevers turn-on immune defenses

"Give me a chance to create a fever and I will cure any disease," said the great physician, Parmenides, 2,000 years ago. In his book, SOLVED - THE RIDDLE OF ILLNESS, by Stephen E Langer M.D. (Keats Publishing, New Canaan CT), writes: "Experiments done by G. W. Duff and S.K. Durum showed that at a two degree centigrade increase of fever, certain immune defenders - T-cells and antibodies - increased by 2000 percent over their number at normal body temperature... Antibody production in the spleen cells has been found to increase dramatically during a fever. Scientists have concluded that the hormone-like substance called interleukin-1, sets off body defense cells to fight infection and also sends brain signals to increase body temperature, which provides an ideal climate for the multiplication of defense cells."

The existence of a fever indicates the immune system is active and working to produce white blood cells and antibodies to neutralize the invading virus, toxin, fungus or other pathogens. A fever is a reactive phase of immune defense, and in this phase, nutrients are used up at a rapid pace. The rate of metabolism is faster and the pulse is elevated. Fevers usually triumph over infections, and then the fever subsides and the metabolism returns to normal. Sometimes the immune response in a fever is not adequate to clear the infection. In some cases, fevers get so high (over 106_ F) that they damage the brain and heart. Generally, fevers of 103_ F or less are best left to run their course. Most people with chronic immune dysfunction, however, rarely get a fever and, instead, have a different problem: an inactive immune system due to chronic low body temperature.

Chlorella, spirulina, royal jelly, molasses increase body heat

Blackstrap molasses provides an energy lift that is sustained, because of its very high mineral content, in contrast to white sugar, which lifts you up and then lets you down. Foods high in white flour and white sugar stress the adrenal glands, which ultimately leads to fatigue, because they do not contain potassium, iron, magnesium and copper, minerals that have a critical role in metabolism. Whole grains, fruits and vegetables create a higher sustained level of energy, because their balanced composition releases more electrons and produces more ATP in the cells. Whole foods contain potassium, that is completely missing in white flour and white sugar. Caffeine found in tea and coffee stimulates the production of ATP and increases energy levels. However, these may over stimulate the adrenal glands in some persons leading to adrenal exhaustion. Green tea and Ginseng tea, combined with honey, are recommended as they are milder stimulants and give a gentle sustained energy lift. Even better is Chlorella and Spirulina as superfoods that support energy production in the cells.

Royal Jelly – Experiments in mice found antifatigue effects, improved macrophage function, IL-12 production, reduced histamine and IL-6 and decreased PGE2 prostaglandin. Shifted TH2 dominance to TH1. Other effects reported are reduced cholesterol levels and serum lipids, normalization of HDL and LDL, improved adrenal function; effective treatment of warts. Some persons allergic to wheat and yeast are also allergic to royal jelly. (1,2, 3, 4)
1. Antifatigue effect of royal jelly in mice, Kamakura et al; J Nutr Sci Vitaminol (Toyko).

2001 Dec;47(6):394-401
2. Restoration of macrophage function and improvement of Th1/Th2 cell responses, by Oka H et al; Int Immunopharmacol. 2001 Mar;(3):521-32
3. Effects of royal jelly on serum lipids, Vittek J et al, Experientia. 1995 sep 29;51(9-10):927-35
4. Effects of royal jelly on exertion of corticoids, Kreze A et al. Vnitr Lek. 1969 Apr;15(4):341-6

Vegetables that may lower body temperature and reduce thyroid function include most soy products

A newsletter published by Biotics Research Corp, Ogden, UT, March, 1994 indicates the following vegetables may depress Thyroid function: Bok Choy, Broccoli, Brussels Sprouts, Cabbage, Rutabagas and Turnips. No more than two servings per week are recommended for persons with low body temperature. In animal experiments, Brussel sprouts and cabbage were associated with reduced thyroid function. Excessive use of soy products has also been associated with low thyroid function. Adults who are hypothyroid should limit soy use to Miso or Tempeh only and growing children should avoid soy products altogether. A severe allergy to peanuts in adults is now thought to be associated with their having been feed soymilk as babies.

Both grapefruit and licorice interfere with an enzyme (11-beta-OHSD) that oxidizes cortisol into cortisone, thus elevating cortisol levels. Grapefruit can also interfere with the P450 liver enzyme detoxification pathway. When low thyroid function is present, grapefruit should be used only in the morning. On the other hand, if blood pressure is low or normal-low, small amounts of licorice in the form of tea given two or three times each day can strengthen the adrenals. There is no information indicating any problems with using oranges or tangerines and there are ample case reports of benefits from the use of lemons or limes in detoxifying the liver that helps normalize body temperature. .

Seafood, grass-fed beef and free-range organic poultry, whey protein and plants from the sea are highly recommended along with spicy foods (cayenne, African bird pepper and chili) to enhance thyroid function and increase metabolism.

Recommended article on Thyroid on the Internet from Australia – 24 pages with 102 scientific references. Found at www.holistichealthtopics.com/HMG/thyroid.html.

Estrogen and plant phytoestrogens in human health

Synthetic estrogens like Premarin have been prescribed to women for decades to alleviate symptoms of menopause. Recently, the FDA has determined that prescribed estrogen is carcinogenic (cancer causing). There is a substantial body of research that estrogens are linked to some forms of cancer, particularly breast and ovarian cancer. In fact, one treatment for breast cancer is Tamoxifin; a drug derived from a tree that blocks estrogen receptors in the breast and ovaries, but not in other parts of the body, where estrogen is needed for important functions like calcium absorption into the bones. Published research indicates that phytoestrogens like genisten found in red clover and

Tumeric (Curcumin) block breast cancer cell proliferation, while Curcumin and Silymarin can inhibit the inflammatory effects of NF Kappa B (1)

Some natural compounds are proestrogenic in some areas of the body and anti-estrogenic in other areas. There are thousands of natural phytoestrogens in plants and their functions vary. There are good estrogens and bad estrogens. The bad estrogens are mainly synthetic compounds, like pesticides and derivatives from plastics that act like estrogens and get inside cells, and then do havoc, paralyzing their metabolic activity. Plant phytoestrogens actually block the bad estrogens from getting inside the cells.

Lignans: The Life Extension foundation (www.lef.org) in an article by Terri Mitchell (Dec., 2002) writes that lignans nullify strong estrogens and get them out of the body. They do this by increasing a protein called "sex hormone binding protein" or (SHBG). Lignans are found in berries and in flaxseed. Flaxseed is very high in lignans and is well known for its anti-cancer properties. Extra virgin Olive oil also contains lignans and has well known anti-cancer properties, as a component of the Mediterranean diet. Resveratrol from the skin of red grapes is a very good phytoestrogen and antioxidant.

1. Natural products as targeted modulators of NF Kappa B; by Bremner P and Heinrich M, J Pharm Pharmacol. 2002 Apr;54(4):453-72

Estrogen in your "boiled" steak? Estradiol added to meats may be linked to low body temperature

Guiroy PJ et al report that, in a study of 13,460 animals (steers and heifers), values in weight gain, after body fat weight averaged 564 kg in steer implanted with "Revalor-S" hormones to promote weight gain, versus controls in unimplanted steers, whose weight averaged 520 kg (1). In this experiment it can be seen that in the animals implanted with the hormones "Revalor-S", the weight gain was an average 44 kg per animal, or about 100 pounds. At current prices, implanting hormones in steers could add a monetary value of about $50 per steer at "on-the-hoof" market prices. For a farmer selling 100 steers, that is an extra $5000 in his pocket.

This past fall (Oct, 2002), I invited some friends over for a Stir-Fry. At the time I was unable to locate any organic beefsteak, so I decided to purchase some round steak at a local grocery store. I was amazed, as I began to fry the 2.5 pound steak and noticed water getting into the frying pan in an unusually large quantity. I estimate at least a cup of water ended up in the frying pan. I knew the ceiling wasn't leaking and I surmised that I would end up with a boiled steak stir-fry. I could see it wasn't actually blood, but water, and lots of it, and it was coming out of the beef. I wondered how it got there. A few weeks later, I again bought some beef steak for another stir-fry and noticed the pan fill up with water again. I started to wonder if the grocery store was injecting water into the beef, or if hormones, given to cattle for weight gain before being sent to the slaughterhouse, were responsible for all this water. After all, it is known that estrogen causes sodium and water retention and weight gain in women. Meanwhile, for the second time, I observed the "incredible shrinking steak" surrounded by all this water.

To resolve the question that hormonal estrogen might have been given to the cow to increase its weight (water weight) before slaughter, (and therefore its dollar value), I searched for and found some organic beef steak in a local health food store. In this 3rd stir fry, I was amazed, as I fried the steak, that no water at all came out of it, and there was far less shrinkage; in fact, very little shrinkage, compared to what I now believed was the estrogen-enhanced store steak. Not only was there no water, the meat tasted one heck of a lot better. Those cheap sales on beef and steak, that come to your door with coupons, may look more attractive than the higher cost organic meats, but they are not as good-a-buy as once thought. You have to subtract the water from the steak to see what you really bought.

The FDA rules prohibits the use of hormones being fed or injected in poultry or pork, I have seen, on occasion, an incredible amount of water coming out a chicken or turkey being roasted. This was caused by an injection of up to 8% sodium phosphate. I avoid these birds also.

Terri Mitchell, writing in "Life Extension" Dec 2002, states that "eating hormone-treated meat may increase estrogen levels hundreds of times over what a body normally produces. It's disputed at this point just how much synthetic estrogen ends up on the dinner plate. Beef cows in the U.S. are implanted with multiple synthetic hormones, including estradiol, to make them put on weight. There is no withdrawal period for these implants, which are in the cows at the time of slaughter."

Aug 2002: I talked to Mark, a local Wisconsin farmer, who told me about his neighbor who recently sold 24 of 25 steers he had. He claimed that he had injected hormones and increased the weight of 24 steers about 75 lbs each that he then sold to the slaughterhouse. The farmer, (his neighbor), had no qualms about injecting the hormones into the steers, as long as the government allows it and it puts money in his pocket, but he did not want to eat the hormone-injected beef himself. Mark stated: "The 25th steer that he kept was not injected with the weight enhancing hormones…that's what he told me." Mark, who owns a dairy herd for milk production, said he has never used any hormones including Monsanto's bovine growth hormone, to increase milk production or weight gain, because he believes this is plain wrong and unhealthy for the cows. I would not want to eat meat or drink milk with hormones added, so why would I want to sell it to others?

Mark is a farmer with a conscience. Yet, what about the farmers desperate to make their next mortgage payment? These farmers may not even realize how they are harming the cows and the people who eat this meat, when they inject these hormones into the animals for more rapid weight gain. The public buys steak and milk and does not know from whose farm it came, Mark's or his neighbor's.

A commercial hormone, estradiol, is being fed to the unknowing public. This is a drug that is being given to the public in the meats they buy at their local stores and at the fast food restaurants, like McDonalds and Burger King. Meanwhile, our government has its head buried in the sand over the link between meats fed to the public that are loaded with estrogen and the national obesity epidemic. It is an outrage. Where are the lawyers?

Finally, when you consume excess estrogen in your food from commercial beef, pork and poultry injected with growth hormones, the estrogen binds with thyroxine and lowers your metabolic rate. This lowers your body temperature. The estrogen also causes sodium and water retention. This can raise your blood pressure and lower energy production in the mitochondria of the cells. Collectively the effects of excess estrogen from meats in your local grocery store and fast food restaurants are contributing to low body temperature, lowered immune responses to all infectious disease and this includes cancer.

Besides all this, excess estrogen in meats is contributing to obesity, high blood pressure, insulin resistance, heart disease and diabetes. The use of hormone injections in cattle and poultry is banned by the European Union and in many foreign countries. Young girls are having puberty at younger and younger ages. Many children, along with over half the adult population of the United States, are now seriously overweight or obese, and about the same number are hypothyroid, with low body temperature, and suffer from all the accompanying health-related adverse effects. For anyone serious about regaining or maintaining their health, it is time to say "goodbye" not only to junk food, but meat contaminated with growth hormones. It is time to get back to basics and buy Organic.

1. The effects of implant strategy on finished body weight of beef cattle, by Guiroy PJ et al., J. Anim Sci. 2002 Jul;80(7):1791-800

The alternative – buy organic grass-fed beef and free range organic poultry direct from the farmers

A book on the health benefits of grass-fed beef, "Why Grass-fed Beef is Best," by Joe Robinson is available at www.eatwild.com or at www.acresusa.com. You can also call the publisher Vashon Island Press at 206-463-4156. (The book contains the names and addresses of nearly 100 farmers who raise grass-fed beef, pork and poultry).

Essentially, grass-fed beef is high in Omega 3 fatty acids and low in omega 6 and 9. This makes the fat profile of grass-fed beef and poultry similar to cold-water ocean fish. Grass-fed beef and poultry are good for energy and a heart-healthy lipid profile. In contrast, the fat in corn-fed or soybean-fed beef is deficient in omega 3, high in omega 6 and 9 and is lacking in these heart protective ingredients. If the cows or steers ate some corn and soybeans, I wouldn't be overly concerned, as long as the bulk of what they ate was grass or (in the winter) hay. You won't get the same marbled fats with grass as you do with corn-fed steers, but the meat will be leaner and healthier, when you cook it in a Crock Pot at low temperatures, it will be just as tender as the corn fed beef.

Links and sources: www.organictrader.net. National Organic Directory – 1-800-852-3832 or www.caff.org. 346 pages. Lists farmers and wholesalers nationally. Check with your local library to see if they have or will purchase a copy.

Local resources: Check with several local health food stores and co-ops. Prices for organic meats, dairy products and vegetables vary widely. Go to www.google.com and search for "organic beef" and your state. Examples of search terms: Organic beef NY Organic poultry WI   free range chickens TX   Beef no hormones FL. I think you get the idea. If you receive too many leads, insert the name of a local county in your search terms and this will limit the number of search results.

My experiences: I found that in websites where the meats are "Certified Organic" the prices are $1 to $2 per pound higher than transitional sites or from farmers who have grass-fed beef, have never used hormones or antibiotics but have not gone through the Organic Certification process. I found a local farmer who states he does not use hormones or antibiotics and a quarter side of beef (about 180 pounds) costs $2.00 per pound, cut to your specifications. Although not certified, that is just as good as organic to me, and it costs less than the estrogen and antibiotic contaminated stuff in the local grocery store, that I refuse to purchase or eat any longer. They can offer it free, and I would refuse it. The uninformed public actually pays real hard earned dollars to ruin their health eating this stuff.

10

Free radicals and anti-oxidants
What are free radicals?

Most scientific publications refer to "free radicals" as reactive oxygen compounds that have an unpaired electron in their outer ring. That is to say, they are missing an electron. Two free radicals that have been identified are Super oxide and hydroxyl. Hydroxyl is (OH) and is very reactive. When it reacts with a cell membrane, it can cause severe damage by setting off a chain reaction that produces more free radicals. Anti-oxidants (oxygen modulators), protect cell membranes from free radicals and are believed to destroy free radicals by donating electrons to them which changes their chemical structure into more stable compounds like hydrogen peroxide (H_2O_2).

For example, two OH- (hydroxyl free radicals) that absorb electrons will join together to from H_2O_2 which is far less reactive. The enzyme catalase then breaks H_2O_2 down further into oxygen and water. Raw potatoes contain catalase and when a slice of potato is placed in a glass of H_2O_2, bubbles of oxygen are given off.

At the IBOM convention in Dallas, TX on 3/25/94, H_2O_2 and ozone were shown to increase PO_2 levels and increase ATP production in the cells by up to 40%. In other words, some anti-oxidants convert free radicals into oxidative byproducts and produce energy in the cells. In this way, anti-oxidants enhance the oxidation process and stop the damage caused by free radicals. Free radicals are unstable electron deficient molecules. They can react with cell membranes and destroy them. Anti-oxidants, which I believe is a misnomer, since they are really oxygen modulators, cause the oxidative reactions to occur in the Mitochondria of the cells, instead of in places where they do damage to the cells (i.e. the membranes). Selenium has been shown to help prevent lipid peroxidation and damage to the membranes of cells. The mineral potassium has an antioxidant role in the body as it donates electrons to help produce energy in the mitochondria. Whether a mineral or element is pro or antioxidant depends on whether it has electrons to donate or is in need of electrons.

There is disagreement among the experts as to whether or not oxygen itself is a free radical. I am of the opinion that oxygen, what we breathe (O_2) is not a free radical, since it is not normally electron deficient and it is required for the life of the cell and for the production of both heat and energy in the body. Oxygen is one of several ingredients required for the mitochondria in our cells to produce ATP - Adenosine Tri-Phosphate. However, in the presence of pollutants and certain chemicals in the air that steal electrons from oxygen in the air, the oxygen would become unstable, electron deficient and would become a free radical.

Effects of free radicals

The following are a list of symptoms and conditions that are believed to be caused, in

part or in whole, by excess free radicals in the body. They include:
1. Damage to cell membranes leading to cell destruction (aldehyde release from lipids)
2. Damage to the DNA of cells, causing pre-cancerous conditions in some persons.
3. Chronic fatigue.
4. Sleep disorders and disturbed sleep patterns.
5. Inflammation of the large intestines, leading to malabsorption of nutrients.
6. Aging of the skin, with wrinkles and loss of elasticity, due to destruction of collagen.
7. Inflammatory reactions that produce histamines.
8. Increased inflammatory prostaglandins.
9. Susceptibility to bruise easily, indicating weak capillaries and a weakening of the veins and arteries.
10. Neurological damage in some persons.

Testing for free radicals

A 5 minute test for free radical damage is available that uses a small sample of urine. It measures released aldehydes from free radical oxidized lipids. A color chart is provided to measure the extent of free radical activity. It is called the Oxidata Test and is manufactured by Apex Energetics, 1701 E Edinger Ave A-4, Santa Ana, Ca 92705. Sold to health care professionals 1-800-736-4381. www.apexenergetics.com. Apex Energetics has other test kits and a unique range of original homeopathic formulas.

S.O.D., manganese and fresh greens

Super Oxide radicals, considered the most damaging of all free radicals, are converted into usable oxygen by S.O.D. (Super Oxide Dismutase). Manganese is a trace mineral that is used in the production of S.O.D.. Excess iron in the body increases production of the damaging Super Oxide radical. Avoid dietary supplements with iron added. Avoid white bread with iron added. The form of iron added to vitamin and mineral supplements produces dangerous free radicals. Children die each year from eating iron pills intended for their mothers. If you need iron, obtain it from foods like spinach and other dark green vegetables, whole grains or blackstrap molasses, liver and oysters. For manganese, oat bran and pineapple are your two highest natural sources.

SOD is found abundantly in Spirulina, Chlorella, broccoli and most fresh raw green plants. SOD and catalase are enzymes that are also produced in the body. Cooking destroys all enzymes including SOD and catalase. Parsley, watercress, cilantro, spinach or other dark greens supply you with S.O.D. Oh, what value there is in a daily salad. Presently, there is inadequate information as to whether these same vegetables also contain catalase, an enzyme that is known to exist abundantly in raw potatoes but likely found in other raw vegetables.

Ozone – two types. Ozone as an electron donor (antioxidant) or as a free radical

Ozone (negatively charged) is produced with an electric arc or in a lightning storm. It is not a Free Radical, since it has excess electrons to give up. It reacts with body fluids to produce ozonides that are not electron deficient. People breathe easier and experience higher energy levels in the presence of negatively charged ozone. On the other hand, ozone (positively charged) is produced with pollutants in the presence of the suns ultraviolet light. The type of ozone that is formed in the presence of polluted air and sunlight is electron deficient. This (positively charged) ozone is very much of a free radical and will steal electrons from your lungs and blood cells and make you short of breath as well as cause fatigue. This is the only kind of ozone people hear about and they think all ozone is the same; it is not. The bad ozone (positively charged and electron deficient) reduces the production of energy in your cells and makes you feel weak and tired whereas, the good ozone with electrons to donate, increases the production of ATP in the cells and makes you feel energized and strong.

Free radical scavengers

Nutrients that are anti-oxidants and free radical scavengers include D'Glucaric acid, proanthocyanidins, Carotenoids, Vitamin A, C, E, Selenium and Manganese; other naturally occurring flavinoids (i.e. Citrus rinds) that protect cell membranes from free radicals. Among 19 fruits tested in 2002, cranberries had the highest level of antioxidant activity, with high levels of antioxidant phenols.

There are ample amounts of clinical studies that show the protective effects of Beta-Carotene and Vitamin A in the prevention of cancer. In HIV, Beta-Carotene has shown an ability to either stabilize T cell counts or increase them in most persons.

Proanthocyanidins found in grape seed extract are called "OPCs" and are labeled as such in their health food stores. Their anti-oxidant properties are essentially the same as Pycnogenol, a trade name for proanthocyanidins found in pine bark. Proanthocyanidins are easily assimilated, when taken orally, even in persons with severe malabsorption problems and are known to cross the blood-brain barrier. Proanthocyanidins are extracted from the bark of the Maritime Pine trees that grow in the coastal region of southern France. Richard Passwater, Ph.D., in his book THE NEW SUPERANTIOXIDANT says that Pycnogenol is the most potent free radical antagonist known to medical science and is a Vitamin C potentiator. Proanthocyanidin are also found in bilberries, elderberries, blueberries and cranberries.

A case report - benefits of using Pycnogenol

Jim, from Milwaukee and living with HIV, reported the following benefits from using Pycnogenol for one week
1. Increased thirst for liquids and frequent urination.
2. Fatigue reduced - energy levels up.

3. Normal sleep patterns restored for the first time in 2 years - no more interrupted sleep.
4. Thinking was clearer.
5. Lymph nodes were no longer sore.
6. Stool diameter increased in size, indicating an anti-inflammatory effect on the large intestines.
7. Stools floated for the first time and were normal color.
8. Shortness of breath was gone.
9. Histamine production that caused a reflux reaction in his stomach stopped. He no longer needed to take H2 blockers.
10. Stomach gas stopped.
11. A sinus infection that had started at the beginning of a trip had cleared up, without the need for antibiotics.
12. He felt lighter on his feet while walking.

At one point Jim said: "I have never taken a supplement or any medication in the past 5 years that has so many benefits and results in such a short period of time." As we drove along, I remarked to Jim that I thought my eyesight had improved. On the second day of the trip, I said to Jim: "I can't believe how far I can see and how clear everything is. In the past two days, my eyesight has improved 100%. Could it be the Pycnogenol"? I remarked that Dr. Passwater said in his book that Pycnogenol improves visual acuity.

Anyone can start off with the maximum dose. However, some persons may need to start at a lower dose than the 1 mg per day per pound of body weight formula. Because this product is so powerful, it may set off a healing crisis in some parts of the body that could temporarily increase pain in some persons. If this happens, I suggest you start off with 20 or 30 mg the first day and increase in increments, until you reach the desired level.

Bilberry reduces eye floaters.

A person in Houston, TX told me that he completely got rid of eye floaters (little brown spots or specks that sometimes look like fruit flies) by taking 500 mg of Bilberry daily for 30 days. A sudden increase in eye floaters has been linked to either HHV-6A or CMV retinitis or free radicals. Bilberry, a potent source of proanthocyanidins, may be a better choice than Pycnogenol for persons with eye problems.

Glucaric acid – major detox pathway - binds estrogen & carcinogens

In their book, "D'Glucarate Against Cancer,"(1) Thomas Slaga and Judi Quilici-Timmcke M.S. publish research that demonstrates that Glucaric acid found in numerous fruits and vegetables, and now available in supplemental form, is a major detoxifier of toxins and carcinogens in the body and prevents and stops cancer growth. Glucaric acid is also produced in small amounts in the body. An enzyme called Glucuronosyl transferase binds the toxins to glucaric acid, and then they are excreted from the body through the bile or the kidneys.

In a reverse process, an enzyme called Beta-glucuronidase can separate the toxin from the glucaric acid and release it into the body. This is especially dangerous, and often happens in cancer, viral hepatitis and liver necrosis. Slaga also reports that when beta-glucuronidase is elevated, it increases the number of estrogen receptors. Lack of glucaric acid and increased beta-glucuronidase has been found in breast, ovarian, lung, colon, liver, bladder and prostate cancer. Slaga reports that based on scientific studies, an effective dosage of glucaric acid would be from 200 to 2000 mg daily. Glucaric acid is found in some fruits and vegetables. Calcium D'Glucarate is available as a dietary supplement. Persons under a toxic overload should try to consume 1500 to 2000 mg of glucaric acid daily. Because it is processed quickly out of the body, it is best to consume a food with glucaric acid once every 3 or 4 hours throughout the day. Apples low in sugar, like Granny Smith or Winesap, are highly recommended. Dietary Supplement: D'Glucarate – 2 capsules twice daily or one every 4 hours.

1. D-Glucarate – A Nutrient Against Cancer – Thomas Slaga, A Keats Health Guide, (found in health food stores).

Food sources of glucaric acid

Whole Apple – about 300 mg
Oranges and grapefruit – 300 to 400 mg
Broccoli – raw about 500 mg per cup
Cherries about 200 mg per cup.

Example: one half grapefruit and one orange for breakfast and 3 apples all day provide about 1500 mg of glucaric acid. Eat a serving of a food high in glucaric acid about every 4 hours throughout the day.

Cranberries – rated the highest in antioxidants of 19 fruits tested. Bad cholesterol lowered – inactivates bacteria

In an article published in the Journal of Agric Food Chem, 2002 Oct 9th, by Joe Vinson et al at the University of Scranton, Scranton, PA, researchers tested 19 common fruits in the American diet gram for gram for phenol content and found cranberries to be the highest, followed by red grapes. On the basis of antioxidant phenol content, raw cranberry is best, with pure cranberry juice found in health food stores having the highest content of antioxidants of a prepared drink. This is followed by cranberry sauce, while cranberry cocktails have the least. Mixing pure cranberry juice with pure red grape juice or apple juice on a 50/50 basis makes an enjoyable drink. Research has shown that cranberries reduce the oxidation of LDL and decrease total cholesterol levels. Drinking 8 ounces of pure cranberry juice daily should have profound benefits on raising antioxidant levels in the blood. Cranberries contain several types of antioxidants besides phenols. These includes 3 types of quercitin, 7 flavonol glycosides and anthocyandins. Vinson reported that the flavonal glycosides showed equal or greater free radical scavenging ability than vitamin E. Apples were also reported to contain phenol antioxidants. In terms of total antioxidants, cranberries even rated higher than broccoli, the vegetable with one of the highest antioxidant rating and well established anticancer properties.

Researchers (1) have also found that cranberry juice concentrate completely prevented the growth of a number of bacteria and fungus in an in-vitro experiment including candida albicans, klebsiella pneumonie, e-coli, staphylococcus aureus, pseudomonas aeruginosa, and salmonella enteritidis. However, antibacterial activity was found with dilutions of 1:32 parts cranberry juice. While no treatment protocols have been proposed, one or two ounces of pure cranberry juice, taken straight or diluted, with an equal amount of water or added to apple juice, taken every 4 hours, should be sufficient, in my opinion, to demonstrate some antifungal and antibacterial effects. From folk legends, cranberry juice has been known to prevent and clear urinary tract infections. However, if we can believe the latest research, cranberry juice used in a sufficient amount, and used consistently, may inactivate numerous kinds of infections elsewhere in the body besides the urinary tract.

1. JAMA, Vol 283, p 1691, April 5, 2000

Natural sources of antioxidants

1. D'Glucarate is found in – Apples. Broccoli, Apricots
2. Glutathione - winter squash and avocado. Promoted by cold processed whey proteins, cottage cheese and ricotta cheese, eaten as a late evening snack.
3. Carotenoids –rinds of lemons and oranges or lemon/olive oil drink, garlic and onions, carrots, yams, squash, sweet potatoes, pumpkin, dark green vegetables, red and concord grapes and many other whole unprocessed fruits and vegetable. Note: The darker the color of the fruit or vegetable, the more antioxidants it contains.
4. Vitamin A - cod liver oil - 1 or 2 tablespoons daily. If it tastes stale or rancid, do not use. Buy cod Liver oil from a store a store that keeps it refrigerated.
5. Vitamin C Food sources: Acerola cherries, rose hips, oranges, lemons, limes, berries, bean sprouts, most fruits and green leafy vegetables. Note: Most vitamin C sold today is synthesized from corn, and persons with multiple allergies may not tolerate this synthetic form of vitamin C.
6. Vitamin E - 400 IU daily – wheat germ and wheat germ oil.
7. Selenium –400 to 800 mcg daily - Food source - Brazil nuts, Brewer's yeast tablets.
8. Cold-processed whey proteins (Immunepro or Immunocal). Use only late in the evening or before bedtime – 5 to 10 grams once a day. Promotes deep restful sleep, glutathione, increases human growth hormone and DHEA levels, lean muscle mass and reduces stress on the adrenals. Whey protein is a perfect match with a glass of tart cherry juice that is a source of natural melatonin.
9. Manganese - needed to produce SOD. Pineapple, oat bran, whole grains.
10. Alpha Lipoic acid (ALA) and Catalase – (Natural source – raw potatoes – rich in ALA and catalase). Slice a raw potato and eat the chips plain or dipped into a yogurt herb base. ALA increases glutathione levels and catalase breaks down hydrogen peroxide into oxygen and water. Avoid ALA in pills – it is made synthetically.
11. Proanthocyanidins and phenols - found in Pycnogenol (pine bark), grape seed extract, bilberries, elderberries, blueberries and cranberries. Elderberries, like cranberries, are a powerhouse of antioxidants. Cranberries are very high in the antioxidant phenols.
13. Foods high in antioxidants: carrots, squash, sweet potatoes, raw white potatoes, pumpkin, citrus rinds, onions, garlic, blue green algae, chlorella and spirulina. Yellow onions

are high in quercitin and garlic contains many antioxidants.

How to make elderberry extract

To make an alcohol-free extract, you first need to use alcohol to liquefy the active ingredients in the elderberries and then use low temperature evaporation to remove the alcohol.

1. Place 1 pound of dried elderberries or (13 ozs dried elderberrries and 3 ozs of elder flowers) in a porcelain, glass or stainless steel bowl (do not use aluminum) and add one liter of Vodka (80 proof) and 2 liters of water.

2. After 24 hours, place the mixture (before straining), berries and solution into a "slow cooker", "crock pot" or "Nesco." Note: Adding Elder flowers to the batch improves taste (sweetens) and aroma and is reported to benefit the eyes and kidneys.

If using the Rival brand Crock Pot, set at "low." Leave cover off and insert a candy thermometer in the solution. Check temperature every half hour until it reaches 125_ F (about 1 hour with a crock pot). Then mark your clock for 3 hours hence, when all the alcohol should have evaporated.

3. With the Rival brand crock-pot set on low, it took exactly 4 hours total to evaporate all the alcohol from the solution. If using a Slow Cooker or Nesco, you might initially set the temperature to 160_ F until the solution temperature reaches 125_ F, then reduce the temperature setting to 125_ F or to a setting that keeps the solution between 125_ F to 130_ F for 3 hrs.

Three hours later, turn off heat and place cover on and let stand for 2 hours. Use a cup or small bowl to scoop out berries and solution and strain through a fine screen strainer. You may also do a second straining through cotton terry cloth placed over a large funnel to remove fine sand and pulp. Your finished product will be smooth and have the deep purple color of ink. Pour into a pint glass jar, refrigerate it and use within 7 days. You should end up with about 2 quarts or liters. To store long term, freeze balance (about 3 pints) in ice cube trays. When frozen, remove and store in plastic bags in the freezer.

Adult dose: Two tablespoons or the equivalent in ice cubes of extract twice daily with the last dose before bedtime. Mix with orange, concord grape juice or filtered water. Note: if diarrhea results, stop using it until your conditions stabilize, then gradually reintroduce it and increase use gradually, until you are at the ideal dose.

11

Detoxification of the liver and colon Whole lemon/olive oil drink

Detoxification of the liver and lymphatic system and significant improvements in how persons with AIDS, CFIDS, GWS and cancer feel is why it has become so well known. This is the first drink anyone reading this book should try. The drink is made by combining in a blender the juice of a whole lemon, the rind of half a lemon, one tablespoon of extra virgin olive oil and a glass of water or fruit juice. Strain and drink one or more times weekly. Some people use it daily. It tastes even better made with grape juice.

The miracle of the whole lemon/olive oil drink

Neuropathy is a painful disorder of the nervous system which causes numbness, burning or aching sensations in various parts of the body. Swollen lymph nodes (lymphadenopathy) affects 80% of all persons with AIDS, at some point in the disease progression. Wasting syndrome is a progressive loss of muscle mass. In Africa, AIDS-related wasting syndrome is called "Slim's disease."

In Dec., 1994, I reported in Positive Health News (1) on the case of a friend who reversed neuropathy, lymphadenopathy (swollen lymph nodes) and wasting syndrome with a home drink made from whole lemons, fruit juice and cold pressed extra virgin olive oil with lecithin added. After 10 days, my friend said his swollen lymph nodes and neuropathy were 90% gone. He no longer needed his cane.

Since this initial report was published, I have talked to countless HIV+ persons who have used the drink daily. They have all reported a complete cessation of swollen lymph nodes in 5 to 7 days and neuropathy in about 2 weeks. To date, only one person failed to reduce lymphadenopathy with the whole lemon drink. In addition, 11 of 13 persons with wasting syndrome have reported a weight gain of 1 to 2 pounds per week. Persons who were of normal weight, or who were overweight when they started the lemon drink, have not reported any weight gain. One PWA from Ft. Myers, Fl, who was 30 pounds underweight, recently wrote that he has gained 21 pounds in 8 weeks, using the whole lemon/olive drink daily. Two additional persons with neuropathy have reported that 90% of the symptoms were gone within two weeks and completely gone within three.

Other benefits being reported are an increase in energy, increased appetite and a more normal body temperature. Persons with CFIDS are nearly unanimous in reporting benefits.

Certainly, no claims are being made that this simple home remedy will cure anyone of AIDS. A single anecdotal case that is successful is no basis for thousands of people to try a new treatment. However, from all reports I have received, the treatment is safe and effective. The number of persons reporting benefits is becoming statistically significant. This treatment is not patentable. No pharmaceutical company will make money on this simple and inexpensive discovery.

How to make the lemon/olive oil drink

1. In a blender place the juice of one lemon and the rind of 1/2 lemon (cut up).
2. Add 1 cup of orange juice, red grape juice, other fruit juice or water.
3. Add one tablespoon of (cold pressed) Extra Virgin Olive Oil (from your health food store).
4. Optional -add about a one-inch piece of raw ginger root.
5. Optional - to inhibit herpes, CMV or HHV-6A infection; add the powder from one 250 mg capsule of BHT to the blender.
6. Blend at high speed for 1 minute.
7. Pour mixture through a strainer to separate the juice from the pulp. Discard the pulp. Note: if you remove the lemon seeds before placing the lemon in a blender, you may drink pulp and all and forget the straining. The ginger root is optional, but helpful, to digest the olive oil.

The drink may be consumed all at once. A few persons have been unable to use the drink, as they are allergic to citrus fruit. However, they will still obtain benefits from the cold pressed olive oil and should use 2 to 4 tablespoons daily.

Note: if neuropathy is present, add one tablespoon of lecithin granules to the drink or take 2 lecithin capsules twice daily with the drink, divided into two portions. I recommend triple strength lecithin. Consider PC35 by Jarrow formulas. If you use whole leaf aloe vera juice daily, you can add one tablespoon daily to the whole lemon drink. If you have low body temperature, take 2 or 3 cayenne capsules with the whole lemon drink.

Note: Don't use cayenne, if you have acid-reflux syndrome, as it might make this condition worse.

In Dec. 1995, a PWA from Brooklyn, who had used the whole lemon drink daily for 13 months and a product called Clarkia-100 for the past 4 months, says he is now PCR negative for HIV. However, he says if he stops using the whole lemon drink for 3 or 4 days, some soreness in his lymph nodes returns indicating that the other AIDS virus, HHV-6A is still there. He only recently started using Naltrexone. He admits to being on a poor diet, high in grains and eats little vegetables. Symptoms relieved suggest that this drink may do more than flush the liver and lymph system, but may also be having a direct antiviral effect against HHV-6A and HIV.

I have observed over the past few years that more expensive brands (Monks, Krinos) not only taste better, but also are more therapeutic. If you can find cold pressed olive oil in a darkened jar or can, it will have a fresher taste. Exposure of oils to ultraviolet light in a clear jar causes lipid peroxides to form. In other words, the oil becomes rancid.

Whole lemon drink flushes toxins from the liver and lymph – anti-viral and immunological benefits

Lymph fluid drains into the liver, which is why movement of lymph out of the liver is necessary for clearing infections from the lymph system. The movement of lymph fluid is crucial in AIDS and CFS. Moving toxins out of the lymph system also helps bring new immune cells, NK and Killer T cells to the lymph nodes from the blood supply, where they can attack HHV-6A. HHV-6A is the primary cause of viral damage to the newly formed

Antigen Presenting cells in the Lymphoid tissue. These cells are needed to restore cell-mediated immunity. The reduction in swollen lymph nodes, widely reported, strongly suggests that the lemon/olive oil drink has a direct antiviral effect against HHV-6A. Lemon oil (from the rinds) is an essential oil reported by several sources to be antiviral. Cleansing the liver and reducing toxins in the blood and lymph also reduces Th2 cytokine levels.

Lemon drink aids in absorption of essential fatty acids

It is common knowledge that in HIV progression, fat and essential fatty acids are not well absorbed. It is also well known that any normal overweight person, who goes on a very low fat diet, will lose weight - mostly fat. Fats and oils raise saliva pH, while grains lower the saliva pH. Essential fatty acids are needed by the body for the production of various hormones (Preston). Pectin from citrus rinds and from apple sauce (not the juice) helps in the assimilation of fats and oils. When oil is added to water, it will not mix. However, you will notice that the Lecithin and Olive oil is totally dispersed throughout the Whole Lemon-drink. The pectin in the rind of the lemon causes this dispersion of the oil. The proof of absorption of the oil could come from a blood test, but it is also indicated by the rapid return of saliva pH to normal-6.4.

In all three conditions, neuropathy, lymphadenopathy and wasting syndrome, I have found saliva pH to be on the acid side (5.5 to 5.8). pH is a measure of the degree of acidity or alkalinity of a substance. The whole lemon/olive oil drink usually causes saliva pH to return to a normal range of 6.2 to 6.4 within 2 to 3 days. In 6 cases I observed, weight gain started when saliva pH reached 6.2. The whole lemon drink quickly brings very tangible benefits to its users that improve the quality of their lives.

When taken with meals, the lemon juice acts on proteins to break them into a free form, which is more easily assimilated. Also, the lemon juice helps to dissolve minerals in the food for better assimilation. This drink should be used with all dietary supplements to improve their assimilation.

Olive oil also increases the production of bile in the liver. Bile helps emulsify fats and also helps the liver get rid of toxins and waste products of metabolism.

The Whole Lemon drink has produced dramatic results in normalizing saliva pH values, detoxifying the Liver, reducing swollen lymph nodes, increasing absorption of nutrients, restoring normal weight and building up the White Blood Cell count. It seems only logical to use it in conjunction with the daily Castor Oil packs. Dr. Philip Princetta of Atlanta, GA told me that when the liver is flushed out with the Lemon/Olive Oil drink, the lymph fluid moves into the liver to be processed and eliminated from the body. He said that "swollen lymph nodes are always a sign of liver congestion and the lymph nodes will reduce in size when the liver is cleansed."

Coffee retention enemas

The Gerson Cancer Institute has been recommending coffee retention enemas for the past 50 years. According to Charlotte Gerson, the coffee enema has a specific purpose - to lower blood serum toxins that are flushed out of the liver into the colon to be eliminated. According to Dr. Peter Lechner, palmitic acid in coffee enemas promotes the activity of glutathione S-transferase to detoxify the liver, which reduces toxins in the blood serum. The Gerson Institute reports that cancer patients have a 90% reduction in pain, when they use the retention enemas.

The coffee is made by adding 3 tablespoons of regular grind coffee to a quart of distilled water and simmering for 10 minutes. Cool to room temperature. Strain. Admit to colon, while lying on your back, then, lay on the right side. Retain for 12 to 15 minutes. Persons who are very ill may do this daily or less often as needed. More information can be found in "The Gerson Primer," which can be obtained by calling 619-585-7600.

EDTA removes heavy metals and opens clogged arteries – an alternative to bypass surgery

Heavy metals like lead and mercury and other toxins can depress body temperature, suppress activity of the glandular system and slow down the immune system, making people susceptible to chronic infections, yeast overgrowth and even cancer. To determine whether heavy metals are a problem for you, have your physician test for the level of lead, mercury and other heavy metals. Hair analysis can be helpful in making this determination.

EDTA is a man-made amino acid, approved by the FDA, for treating lead poisoning. EDTA chelation therapy removes lead and other heavy metals and has been reported to significantly lower susceptibility to cancer. Many people have chosen EDTA chelation therapy over bypass surgery to remove calcium plaque from the arteries and improve blood circulation to the heart. Mercury filings (Amalgam) in teeth have been reported by several sources to depress the immune system. Chemical additives in food and insecticide residues on fruits and vegetables also add to the toxic overload, as does smoking cigarettes.

For a national list of physicians offering EDTA chelation therapy, contact ACAM in Laguna Hills, CA Fax 949-455-9679, or find a local physician who offers EDTA chelation therapy at www.acam.org. IV EDTA has been prescribed by physicians and used on nearly half a million persons as a treatment for partially blocked arteries, and arteriosclerosis and as a low cost non-invasive alternative to bypass surgery. Some people have been helped by an oral EDTA product called "Formula 1" from Golden Pride Raleigh in West Palm Beach, FL (available in capsules or mixed with honey) www.goldenpride.com or 561-835-0075.

Removing heavy metals

One manufacturer of health food supplements told me that pectin is good to remove heavy metals. Pectin is found in apples and in the rinds of lemons, oranges and grapefruit. Apple pectin and citrus pectin is sold in health food stores in both tablet and powder form. Drinking a cup of a combination of Buckthorn and Red Clover twice a day may be beneficial in lowering heavy metals. Heavy metal toxicity is believed to lower body temperature. Tuna fish, which is high in mercury, should be avoided, if hair analysis shows high mercury levels. Having your dentist remove Amalgam (Mercury) fillings from your teeth, and replacing them with a white composite plastic material, will also reduce toxicity from mercury. The whole lemon/olive oil drink will certainly help

Inner cleanse - the value of colonics and enemas
Garlic, vinegar and chlorophyll enemas for lower bowel

Bad bacteria in the colon produces ammonia, which raises the pH of the colon (an alkaline direction), and also produces several toxins, which can cause many symptoms - even cancer. The friendly bacteria produce lactic acid, which lowers the pH of the colon (an acid direction) and which kills the bad bacteria. Some of these friendly bacteria are lactobacillus acidophilus, plantarum and B Longum. Besides lactic acid, the friendly bacteria may produce digestive enzymes and many of the B vitamins, including B-12.

To remove HIV, Candida and other pathogens from the colon, consider Colonics and enemas, also special colon cleaning drinks that may be taken orally. Professionally administered Colonics are the most effective, as they reach the Transverse colon, the last segment of the colon that home enemas may not reach. While infections in the Ascending and Transverse colon are not common, persons, who are HIV+, and who have symptoms, would benefit from a colonic. To locate a Colon Therapist near you, look in the Yellow Pages under "Colonics" or call your local health food store for a reference. Colonics remove a lot of toxins from the body. One long-term survivor of HIV told us that a monthly colonic, that he has had done for several years, has been very beneficial for his health.

It is best to clean out the lower colon area with a pint of warm water before retaining the Garlic and Chlorophyll enema. To one pint of water in a blender, add 2 cloves of raw garlic, 2 to 4 tablespoons of apple cider vinegar and 2 tablespoons of liquid chlorophyll. Beat until blended. Pour into enema bag and use either early in the morning or late in the evening once a day. Try to retain the mixture in your colon for at least 5 minutes before releasing it. Adding 2 or 3 capsules of Black Walnut may make this mixture more effective in killing parasites. Open capsules and pour powder into enema bag.

Enema kits may be purchased at your local drugstore. The Kits come with a small plastic shut off value that should be depressed (shut off) between bowel movements. Enemas are effectively administered in a bathtub. Suspend enema bag about 18 inches above the top of the bathtub. Use a self-adhesive hook you can find at any hardware store. Lie on your left side and allow water to fill colon until it feels full, then lie on your back with knees drawn toward chest and continue to allow more fluid into the colon until it feels full again. Shut off water flow with finger control valve. Retain for as long as possible or up to 5 minutes before releasing.

Enemas are recommended once a day early in the morning. You will notice tremendous benefits. Note: Enemas should not be given just after eating, but about 4 hrs after your last meal. Use enemas once a day for the first month, then 2 or 3 times a week after that, as needed.

Caution: The very first enema should be administered using only clear lukewarm distilled, boiled or purified water. Water should be at room temperature or slightly warm before using. The water should be filtered and free from chlorine. Note: City tap water is sometimes contaminated with cryptosporidium. A home filtering system must remove particles down to 1 micron or less to remove cryptosporidium, a protozoan that can cause life-threatening diarrhea in persons immune compromised.

Self-test for friendly flora - floating stools & yellow urine

An ancient Chinese belief was that, when your stools are sinking, your health is deteriorating. Stools will float on water, when friendly flora in the colon area produce a type of lipid, that makes the stool weigh less than the water in your toilet. Stools that sink indicate the absence of friendly flora. In addition to producing gamma interferon, which builds up T cells, friendly flora like acidophilus, produce a wide range of B vitamins, which cause your urine to be yellow. Sinking stools and clear urine are bad signs. Floating stools and yellow urine are good signs and indicate a healthier colon. However, if you are taking B vitamin, the yellow urine test does not count, as the B vitamin supplements will cause your urine to turn yellow. To gauge this test properly, stop taking all supplements with B vitamins for 2 days and check the color of your urine on the third day. If your stools float, are large in diameter and your urine is yellow (without B vitamin supplementation), it means your colon is normal with a healthy colony of friendly flora.

Water, fresh vegetable and fruit juices

Drinking lots of good clean water helps the body remove most of its toxins and poisons. You could imagine how dirty your clothes would look, if you tried to wash them with just half the water you normally use. People with low rates of metabolism and body temperature do not crave water, and this causes the toxins to build up in the blood and in the cells. Increasing body temperature increases thirst for liquids. This urge should be satisfied, as water is necessary for the kidneys to function, removing toxins from the blood. Freshly made carrot, celery and parsley juice will speed up the removal of toxins from the body. As a rich source of nutrients and electrons, they will increase energy levels quickly. I would suggest 2 to 4 glasses daily. When a person does not have a juicer, I would suggest a glass of low sodium V8 Juice, with a spoonful of Barley Green, kamut or wheat grass powder added, along with some Tabasco sauce and a little lemon juice.

Exercise, steam baths and sun tanning. Ultraviolet light builds up WBC's and improves calcium absorption

Walking or light exercise is an excellent aid to digestion. It is especially recommended after a heavy meal. Walking one to two hours each day is vitally important to restoring your health. Walking helps move lymph fluid that contains toxins, that must be excreted. Sweating and urination, which result from walking and mild exercise, remove toxins and waste products from the body and oxygenate the blood. It is just as important as anything else you do in your recovery program. Walking after you eat a meal is a tremendous aid to digestion. Swallowing your saliva, while you are walking, will also help with the digestive process. Sipping on lemonade or grapefruit juice can stimulate the flow of saliva.

Steam baths, not saunas are recommended. Too many chemicals are added to saunas that can cause problems, particularly allergic reactions. If you belong to a local fitness and health club with a steam room, use it two or three times a week for about ten minutes each time. It opens the sinuses and the pores of the skin and stimulates the removal of toxic waste matter from the body.

On the contrary, a technique known as "photopheresis," where HIV infected blood has been exposed to ultraviolet (UV) light, shows nearly complete destruction of the HIV virus and no harm to the blood cells. The technique is described in Dr. Wm. Douglass's new book, "Into The Light." It is also described in Ralph Moss's book on "Cancer Therapy" (Equinox Press, NY) and in the book on "AIDS, Cancer and the Medical Establishment" by Raymond Brown, MD. In Ralph Moss's book, he quotes a study done at Henry Ford Hospital in Detroit, where UV treatment of the blood led to partial remission of AIDS-related Kaposi Sarcoma.

This book describes the positive results of several HIV+ persons, whose blood was treated with UV light. Several of the cases used combination therapies of UV light along with ozone or H_2O_2. Total white blood cell counts increase with sun tanning (The Swannanoa Report, Ivy, VA).

Sun tanning twice a week for about 15 minutes duration each session is recommended. A tan skin is a good sign of a healthier body inside. Ultraviolet rays destroy viruses and germs on contact. Sunglasses should never be worn continuously outdoors. Take them off and let your eyes get exposure to the natural ultraviolet light of the sun that stimulates the pineal gland. It will strengthen your eyes and your immune system. Vitamin D is produced when the skin is exposed to ultraviolet light. Vitamin D is necessary for the assimilation of Vitamin A and calcium. Without sufficient calcium in your blood, your body will not be able to carry nutrients across cell membranes. Without proper calcium utilization, you won't benefit from vitamin or mineral supplements. Calcium is like the mailman for delivery of amino acids, vitamins and minerals to cells. Without it, cells will starve from malnutrition. People who sun tan will sleep more soundly at night. Update: In a sun Tanning Salon, ask for a bed that emits only UVA and avoid UVB. UVA promotes Th1 cytokines, while UVB promotes Th2 cytokines.

The form of Vitamin D created by sunlight is D3 (Calciferol), and not D2 (a plant sterol). D2, the form added to milk and many supplements, has caused some researchers like Raymond Brown; M.D. to say it may be potentially harmful. Raymond Brown writes: "Synthetic D-2, used in many vitamin supplements, may cause disturbed calcium metabolism and cholesterol metabolism and conditions related to magnesium deficits." From his book: "AIDS, Cancer and the Medical Establishment," (Robert Speller Publishers, NY).

Colon implants of raw garlic clove "a ten-cent miracle"

In Italy, colon implants of raw garlic are being used as an effective treatment for diarrhea. The technique is simple. Before bedtime, cut and shape a small clove of raw garlic and, with a knife, make several small incisions into the garlic clove. Pour olive oil over the clove, then insert into the colon just like you would with a suppository for hemorrhoids. While you sleep, juices from the garlic clove directly enter the blood stream and do a wonderful cleansing of the blood - killing worms, parasites, yeast, fungus, germs and viruses. Colon implants of raw garlic are good to reduce colon inflammation, for anyone with weight loss or wasting syndrome, night sweats, herpes, and help induce a good nights sleep.

Note: if the clove burns the anus, try using "GOOT" - a Garlic ointment made by blending raw garlic with olive oil and coconut oil. GOOT should be made fresh every 14 days. It is both gentle and effective. The recipe is found at the end of the chapter on "Symptoms and Remedies."

Kombucha tea

One of our readers reports that after drinking a 1/2 glass of Kombucha Tea for 2 and 1/2 months, that he has better digestion, appetite and improved skin integrity. The tea is a fermented drink made from green or black tea, brown sugar and water and a species of fungus called Saccharomyces ludwiggi in symbiotic growth with other species such as Bacterium xylinum, Bacterium gluconicum (Tea Fungus Kombucha, by Rosina Fasching).

A book on "Kombuchu" by Gunter Frank tells of Kombuchu tea being used for stomach ulcers, rheumatism, hemorrhoids, gout, hardening of the arteries, arthritis, detoxifying the liver, high blood pressure, inflammation of the large and small intestines and sclerosis. Kombuchu tea contains glucuronic acid, a precursor of polysaccharides, which have a detoxifying effect on the liver and other organs. It also contains lactic acid, and usnic acid - an anti-bacterial agent.

How to make Kombuchu tea. Bring 3 quarts of filtered water to a boil. Remove from heat. Add one cup of light brown sugar and five tea bags (black/orange pekoe or green tea) or one tablespoon of bulk tea. Steep for 15 minutes. When solution is cool, remove tea bags or strain. Pour solution into a glass, china or glazed earthenware container. Do not use metal. Add 1 cup of Kombuchu tea from a previous batch or a Kombuchu mushroom. Place a cheesecloth or similar cloth over the pan and a rubber band around it. Place in a warm dark room. After 7 to 10 days, remove the Kombuchu mushrooms, wash them and refrigerate in a plastic bag until you are ready to make your next bath. With each bath, you will gain one new mushroom. The Kombuchu beverage is now ready to consume. Pour into a glass jar and refrigerate it. Drink 4 ounces with each meal. Consume within 3 weeks.

A Kombucha mushroom and instructions are available from your local health food store or Laurel Farms, 13470 Washington Blvd., PH, Venice, CA 90292. Ph No. 310-289-4372. Note: There is one report that two persons got ill after drinking a batch of Kombuchu that got contaminated, but there have been no other adverse reports since.

Pectin removes heavy metals

Dr. James Balch MD, reports that pectin is good for diabetics, removes toxins and heavy metals, lowers cholesterol and reduces the risk of gallstones. Dr. Balch reports that **pectin is found in apples, bananas, the rinds of citrus fruits (lemons, oranges and grapefruit), carrots, beets, cabbage and okra.**

In 1998, I talked to a former drug addict who told me he could remove all the street drugs he ingested by drinking a package of liquid pectin he would buy at the local grocery store. He would mix it with water and drink the whole thing at once. He said, "In about 2 hours, all the drugs in his blood were gone." He told me this included everything from marijuana to heroin to cocaine.

Pectin in the rinds of lemons, used in the whole lemon/olive oil drink, may partly explain its many benefits, including removal of heavy metals. Heavy metal toxicity affects persons with Hypothyroidism, HIV, Hepatitis, CFIDS, Cancer, Multiple Chemical Sensitivity and anyone with depleted Glutathione levels. Pectin to the rescue.

How much pectin to use?

There are no known limits to how much pectin is safe to use and there are no known side effects for using it in large quantities. Applesauce contains 4 grams of fiber per cup much of it in the form of pectin. Green apples of any variety, but especially Granny Smith variety, are very high in pectin. For someone very toxic, I would suggest 4 to 6 servings daily of any of the following: apples, bananas, carrots, beets, cabbage and okra. Apples can be eaten in the form of natural applesauce (without sugar added). If you can eat 3 cups of applesauce daily and 1 serving of 2 other choices, like bananas, carrots, beets, cabbage or okra, you should see measurable results in lowering the heavy metals in about 10 days. Both apple pectin and citrus pectin are also sold in health food stores in powder form. Suggested adult dose: about 5 grams (5000 mg daily) once or twice daily. Remember, apples are also very high in glucaric acid, another major detox pathway.

Suggestion: Cook up your own applesauce. Cut up pieces of apples with the skins. If you use Rome, Jonathans or other red apples, find the ones that are the most green in color. Adding sugar is optional, but should be avoided, if you have a yeast problem. Add about 1/2 inch of water to the bottom of the pan and a dash of cinnamon and ginger, while cooking it. With red apples, you can make a most delicious red-colored applesauce. Do not overcook. Chunky applesauce is just plain tasty. Serve it hot with slices of ripe bananas, topped with a little coconut milk or Haagen Daz ice cream. Now, that is a treat and a healthy one at that!

Now that you know what to eat to detoxify your body and promote a healthy colon, and how to eat, what else can you do to promote the kind of friendly flora that will lower the pH of the colon, produce B vitamins, digestive enzymes and factors that fight cancers, viruses and fungus? Answer: When the soil is right, plant the right seeds - the strains of intestinal flora that will go to work for you.

Castor oil packs detoxify the liver, shrink tumors, dissolve scar tissue and increase white blood cell counts

By Mark Konlee - Nov. 2, 1994:

On October 7th, I spoke with Robert M from Brooklyn, NY. He told me that after using castor oil topically on his lymph nodes for just 10 days, his T4 counts increased from 360 to 420 and his T8's increased from 670 to 1050. He attributed the increase solely to the use of the castor oil. Robert then told me of his interest in castor oil, when a friend of his had 100% success with castor oil on his cat that had a large cancerous tumor growing on the outside of its body.

The friend's veterinarian told him to try rubbing castor oil on the tumor and said it might shrink it and added that castor oil stimulated the immune system. Robert told me he had seen the cat before the castor oil treatment started and that the large tumor had completely shrunk and disappeared in just 30 days. All my friend did was to rub castor oil on the tumor each day for one month. "It sounds unbelievable, but the tumor is completely gone. I decided to try rubbing the castor oil on my swollen lymph nodes on August 15th to see if it would reduce the soreness and swelling. Ten days later, I still had swollen lymph nodes, although slightly reduced. However, the blood test results of August 25th showed this rather sharp increase in both T4 and T8 cells."

Update: On Jan 31, 1995, Robert M. called to tell me that for the first time in 2 years, his swollen lymph nodes had completely returned to normal. He credited the Whole Lemon/Olive Oil drink for the reduction in lymph node size. "This drink returned my saliva pH to normal (6.4) in 2 days and in 4 days, my swollen lymph nodes were gone." On Feb. 18, 1995, Robert M called me on the test results of the first 30 days of doing both the Whole Lemon/Olive oil drink and the daily castor oil packs. He reported his CD4 count increased from 294 to 338. His CD8 count dropped from 1400 to 1300. His WBC was 6,100; RBC - 5,280 and HGB - 16.3. He said he was very pleased with the results.

That evening (10/7/94), I told Jim, who has HIV, about Robert's experience with castor oil. I said: "Jim, I don't know much about castor oil, except that it comes from the castor bean plant. Do you know anything about it?" Jim replied: I never used castor oil myself, but in 1991, several PWA's in Houston, TX were using castor oil packs and reported that they were feeling better."

Mark: "Tell me everything you know about PWA's who used castor oil and the benefits they received."

Jim: "I'll tell you about a friend of mine, Dean. Dean heard about castor oil from Ed Jamail, who belonged to A.R.E. (Assn. for Research and Enlightenment). A.R.E. has a library in Virginia Beach, VA with all the reading on the late psychic, Edgar Cayce. Cayce frequently recommended castor oil packs and a heat pad applied topically for wide range of health related problems. Dean had heard that persons doing the castor oil packs were reported to be feeling better. So he decided to give it a try. He had impressive results. In 30 days, his T4 counts increased significantly.

Mark: How much?

Jim: I believe from 140 to 263. At the time, he was under the care of Dr. Patricia Salvato, M.D. His T4 counts had been continuously dropping for several months and Dr. Salvato thought the test results were in error and ordered a second test. The second test confirmed the T4 count increase was correct. Dean never told Dr. Salvato that he was doing the castor oil packs.

Mark: Did Dean take any drugs, supplements or follow any special diet?

Jim: No, he ate whatever he felt like - no special diet. He was not on any drugs or medications. He had been taking some vitamins and anti-oxidants, but had been on them for some time while his T4 counts kept dropping.

Mark: How did Dean do the castor oil treatments?

Jim: He used the method recommended by A.R.E., the Edgar Cayce Foundation. Edgar Cayce was a psychic who would go into a trance like sleep and give readings on a person's health problem. It would be best to call Ed Jamail in Houston, TX. Ed was a member of A.R.E. for several years and worked with Dean to design the protocol

Mark: (To Ed Jamail): Jim told me about Dean's use of castor oil packs in 1991. Can you tell me the protocol he used with the castor oil packs?

Ed: I'd be glad to. It was in September 1991, that Dean tried the castor oil packs for one month. He did 28 treatments total over a 4-week period. Four days each week, the castor

oil packs were done over the abdomen area and 3 days each week, they were done over the thymus gland area - the upper part of the chest. It was thought that the castor oil would detoxify and stimulate the Thymus gland to maturate T cells produced in the bone marrow.
Mark: What results did Dean have?
Ed: Dean was not looking very well at all when he started on the castor oil packs. In 30 days, he looked and acted like a new person. He told me his T4 counts increased significantly (140 to 263).

"Castor Oil – The Oil that Heals" by William A. McGarey, M.D.

Dr. William McGarey founded the A.R.E. Clinic in Phoenix, AZ over twenty years ago. In his book, Dr. McGarey relates to the reader experiences using castor oil in his clinical practice over the past two decades. He is the author of an earlier monograph on the medicinal properties of castor oil called EDGAR CAYCE AND THE PALMA CHRISTI.

Dr. McGarey states that castor oil contains a unique fatty acid found nowhere else in nature - Ricinoleic acid. It has a "hydroxyl group on the twelfth carbon"....This relationship of hydroxyl group and unsaturation exists only in castor oil." In his book, Dr. McGarey states the following medicinal properties of castor oil:

Increases eliminations; stimulates the liver and all organs and glands including the colon; reduces toxemia, inflammation, pain, nausea and swelling; dissolves adhesions, lesions and gallstones; increases lymphatic circulation, relaxation and lacteal duct circulation. This is only a partial listing. Dr. McGarey cites experiences of skin cancers disappearing with topical applications. On the immune system he writes: "From our own research at the A.R.E. Clinic, the major findings included: (1). Total lymphocyte count increased significantly in the group using castor oil packs; (2). T -pan lymphocyte count (T-11) increased significantly in the group using castor oil packs...Our clinical experience with the castor oil packs applied over the abdomen led us to understand that the packs enhanced the function of the thymus gland and other components of the immune system."

Dr. McGarey also discusses the beneficial effects of castor oil on the Autonomic Nervous System and its properties in relaxing the autonomic nerves, the majority of which are concentrated in the abdominal region. Dr. McGarey has prescribed castor oil packs for persons with cancer, colitis, ulcers, gallstones, hepatitis, neuritis, lymphitis, uremia, gastritis, Hodgkin's disease, sluggish kidneys and cirrhosis of the liver.

Dr. McGarey's book - THE OIL THAT HEALS (232 pages) is published by A.R.E. Press in Virginia Bch, VA.

New protocol discontinues the reuse of preheated castor oil

August 1, 1995

The original Edgar Cayce procedure for doing castor oil packs was to add fresh castor oil to the wool or cotton flannel and to wash the cloth once every 21 days. However, when 3 PWAs did this daily for 8 months and we began observing declines in the WBC counts, we modified the instructions to reduce treatments to 3 per week over the three target areas - liver, thymus and spleen. In addition, the cloth is washed out after each treatment. So far, 9 out of 10 persons following the new protocol have reported increases in White Blood Cell counts.

First time users: Lay heat pad on table. Cut a piece of plastic to the size of the heat pad and place on top of pad. Cut one layer of white cotton or white wool flannel to the same size and place on top of the plastic. Turn heat pad on high. Pour 1/3 cup of cold pressed castor oil in center of flannel and spread manually up to 2 inches from edge of flannel. After five minutes of preheating, lift up pad and place against the area of the body to be treated. Wrap a large bath towel around the body and over the heat pad and pin in place. Reduce heat to medium if it feels too hot. Let it remain in place for 1 hour.

When the hour is over, remove pad, plastic and flannel and place aside. Massage oil into skin and then rub skin dry with a dry hand towel. Once the treatment is finished, the castor oil in the flannel that has been heated is not to be reused by adding more castor oil to it. You must wash the oil soaked flannel in warm water with baking soda before using the flannel again. Add 1/4 cup of baking soda to 2 quarts of warm water. Soak flannel in water and squeeze out the castor oil. Rinse thoroughly with clear warm water before reusing the flannel for another treatment.

A convenient alternative to wool or cotton flannel: One PWA told of satisfactory results using white cotton terry cloth purchased from a local fabric supply outlet. He buys 2 yards at a time, cuts a piece to the size of his heat pad. When he is done with the castor oil treatment, he throws the terry cloth away and uses a new piece for his next treatment.

First time users weekly schedule: Do the castor oil packs once a day for 3 days over the Thymus area (just above the heart); twice a week over the liver area (under right rib cage to right of naval) and twice a week over the spleen area (at the bottom of left rib cage). After 4 weeks, reduce treatment to 3 times a week - once over the three target areas- liver, thymus and spleen.

Some manufacturers of over the counter castor oil use high temperatures to extract more castor oil from the castor bean. High temperatures induce lipid peroxidation rendering the product ineffective as an immune stimulant. I have had three confirmed cases where castor oil extracted by a high temperature process failed to increase T cell counts. In all instances, the words "cold pressed" did not appear on the label. Once the castor oil bottle is opened, store it in a cool dark place or in a refrigerator.

Where to obtain "cold pressed" castor oil

Local sources: health food stores. Woolen flannel - fabric shops; heat pads - drug stores and department stores. Wholesale or retail order source for cold pressed castor oil, wool or cotton flannel is Heritage Store - 800-862-2923 or 804-428-0100.

What about taking castor oil orally?

Castor oil is sold in drug stores as a remedy for constipation. You would think that the last thing that someone with diarrhea would want to take is a product with laxative properties. However, if the castor oil knocks out the pathogen that is causing the diarrhea, then truth may be stranger than fiction. One person told me he stopped his diarrhea by taking orally one tablespoon of cold pressed castor oil daily for 3 consecutive days.

At least 4 people I spoke with this month have told me their mother or grandmother would make them take a teaspoon of castor oil by mouth whenever they came down with a cold or flu. One person told me his great grandmother, who is over 100 years old and still going strong, takes one teaspoon a day and has for several years.

A local person told us that as a child, she had Tuberculosis, and her parents made her swallow 2 Tablespoons of castor oil daily with orange juice. She vomited some of it up, but credits the castor oil for her recovery.

When castor oil is used orally, I recommend taking it before bedtime. Cold pressed castor oil capsules are manufactured by NCA, 1725 E Fowler Ave, Tampa, FL 33612. Ph No 813-977-1000. 5 or 6 capsules before bedtime once a day is a suggested dosage.

Letter from a PWA who used castor oil for 4 years

Nov. 14, 1994

In 1990, I came down with scarlet fever, severe colitis, lung infections, nail infections, asthma and lost 35 lbs. I also had severe nausea. My lymph glands were swollen. Doctors tested me for HIV after 1.5 years on antibiotics. They told me I was HIV+ (Oct., 1990) and suggested I start taking AZT. They also gave me Bactrim for P.C.P. I reacted to the Bactrim violently and took it only once. My T4 cells were 230 at the time.

I decided to look elsewhere - on my knees - then the pathway to my journey began. I must stress that everything I found I believe was a result of prayer and God's personal love for us all. This is what I did:

I became a vegetarian, but do eat some deep-sea fish. I started taking oral $H2O2$ drops - one month on and then two weeks off. The dose was 5 drops of 35% $H2O2$ in distilled water 3 times a day taken on an empty stomach. I increased the dosage by 3 drops per day until after 15 days I was taking 20 drops 3X. I then gradually reduced the dosage over the next two weeks and then stopped for two weeks before resuming the cycle. I also took CO Q10, Garlic, Citricil (grapefruit seed extract), Primrose Oil, Bilberry, Hepisil, EPA 1000, Cell Guard and Herbal Fiberblend (by AIMS - makers of Barley Green).

Two months later, my T4 cells were 430. Six months later, they were 460. Over the next three years, my T4 cells ranged in the 450 to 550 range. However, I frequently had genital Herpes outbreaks. In 1993, I heard about Castor Oil. My method of using it was as follows: I used a bathtub Jacuzzi setup. I filled the tub about half full of hot water. I rubbed castor oil all over my body and on my lymph nodes. I stayed in the hot tub with the castor oil rub down for 30 to 40 minutes each day. I did not use any soap until at the end of the session. After two months of doing this, I was tested and my T4 Cells had risen to 780. Since this, I have been doing the complete castor oil rubdown 2 to 3 times a week along with the hot water soak.

In September 1994, I started using ozone at home - Rectal insufflation, Sauna Bag and drank ozonated water. I feel wonderful! My weight is normal now. My Herpes is gone as of Nov. 1994. I have ten times more energy and strength than I had before. My eyesight has improved - no more night blindness. I'm excited about working again. I feel perfectly normal. My ozone machine is a double corona from Cleanwater Systems (800-837-8655). I will work on this and get some new numbers to share with you.

Respectfully,
Gerry K Laguna Bch, CA

PS: My lymph nodes were swollen until I started on the ozone, Now, they have gone all the way down.

Editor's Note: Gerry credits God with giving him direction for his recovery. He said that he has incredible energy and can run all the way up a small mountain in his backyard. He no longer uses the oral H2O2 since starting on the ozone. He said the castor oil rubdowns have removed all the brown spots from his skin and that his skin is beautiful. I'm 35 years old, but many people think I am 21.

12

Good and bad immune profiles

In January, 1993, seventy persons with HIV responded to a survey questionnaire we mailed out. The information provided did positively confirm certain conditions that exist in persons whose immune responses were improving as well as those conditions that exist in persons whose immune responses continued to decline. With this data, I have created two profiles - one for the person whose immune system is on the mend and one for the person whose immune response was failing. I will call these two profiles "A Good Profile"(G) and "A Bad Profile"(B). In January 1994, body temperature was added to this profile.

A "good profile" (A)
(associated with a stronger immune system)

1. Normal basal body temperature of 97.6 to 98_ F taken before rising in the morning. .
2. Saliva pH is near 6.4 (6.2 to 6.6) before eating. (Indicates pH of blood is neither too acid nor alkaline and an ability to absorb nutrients from food).
3. First Urine pH reading in the morning is 5.5 to 5.8. (Indicates the adrenal glands are working).
4. Good Appetite and eats when hungry (indicates low levels of toxicity and a functioning pancreas and liver).
5. High energy levels (indicates low level of toxicity and normal liver, adrenal, pituitary and thyroid functions).
6. Stools float most of the time (indicates presence of friendly flora in Colon).
7. Stools are large diameter (indicates no inflammation of G.I tract)
8. Urine is usually yellow in color (indicates friendly flora are producing B vitamins and gamma interferon in the Colon. Note: B vitamins supplements will also produce yellow urine).
9. Sex drive is strong (indicates hormone levels are normal)
10. Weight is normal or increasing (indicates digestion and assimilation is working)
11. Sleeps well at night (indicates adequate calcium levels in the blood).
12. Stress level is low.
13. Smooth healthy skin with few eruptions (indicates a healthy G.I tract).
14. Cuts and wounds heal rapidly (indicates adequate Potassium and Magnesium levels and a normal liver).
15. Leads an active life with adequate physical exercise (indicates a detoxified body).

A "bad profile" (B)
(associated with low vitality, poor digestion, chronic infections and a weakened immune system)

1. Low Body Temperature (from 1/2 degree to several degrees or more below 98.6) – or

low basal body temperature. Low Body Temperature is related to digestive disorders - stomach heat is too low to stimulate digestive enzymes. People with low body temperature may have difficulty digesting meat, hard cheese and may have problems with wheat. They are prone to suffer from fatigue, have thrush, skin disorders, chronic infections as well as low white and red blood cell counts.

2. Saliva pH is either 6.0 or lower before eating or 6.8 or higher before eating. An acid saliva pH is related to fast movement of food through the digestive tract and inadequate absorption of nutrients and a toxic blood condition - too high in CO_2 and other waste products. See the chapter on "Balance your pH."

3. First urine pH reading in the morning is alkaline, usually 6.2 or higher. This pH profile is associated with elevated estrogen levels, a deficiency of free cortisol, insomnia and stress. Use either Coenzymated B vitamins or betaine HCL, Whole Lemon/Olive oil drink. Drink Red Clover and Ginger tea with your meals and drink a cup of Marjoram and Thyme tea before bedtime in addition to other suggestions to improve adrenal function.

4. Poor appetite - person eats because it is time to eat, not because he is hungry. Indicates a toxic liver, toxins, side effects of some drugs and impurities in the colon and blood, low levels of digestive enzymes and dry mouth syndrome (lack of saliva). Suggestions: Add lemon juice to all your food and make a cup of tea from Gentian Root and Ginger root to sip on with or after meals. Consider the use of lemon juice and cayenne capsules before meals to stimulate appetite.

5. Fatigue - caused by acid blood, toxins, side effects of some drugs, lack of deep restful sleep, faulty digestion and assimilation of nutrients.

6. Stools sink more often than they float - caused by toxins and pathogens in the colon that kill off friendly intestinal flora. Friendly flora produces lipids that cause stools to float. Need Colon cleansing, cultured cabbage juice, lemon juice and follow the Immune Enhancement Diet.

7. Stools are small diameter - caused by inflammation in the colon. Whole leaf aloe vera juice and cultured cabbage juice is good to correct this problem or try Kombuchu tea or use Triphala (Planetary Formulas).

8. Urine that is clear. This is caused by a lack of B vitamins normally produced by friendly flora in the colon. B vitamins cause urine to turn yellow. No yellow color in urine means an absence of good bacteria in the colon. Supplements: Beta-carotene with meals, yogurt eaten with meals, cultured cabbage juice. Foods: Squash, yams, pumpkin, carrots, garlic, parsley and endive.

9. Sex drive is weak - little interest. (Low hormone levels and malabsorption of nutrients, toxins in colon and liver). Supplements needed: Men: Siberian Ginseng, Sarsaparilla, Lecithin, Vitamin E - 400 i.u. daily. Raw wheat germ or Wheat Germ Oil (Viobin brand is best). Women, Damiana, Yam extract. Vitamin E and Red Clover tea.

10. Weight loss - a malabsorption problem with multiple causes - gluten intolerance (avoid wheat, spaghetti or pasta) or food allergies or parasites in the colon).

11. Difficulty getting a good night's sleep (lack of calcium in blood). Helpful supplements: Calcium lactate before bedtime. Take 5 capsules or 1 tsp. of calcium lactate powder in water. Herbal teas before bedtime: Marjoram and Thyme. Steep 1/2 tsp. of each in a cup of hot water.

12. Stress level is high. (Many causes - job, worry about health, lack of money, love, lack of adequate sleep)

13. Lots of skin problems - (dry flaky skin, very itchy, psoriasis, red zits and open sores). Try Sarsaparilla. Helpful ideas for psoriasis: Low fat diet, lecithin, Oregon Grape Root tea, Suntan in a salon, Ozone in a Sauna Bag.

14. Cuts and wounds heal slowly or not at all. (Indicates a sluggish and toxic liver and malabsorption of amino acids and key minerals like potassium, magnesium and calcium).

15. Leads a sedentary and inactive life (couch potato).

Circle the conditions that best describe your self from both profiles and then count scores. If you circled most or all of them in "A", your immune system is in good shape and improving. If Profile "B" best describes you, your immune system is declining. It is now up to you to take charge of your health and reverse your profile.

13

How to heal a leaky gut and implant friendly flora

How to make your own fiber/pectin/probiotic blend

To get stools to float, use a dietary supplement that is a fiber/pectin/probiotic blend or mix your own.

Add one cup of ground psyllium seed or freshly ground flax seed to a bowl. Add 1/2 cup of citrus or apple pectin and 1/4 cup of a blend of probiotics (without maltodextrin added). These must include, at a minimum, L Acidophilus and B Longum. Mix it all together and store in a refrigerator. Use one teaspoon in a glass of water before meals 1 to 3 times daily. Continue using until stools are normal in appearance - large diameter, medium brown and float on water, then reduce to one serving daily as a maintenance.

You can improve the formula by adding L Plantarum (reduces IgE - food allergies) and L. Salivarius (kills off yeast and fungal infections and Salmonella etc.). You can also add glucomannan, wheat, barley or kamut grass or blue-green algae to the formula. Slippery elm - 2 tablespoons of powder help heal a sore gut and adding some yucca helps removes stool odor.

Foods that give you poor quality stools: white rice, white bread, pasta made from white flour, any product made from white sugar or white flour and meats cooked at high temperatures.

Foods to give you healthy appearing stools: Squash, pumpkin pie, carrots, yams, dark green vegetables especially if eaten raw, whole grains cooked at lower temperatures, whole grain breads, hot breakfast cereal (oat bran), pasta from spelt, meats cooked at lower temperatures in a Crock Pot. Raw garlic. Avoid foods with preservatives.

Butyrate, friendly flora and mucosal integrity.

Having friendly intestinal flora is not an option just for a healthy gastrointestinal tract but for a healthy immune system as well. Why observing the quality of stools is so important is that when the stools are not healthy in appearance, neither will be the patient. Restoring gastrointestinal health is a pre-requisite for recovery from most of the illnesses of civilization. Briefly, when you have unhealthy stools and bad flora in the gut, you will have an excess of ammonia produced by those unfriendly flora and this will throw your saliva and urine pH out of balance, and along with it, hundreds of vital enzymes throughout the body - enzymes that not only control digestion, but help in the production of energy in the body and the removal of waste matter and toxins. Toxemia (self-poisoning) is the result of having an intestinal tract loaded with e-coli, candida, parasites and other pathogens.

There is more. You need friendly flora to produce short chain fatty acids like lactic, acetic, butyric and others that create an internal environment hostile to the flora that cause illness and you need these same friendly flora (acidophilus and bifidobacteria) to produce these short chain fatty acids to stimulate the growth of mucus membranes throughout the intestinal tract and mucin, the intestinal lubricant. You need healthy mucus membranes as much as you need healthy skin. The mucus membranes of the gastrointestinal (GI) tract are critical to prevent leaky gut syndrome, acid reflux syndrome, ulcers, allergies, etc. You can't have mucosal immunity without healthy mucus membranes. When the intestinal tract has insufficient mucus membranes, it leads to absorption of foreign proteins (byproducts of digestion) and to a TH2 cytokine immune response (IL-6 and IL-10). The resulting overload of toxins absorbed from the intestines over stimulates your humoral immunity and weakens your cell-mediated immunity.

Failure to have an adequate amount of butyric and acetic acid in the colon impairs the absorption of calcium, magnesium and dozens of trace minerals, leading to endocrine and hormonal imbalances, conditions like insomnia, osteoporosis, high blood pressure and many other imbalances. Bifido bacteria and the short chain fatty acids are virtually non-existent in all persons with AIDS, cancer, lyme, hepatitis, multiple allergies, chemical sensitivities and chronic fatigue syndrome. Because the short chain fatty acids are not in the stools is the reason they sink. Taking yet another multiple vitamin and mineral supplement is not the answer. Most of the fiber supplements and friendly flora supplements on the market are helpful, but the best formula we have discovered is the fiber, pectin and probiotic blends of Acidophilus, Bifidum, B Longum, L Salivarius and L Plantarum.

Diet must be free from a daily intake of hormones in meat or poultry, antibiotics, food preservatives and all antimicrobials that kill off the good bacteria. Kefir and buttermilk are healthier for your colon than yogurt. If yogurt were more sour and less like a sweet pudding, it would be more beneficial.

Some raw vegetables and fruits should be consumed with each meal to provide live active plant enzymes to help the digestive process. Consider parsley or raw ripe pineapple. Honey is a healthy food and a good infection fighter, but to be effective, it must be eaten raw, not added to hot foods or used in cooking. Cooked foods that are easiest to digest are cooked at a low temperature, simmered or cooked at the low setting in a crock-pot or slow cooker.

Urine should have a clear, yet yellow color at least once a day, although if you drink a lot of water, it will be lighter in color. Friendly flora produce B vitamins that turn your urine yellow. For those of you who are not completely sugar-intolerant, a teaspoon of blackstrap molasses in a cup of hot water is a rich source of calcium and over 60 trace minerals. Moreover, these minerals are ionized, that is, completely dissolved in water and completely absorbable, better than most of the calcium supplements on the market. Saliva pH below 6.4 can also be an indication of a calcium deficiency. Without ionized calcium, nutrient delivery across the cell membranes is impaired and fatigue and toxemia result. A small amount of coral calcium powder dissolved in water is a great source of ionized calcium and trace minerals. This is far better than the colloidal mineral supplements on the market that most often have too many toxic metals (lead, mercury) in them. Pectin, especially in the fiber/probiotic blend, removes heavy metals from the body and is a great detoxifier.

Insomnia is related to toxemia, colon toxicity, calcium malabsorption and stress. Insomnia leads to higher IL-6 (Interleukin 6) levels that shift your immune response to the humoral or TH2 side. Exercise - take a walk for half an hour before bedtime, take 5 to 10 grams of Immunepro or other cold-processed whey proteins, eat some cottage cheese, a natural source of calcium lactate, or take 3 to 5 calcium lactate capsules before bedtime. This will help you sleep better.

Recently, two local persons with chronic insomnia have reported the best results with Immunepro – 10 grams once a day before bedtime. Two local persons with chronic insomnia reported deep restful sleep of 7 to 9 hours straight, from using just 10 grams of Immunepro. One person said, "The Immunepro works better than a sleeping pill."

Hops or chamomile tea may be helpful also, but avoid adding any sugar. Sun tanning indoors in a salon for 15 minutes twice a week will help. Also take natural Cod Liver Oil (not emulsified) 3 to 6 capsules daily and this will help as will the whole lemon/olive oil drink. Liquid cod liver oil, on the store shelf, may be rancid. Cod liver oil capsules in a brown or light-proof bottle will give you a fresher product than the liquid oil.

Glutathione levels: Cold processed whey proteins like ImmunePro or Immunocal are very helpful, as are winter squash and avocados for increasing glutathione levels. Whey proteins should be taken only about 1 hour before bedtime to maximize the benefits that include a deeper more restful sleep, human growth hormone, increased lean muscle mass and increased glutathione production. Silymarin (Milk thistle) and alpha lipoic acid (raw potatoes) are also very helpful in supporting glutathione levels. In fact, selenium is critical. In Japan, the average daily consumption of selenium is 600 mcg, whereas in the US, it is less than 100 mcg.

Natural vitamin C from rose hips and Acerola cherries are more beneficial than corn derived or manufactured Vitamin C. Avoid high potency vitamin and mineral supplements sold in drug stores and even in health food stores. Get your vitamins from whole natural sources and not in such high doses. A few exceptions - vitamin E - up to 400 i.u daily is beneficial for heart and circulatory problems, Methyl B12 and folic acid are very beneficial and help reduce homocysteine levels. Dr Christopher makes a whole natural vitamin-mineral formula with no synthetic vitamins added "Vitalerbs." It is found in Health Food Stores.

Note: When choosing between the two forms of synthetic vitamin C on the market, the beet-derived is better. Vitamin C manufactured from beets is available from Nutricology and is better tolerated than synthetic Vitamin C manufactured from corn. Corn is a very common allergen. Alpha Lipoic Acid is a major antioxidant. Rather than taking a pill, I recommend obtaining natural ALA from raw potatoes. Eat one raw potato daily, as a source of natural alpha lipoic acid and catalase. Catalase breaks down hydrogen peroxide into oxygen and water.

Diagnostic tests for leaky gut syndrome

This test is important, as it measures the progress you are making on your diet and protocol to restore normal mucosal integrity and normal absorption of nutrients. To measure progress, you always need two tests; the first is baseline, to find out where your starting profile is, while the second one measures your progress in healing the gut. More information on this test and how to prepare for it is available from Great Smoky Diagnostics Lab at 800-522-4762 or write to Great Smoky Diagnostics, 63 Aillicoa St, Asheville, NC 28801. (Cost is $86 per test).

Leaky gut > allergies, low cortisol and thyroid hormones

Leaky gut syndrome occurs nearly 100% in persons with systemic fungal and yeast infections (candidiasis). Leaky gut syndrome contributes to circulating immune complexes (CIC) that are very immunosuppressive. Immune complexes are clusters of interlocking antigens and antibodies. Normally, macrophages break up these circulating complexes. When macrophages become anergic or lazy, this may fail to happen, and the circulating immune complexes (CIC) may become lodged in organs and tissues and set off inflammatory reactions (1). If the membranes of the intestinal tract are intact, this absorption of foreign proteins, resulting from incomplete digestion, will not occur. Intestinal candidiasis, that punctures small holes in the intestinal tract, can be a source for entry of foreign proteins into the blood supply. Leaky gut syndrome, poor digestion and the resulting absorption of foreign proteins is a major cause of multiple food allergies in persons with CFIDS, and in many cases of early AIDS. The food allergies are the result of an active humoral immune response that causes B cells to produce large quantities of antibodies directed against the foreign proteins.

Dr. Francis Pottinger Jr. has found that meals of entirely cooked foods produce a condition known as "digestive leukocytosis." This condition occurs after ingesting a meal of entirely cooked foods, when there is an increase in white blood cells in response to the lack of digestive enzymes in the food. Eating only cooked foods forces the body to call upon the white blood cells to donate enzymes to assist the process of digestion (2). Many people have also found that enzyme-depleted cooked foods contribute to tiredness and fatigue where enzyme-rich raw foods like a salad or sprouts, produce energy. Recommended: Vegetarian Digestive enzymes (e.g. Absorbaid).

To help heal a leaky gut

Leaky gut syndrome is caused by years of a deficiency of butyrate, that is produced in the colon by bifido bacteria. Butyrate and acetate, by-products of friendly flora, stimulate the rebuilding of the mucus membranes of the entire gastrointestinal tract. Butter and buttermilk are the only known natural sources of butyrate. High fiber diets that promote increased bifido bacteria activity will increase butyrate levels.

Note: Cold breakfast cereals (All Bran) may be toxic to the body, even when they are made from whole grains. This is because most of them are processed at very high temperatures (above 400 degrees F) and have toxic protein cross-linking by-products. Avoid them. Eat hot breakfast cereal only or baked whole grain breads. In general, avoid foods cooked at temperatures above 300° F.

1. Whole leaf aloe juice made from fresh aloe leaves purchased direct from a farmer.
2. Butyren (Butyric acid) by Allergy Research - 2 or 3 caps 3X before meals. Check with your Physician for a Butyrate enema kit. Note: Once your stools start to float, you should not need butyrate supplement any longer.
3. Fiber/pectin/probiotic blend. Psyllium or ground flax seed, pectin, glucomannan, Blue-green algae, coral calcium, slippery elm and at least these 3 probiotics (Acidophilus, B longum and L. Plantarum). Better with Bifidus and L. Salivarius added. Mix together and refrigerate. Use one tsp. in water before meals 3 times daily until stools are normal size and

float on water. Note: A fiber/pectin/probiotic blend called "Perfect Stool Formula" is offered by Vital Health Products at 414-329-0648 www.vhp4.com that has produced normal appearing stool for many people in a few weeks.

4. Drink cultured cabbage juice- 1/2 cup twice daily or eat 2 raw potatoes.
5. Vitamin A - Cod Liver Oil – 3 to 6 capsules twice daily.
6. Food high in L-Glutamine. Cottage cheese and Ricotta cheese are about 4 times higher in glutamine than most other types of cheese. Free-range turkey and grass- fed beef are also high in glutamine. Seeds: sunflower and sesame (tahini). Note - may not be tolerated well by persons with severe food allergies. Free form L-glutamine - use up to 10 grams daily but consider this precaution - test a small amount first if you are hypersensitive. Some people are very intolerant of this free form amino acid.
7. Diet: Cooked orange-colored vegetables (pumpkin, squash, yams) - consume 8 ozs to one pound daily. Also eat raw vegetables, whole grains gluten-free bread and whole grain pasta. Coconut milk. See the chapter on the Immune Enhancement Diet Plan.

1. Enzymes and Enzyme Therapy, by Anthony Cichoke D.C. (Keats Publishing, Inc, New Canaan, CT)

Cultured cabbage juice called "a 50-cent miracle"

Cultured cabbage juice is great for thrush and is especially recommended after anti-biotic therapy. It is an important drink to cleanse the small intestines and colon of multiple infections and to implant friendly intestinal flora. At least two persons have told us that "Cultured Cabbage Juice" is the single most effective healing drink, for all kinds of intestinal problems, that they have ever tried. Raw cabbage is a natural source of Lactobacillus Salivarius.

1. The lactic acid and sulfur it contains will kill pathogens and viruses of all kinds throughout your G.I. tract. 2. The billions of friendly lactobacteria (Salivarius) will become implanted in your colon and produce even more lactic acid, to keep the pathogens out. The lactobacteria also produce B Vitamins and other factors needed by your body's immune system. 3. It will heal ulcers and inflammation of the stomach, small intestines and colon. Besides, this healing elixir costs only pennies a day to make. Cultured cabbage juice should always be taken for at least two weeks after taking antibiotics. Salivarius, L. Plantarum and B. Longum are three of the most important probiotics you can use. (See newsletter in Appendix for more info).

How to make cultured cabbage juice

To make Cultured Cabbage Juice, fill a blender with raw chopped green cabbage and then add distilled water until about 2/3 full. Blend at high speed for 1 minute. Pour into a glass or porcelain bowl. Fill blender with cabbage and water 2 more times and add the mixture to the bowl. Cover with a tightly wrapped piece of plastic or Seran wrap. Let stand at room temperature for 3 days. Then, pass mixture through a strainer or cheese cloth. Throw away the pulp and place the liquid in a glass jar and refrigerate. Drink 1/2 cup 2 or 3 times a day. To make a second batch only requires one day, instead of three. Blend cabbage and distilled water as directed above and add 1/2 cup of the last batch of cultured juice to the new batch and cover with a plastic or cellophane sheet. It will be ready in just 24 hours. This process may be repeated indefinitely.

Home made aloe vera leaf drink - a powerful immune modulator - heals a leaky gut – helpful in CFIDS and cancer

You can make your own whole leaf aloe vera juice at home with fresh aloe leaves. Wash leaves and remove the spines on the edge. The spines contain a laxative. To make one cup of whole aloe juice, cut up one cup of aloe leaves. For whole leaf aloe juice, leave the green skin on the leaf and cut into chunks. Place one cup of aloe vera chunks in a blender. Add one cup of distilled water. Blend at a slow speed for 10 seconds and then strain through a screen-type strainer or cheesecloth. Drink 1 or 2 cups daily. You may make larger batches and store in a refrigerator for up to 5 days. Aloe leaves may be stored in a refrigerator for up to 3 weeks. Source of fresh aloe leaves that can be shipped to your house: Aloe Supply Co., PO Box 93, Belle Glade, FL 33430 (863-467-6200). Using fresh aloe vera leaves is a very cost effective way of healing the gut and detoxifying the lymph system, a better choice than buying processed aloe vera products and costs less than $1.00 a day.

Test to determine if your gut is healing

When you succeed in implanting friendly flora, your stools will begin to float on water. They will be normal diameter - one inch or larger in width and medium brown in color. As your digestion improves, you won't see raw vegetables in the stools either. High fiber diets promote normal pH values in the colon. The pH of a healthy colon should be between 5.5 and 7.0. If it is 8 or higher, it is too alkaline as is usually found in persons with a toxic colon. Healthy stools also have little or no odor.

Finally, after you have had normal stools for about 8 weeks, have a stool analysis to measure butyrate, Bifidus and Acidophilus levels. They should all be in the normal range. Also, a test for "leaky gut and malabsorption" should indicate that this problem has disappeared as well. Stop taking B vitamins for 24 hours, as they turn your urine yellow. Your urine should still be yellow, not clear, indicating the presence of B vitamins produced by the friendly flora.

Carcinogenic "acrylamides" are formed by high temperatures

In experiments on rats, researchers found that whole grain breakfast cereals (processed at high temperatures) caused more cancer than did white flour fed to control group. Avoid a breakfast cereal called "All Bran" and other cold breakfast cereals - they are processed at too high a temperature, often above 400 degrees F. Many of these "cold" breakfast cereals are toxic to the body, as the higher temperature at which they were processed cause the formation a cancer-causing agent called "acrylamide." Arcylamides are known to cause cancer in man and animals. They are the result of cooking carbohydrates at high temperatures. Researchers have found that boiling food does not increase the acrylamide content. Boiled mashed potatoes do not contain acrylamides, but you will find a lot of this cancer-causing agent in potato chips and French fries.

Digestive enzymes reduce "circulating immune complexes"

Circulating immune complexes (CICs) strongly promote antibody and autoantibody TH2 reactions and suppress TH1 cell-mediated immune responses. Leaky gut syndrome is a condition that allows foreign proteins to enter the blood and create these complexes. In gay men, anal sex contributes to CICs. Plant digestive enzymes can reduce these foreign proteins in the blood. Food sources that have high amounts of plant enzymes that can be beneficial when eaten with meals are: ginger root, raw red beets, sprouts, avocados, raw horseradish, fresh raw salsa (cayenne), raw pineapple, kiwi fruit and cultured foods. Vegetarian Digestive Enzymes will be beneficial when these foods are not available. Increasing Bifidobacteria activity in the colon and or taking butyrate supplements will help to heal a leaky gut and reduce future serum levels of the CICs.

14

Complementary therapies from Africa and North America

Neem used to treat terminal AIDS patients

Feb, 2003
From: Abha Light Foundation (Kenya, Africa)
Dear Mark,

About NEEM, I don't know if I could praise it enough. We recommend it to all patients at Abha Light.

We've had incidents of bedridden patients getting up after two-four weeks of using only Neem tea and returning to energetic & productive life. I should add that I don't know of any actual cures at this time. . Some people may discontinue using Neem prematurely when they start feeling better. Perhaps they should pulse the treatment – one month on followed by one month off.

Neem (Azadirachta indica. Melia azadirachta indica. Nim or Neem. Margosa Bark) is a tree native to South Asia (India, Thailand) and has been used in India for thousands of years. It is extremely well researched & documented (mainly from India) see www.neemfoundation.org for more information.

It's been transplanted to Africa, where it grows plentifully. It's Swahili name is "muraurabaini" which means "cures 40 diseases" -- the "40" meaning "so many, all" Its' traditional uses have been as anti-malaria and for skin. It is anti-fungal, anti-bacterial and anti-viral.

Traditionally, in India, it is usual for a housewife to serve with a meal a spoonful or two of the leaves fried in ghee to her family at least once a week.

The leaves, bark and seeds are used in medicine. All have similar properties and all can be used effectively for everything, but traditionally the leaves are primarily used for skin diseases, the bark as anti-malarial, and the seeds for everything & for birth control.

Neem is extremely bitter (like grapefruit seed extract). It is its bitterness that cleans the liver, spleen, kidneys & blood. The bitterness creates a negative environment for malaria & other parasites, killing them off or sterilizing them.

Neem will temporarily cause sterility in eggs and sperm. That is why it's also used as an agricultural insecticide & fertilizer. It doesn't kill the pests, it makes them sterile. Therefore after a generation (a few weeks in an insect's life), one's garden/farm becomes pest free.

Long-term use – internally - of Neem will cause temporary sterility in men & women. One will harmlessly revert to fertility after stopping it. It's been used as a birth control for centuries in India.

Neem oil can be applied inside the vagina and it will work as a spermicide! That is, it will prevent birth. It will cure the vaginitis someone may be suffering from and it probably will prevent the transmission of STDs possibly including HIV. A real 3-in-1!

At Abha Light I make a tincture of the leaves and bark. I find this to be effective & economical for our patients. I would advise taking anything from 10 drops to 1 teaspoon a day. There is no known toxicity of Neem. (though don't be overeager and overdose yourself! It's not necessary & why go looking for toxicity levels!)

To make a herbal tincture you put the powdered leaves & bark with alcohol in a sterile glass jar for 2-4 weeks. Shake the jar daily. Then strain through a cheese cloth or coffee filter. Keep in a cool dark place. Vodka can be used in a pinch. Better would be pure alcohol- ethanol (NOT methanol!) but I don't know if that's available to the common folk. Use 300 grams of leaves (about 10 ounces) to 1 liter alcohol or vodka)

Alternatively, the Neem oil (nasty tasting & bitter!!!) could be put into capsules -- "1" "0" or "00" and 1-3 caps a day would be quite enough. You know, Mark, my clients live on the "lower" end of the economic scale, & we find 5-10 drops (a single "1" or "0" capsule) is plenty.

To make a home-made oil suitable for skin (but nasty smelling & tasting) you could put powdered leaves into ordinary oil (olive, coconut, sunflower, etc) and filter it out two weeks later. This homemade oil can be taken internally if you dare (yechh by taste). For external use, you can deodorize it by adding some tea tree oil to it. This will add to its healing properties. (Use 300 grams of leaves to 1 liter of olive oil)

You can dilute pure Neem-seed oil with cooking oil by 50-70% (1:2 or 1:3 parts) and it will still be effective on the skin. This would be economical. or add it into a base-cream of any kind.

Alternatively, 5 -10 leaves a day either boiled as a tea or powdered in capsules (I'd guess about 6 "0" capsules?) daily would be enough. One could also lightly roast the leaves and eat it at the beginning of a meal (Ayurvedic -Indian way

How to make and use Neem Tea

Chinese way -- that is use 3 cups of water for 10 leaves (2 teaspoons powder) and gently boil it down to two cups. Drink one cup in the morning & one in the night.

Anybody with skin diseases should use Neem soap (surely available at health shops & Indian markets in USA). Tooth disease & gingivitis patients could use Neem toothpaste (also at health & Indian shops) or wash the mouth out with Neem tea.

Neem will purify the liver, spleen, kidneys, blood, skin. It's been used effectively to cure diabetes, high blood pressure, liver ailments and ailments of the pancreas, kidney and spleen too. It used against psoriasis, eczema, HIV septic eruptions. I will take a guess and say it can be effective against Kaposi's. It will destroy parasites of all kinds (through pH factor or sterility) where ever they may be found. I think there is no end to the number of diseases that Neem cures.

HIV+ persons should consider using Neem as a general prophylactic. That is, one could take it daily - for a period --say 1 month - in order to purify the blood. Then take a one month break and resume the treatment for another month.

(Note: unless taken daily don't count on it as birth control). For other questions, ask the Neem foundation (www.neemfoundation.org).

Didi Ananda Rucira
PO Box 6919
Nairobi, Kenya (Africa)
abhalight@eudoramail.com   internet: www.abhalight.org

Editor's Note: Scientific research has found Neem to be a powerful inducer of TH1 cytokines. This was reported in Positive Health News, Report No 18.

Didi gives a lot of recommendations on using Neem so as to almost be confusing. However, her e-mail says that the Neem tea alone has revived bedridden AIDS patients as a monotherapy by drinking 2 cups of Neem tea daily. This is made by adding 10 Neem leaves or 2 teaspoons of Neem leaf powder and gently boil it down to two cups. Drink one cup in the morning & one in the night.

Didi also mentions using Neem bark or Neem seed oil. Neem leaf is widely available in capsules. Neemdirect lists over a dozen manufacturers of Neem capsules and markets several Neem products. One capsule three times daily is a standard dose on some bottles but is this enough or should this dose be about 6 capsules daily as Didi suggested?

For Neem powder or capsules, check with your local health food store, supplement supplier or health care practitioner. I have been unable to find any reports or information on adverse effects of using Neem. This herb long used in Indian medicine appears to be relatively safe.

One article on Neem is found at the NLM by Talwar Gp et al Immunol Cell Biol. 1997 Apr 75(2):190-2. I part Talwar states:

"A transient increase in CD4 and more significantly in CD8 cells in noticed…..a rise in TNF-alpha and IFN-gamma in draining lymph nodes…is observed. Another interesting property is their inhibitory action on a wide spectrum of microorganisms, including Candida albicans, C. tropicalis, gonorrhea, drug-resistant Staphylococcus, e-coli, Herpes simplex and HIV-1."

Pregnant women should not use Neem, as it is known to induce abortions. It is a strong promoter of TH1 cytokine responses (IL-12, IL-2 and IFN-gamma) and may help with many other TH1 deficient conditions like cancer.

Neem credited with remission of KS lesion

CA; Feb 10th 2004. Eli who has self-treated for his HIV for the past 10 years with a current CD4 count of 350 and a viral load of 35K added 6 Neem leaf capsules and 2 guaifenesin capsules to his daily regimen in November, 2003. Within a month, a Kaposi's Sarcoma lesion of his leg began to shrink, change colors and then completely faded from view by Christmas. Because of research that indicates Neem to be a powerful inducer of TH1 cytokines, it most likely contributed to the KS remission.

Neem, Hyssop, the Maitake mushroom and DNCB have all been associated with past or current case reports that their use has resulted in KS remissions in persons with HIV but have not been tested in persons with full blown AIDS.

Among the FDA approved protease inhibitors prior to 2003 for treating AIDS, only Norvir (Ritonavir) has consistently remitted KS lesions, even in very advanced cases of AIDS.

Sep 2004: Letter from Didi on home-made protocol for HIV

Dear Mark,
Hope you are well. Did I give you this recipe?

The sisters working in one of the poorest slums in Nairobi is integrating the Great Health Naturally (derived from Mark's own Immunity Restoration book) protocol into their program. These PLAs are the poorest of the poor. They put 40 patients on the following items and within a month 70% of the patients started gaining weight (up to 2-3 kgs), slept better, small odd pains receded, skin cleared and so on. They are taking:

One Brazil nut a day
One tablespoon of psyllium husks a day mixed in water
Lemon-olive oil drink once a week and 2 spoonfuls of "Hot Stuff Sauce" once a day

Hot Stuff Sauce was invented in order to simplify the delivery of the protocol to poor patients. But it's delicious. Try it.

Recipe for Hot Stuff

One litre vinegar (white or apple cider) - balances the acidity of the body
3 whole garlic cloves - antibiotic
One piece ginger - aids digestion, medicinal for lungs and intestines
25 grams turmeric powder aids digestion, purifies the blood
50 grams chili powder or 100 grams of fresh chilies - increases appetite, aids digestion, raises body temperature, aids in good sleep
100 grams blackstrap molasses (high in minerals and vitamins).

Optional Add-ins
25 grams cinnamon - increases appetite, aids digestion, equalizes blood pressure
10 grams fenugreek - anti-fungal
10 grams thyme - antibiotic, anti-fungal

Crush the garlic and ginger. Mix all ingredients in a clean large glass jar. Let marinate (brew!) for 10 days or longer. Shake daily. After 10 days strain through a clean cloth or filter.

Wow! Great stuff, Great Health.

Take 1-2 teaspoons "dose" daily. Sprinkle over food. Or mix into water and drink. Increases appetite, encourages weight gain, help internal acid-alkaline balance, helps give a better sleep, raises and balances body temperature.

Sincerely,
Didi Ananda Rucira, Director, Abha Light PO Box 6919, Nairobi, Kenya (Africa)
visit: www.abhalight.org tel: +254 20 787310   / cell: 0733-895466

From North America – Essiac or Ojibwa Tea
Case reports of increases in NK cells

Essiac Tea was first formulated in Canada in the 1920's by Renee Caisse, who obtained her original formula from a patient who recovered from breast cancer, and claimed to have been cured by local native Indians. The tea has become a legend in its own time as a cure for

Cancer. It contains Sheep Sorrel, Indian Rhubarb, Burdock and Slippery Elm. Ralph Moss, in his book, "Cancer Therapy," (Equinox Therapy, NY), reports on tests that show Burdock kills HIV in vitro.

In May 1993, I talked to Al of Tampa, FL, who claimed to have three friends who are long term AIDS survivors, who feel well, and he said they - "all used Essiac Tea and have used it for several years." Al told me he has used various brands of Essiac tea for the past 4 years and is very pleased with the results he has obtained from Ojibwa Tea. He reported a T8 count of 1050 and a CD4 count of 922 recently. He takes 1/4th cup (2 ozs) twice a day. He claims this tea is all he has used for 4 years. Al told me he always boiled up his own batches at home.

In Dec. 1995, I received a letter from a PWA who had zero NK cells. She reported that after using Essiac tea for 2 months, her NK function was now in the low end of the normal reference range. Sheep Sorrel, a key ingredient in Essiac, stimulates "complement" activity (1). Complement is a substance circulating in the blood that punctures hole in viruses and makes them more easily seen and identified by immune cells.
1. Hitoshi Ito, Japan J. Pharmacol, 40, 435-443 (1986)

The original Essiac formula, which Rene Caisse received from the Ojibwa Indians in the 1920's, is available from Essiac Int'l - Ph. No. 613-837-3673. Essiac Int'l, 2211-1081 Ambleside Dr., Ottawa, Ontario K2B 8C8. Some health food stores carry the original Essiac formula. It costs about $40 for one ounce, a 12 day supply, or about $100. a month.

A less expensive version of the formula is "Ojibwa Tea." It is available from Ojibwa Tea of Life, PO Box 200041, Denver, CO 80220 Ph No. 303-322-7930. Cost for a 6 weeks supply is $18.00. One person who used the Ojibwa Tea of Life formula reported a condition of chronic candidiasis cleared up after using the tea for one month. The tea has also helped children with Autism.

I would skeptical about buying pre made liquid extracts of Essiac tea or capsules. Case reports indicate that when the tea is made fresh at home it is the most effective. When boiling the herbs, make no more than a 30-day supply at one time and refrigerate it. It is important to follow procedures that are known to be effective and not to go for the convenience of pre made solutions or capsules that are not proven to be as efficacious.

Manganese inhibits HIV's reverse transcriptase - helps thyroid function & control of blood sugar

Johns Hopkins Medical Institutions
www.hopkinsmedicine.org

Johns Hopkins scientists have found that simply increasing manganese in cells can halt HIV's unusual ability to process its genetic information backwards, providing a new way to target the process's key driver, an enzyme called reverse transcriptase. By measuring DNA produced by a related reverse transcriptase in yeast, the Hopkins team discovered that higher than normal levels of manganese, caused by a defective gene, dramatically lowered the enzyme's activity. The scientists then proved that HIV's reverse transcriptase responds to manganese in the same way.

Hopkins graduate student Eric Bolton determined that the defective gene is PMR1, whose protein carries both manganese and calcium out of cells. Using special yeast developed by others at Hopkins, he discovered that manganese stops reverse transcriptase, the team reports in the April 26 issue of Molecular Cell. "These results really point to a never-before-proposed way to try to stop HIV in its tracks -- that simply manipulating concentrations of a metal, manganese, can have a profound effect on reverse transcriptase," says Jeff Boeke, Ph.D., professor of molecular biology and genetics at the school's Institute for Basic Biomedical Sciences. "We expect the human equivalent of PMR1 could be a good target for developing new drugs against HIV."

Retroviruses like HIV use reverse transcriptase to make copies of their DNA from RNA, the opposite of how genetic information is usually processed in cells. Each retrovirus has a distinct version of the enzyme, identical in function but different in form and sequence, says Boeke, also a professor of oncology.

The scientists found that each reverse transcriptase they studied has at least two places where manganese and the similar metal magnesium can "dock." Having these spots filled with the right metal is crucial for the enzyme's activity -- its ability to read a particular set of RNA, the scientists learned. When the metals' balance is out of whack, the enzyme doesn't work properly, they report.

"Most reverse transcriptase's we studied prefer to bind magnesium. At the very least they were more active when magnesium was bound to them," says Boeke. "But a little extra manganese changes the activity of the enzyme."

Normally, charged magnesium ions outnumber those of manganese by the thousands inside cells. Having just three times more manganese than normal can cut the activity of HIV's reverse transcriptase in half, the scientists report, even though there's still much more magnesium.

HIV's ability to adapt and overcome drugs means that current treatments like AZT, which target reverse transcriptase directly, generally stop working over time. Using a combination of drugs helps block the virus on many fronts, but finding new drugs or a new class of drugs is needed to help keep the virus at bay. The new work suggests that targeting a cell's manganese transporter could be an effective way to stop HIV from replicating, without targeting HIV's reverse transcriptase directly.

"We've been working under the idea that studying reverse transcriptase in yeast may help improve understanding of retroviruses and lead to new ways to deal with HIV," says Boeke. "By studying yeast genetics we made an important discovery about how HIV works and have identified a target for a new class of anti-retroviral drug. It was completely unexpected, but very satisfying."

The yeast that were missing PMR1 appeared fine, suggesting that targeting the manganese transporter in humans may be relatively safe, the scientists suggest. It's not known whether targeting manganese levels will have a therapeutic benefit, but the mantra of HIV treatment is to reduce the number of copies of the virus.

The studies were funded by the National Institutes of Health. Albert Mildvan, M.D., professor of biological chemistry, is also an author of the report. Food sources: Pineapple and oat bran have the highest amounts of manganese. A glass of pineapple juice has about 2 mg of manganese, the minimum amount recommended for daily intake.

If taking supplements, 10 to 15 mg daily should be sufficient. I would try manganese oxide or citrate capsules, but would avoid any "amino acid chelates" due to the failures of the so-called selenium as an amino acid chelate unless manufacturer can prove actual absorption takes place and has lab results to back up their claims. Thorne makes a

Manganese Citrate with 30 mg in each capsule, the highest I have found.

Case Study Suggestion for HIV: Take one capsule with 30 mg manganese (Thorne brand) every other day or 3 days per week (i.e. Mon, Weds, Fri) and have your physician monitor blood manganese levels. Increase to one capsule a day, if needed, until blood serum levels of manganese have tripled. At this point you can determine its effectiveness by monitoring the viral load at the same time.

Garlic increases NK cell function

A study published in the German Medical Journal "Deutsche Zeitshrift" in Oct, 1989 by T.H. Abdullad, D.V. Kirkpatrick and J. Carter, reports on the results of 7 AIDS patients taking 5 grams of garlic daily as an aged extract, similar to Kyolic garlic. They said that 6 of the 7 patients had normal NK cell activity after 6 weeks and that all had normal NK activity after 12 weeks. Five of the 7 had significant improvements in their T4/T8 ratios after 12 weeks with 3 returning to normal reference ranges of 1.0 or higher. They also reported a lessening of diarrhea in one patient with Cryptosporidia, fewer outbreaks of Herpes, Thrush, Candidiasis and Sinus infections.

If raw garlic does not cause intestinal distress, then 2 to 4 cloves daily is recommended. Never eat it straight, but with something like a salad or on rye crisp. Eight capsules of the Kyolic brand of garlic taken twice a day gives you about 5 grams. For enhancement of NK cell function only, an aged garlic like Kyolic works as well as fresh raw garlic. However, as a natural antibiotic, raw garlic is the most effective.

Garlic's enhancement of natural killer cells make it a very important supplement for persons with AIDS and CFS. Garlic's effect on CD8 cells is unknown at this time. Kyolic Formula 100 in the 300 capsule size bottle is the best buy for the money. There are cheaper brands of garlic available, but I don't know if I believe in their efficacy or their claims.

Raw garlic is even more effective than aged garlic extract in killing fungal and bacterial infections and it also activates NK function. However, persons with sensitive intestinal linings may find it too harsh. The best way to eat raw garlic is with rye crisp or bread to buffer the sulfur based compounds it contains. Suggested dose: 2 to 3 cloves daily.

Note: Avoid using more than the recommended daily dose, as too much raw garlic can stress the red blood cells. Aged garlic extract does not have this effect. However, raw garlic is far superior to aged garlic as an anti-viral, anti-fungal and antibacterial food. To reduce odor, eat fresh parsley with raw garlic. Notes: Kyolic Formula 100. Use 8 caps twice daily.

Bitter melon enemas for HIV - helps balance blood sugar

The use of Bitter Melon to treat HIV was discovered by an American of Filipino descent, Stanley Rebultan of Los Angeles, CA. Stanley was diagnosed HIV+ in 1987. By 1988, his CD4 (T4) count had dropped to 480. Aware of Bitter Melon's use in treating leukemia, he started using the plant in 1988. His experiences have shown that bitter melon (a native Asian fruit) was more effective used in enemas than taken orally. He has been giving himself daily enemas with bitter melon since 1988. His T4 count has increased upwards to 1086, as of April, 1986. In Sept., 1993, his latest T4 count was 1122.

Note: It may be significant that the bitter melon mixture Stanley uses each day is raw..

Other cases I have followed, where all the bitter melon used was boiled, failed to provide any benefits. This indicates to me that heat destroys the active ingredients in the bitter melon, but it leaves open the possibility that a freeze-dried product, used in high enough quantity, might work.

Updated information: Since I first wrote about this story, several people have tried Bitter Melon Therapy and have not had increases in T4 counts. Many have used powdered packets or cooked Bitter Melon. Stanley originally used only raw Bitter Melon for enemas, when he obtained very favorable results. Possibly, cooking or processing Bitter Melon causes destruction of some of its active ingredients. I advise anyone doing Bitter Melon to do it as Stanley originally did it or not to do it at all. Stanley originally used only raw Bitter Melon. Later, he used a mixture of 1/2 raw and 1/2 cooked. By the time this fragmented story circulated around the country, people were using only cooked Bitter Melon for enemas. In theory the freeze-dried bitter melon should have worked. It is possible that the dose used was too small to produce the desired results.

Purchase bitter melon vines, leaves and fruit from local Asian marketplaces. The season for availability starts in May and runs through October. In the off-season, freeze a large quantity for use. Freezing does not destroy the active ingredients. You can buy a freezer and fill it up with Bitter Melon, if need be. To make Bitter Melon for a retention enema, first wash all plants in distilled water. Fill a blender with about 1 quart of chopped leaves, stems and fruit and add distilled water until it is about 2/3rds full. Blend at high speed until it is very smooth. This gives you enough for 2 days of treatments. Place 1 and 1/2 cups in an enema bag. While lying on your left side, let Bitter Melon into your colon, then lie on your back with a pillow under your buttocks. Continue until the entire cup and one-half is in your colon. Retain for 20 minutes, and then evacuate contents in the toilet. That is all there is to it. Do this once a day. That is all Stanley has done since 1988. He has never taken any drugs or other medications for HIV.

More cases of results with raw bitter melon therapy

Jerry is from San Diego, CA. He told me in November, 1993, that he has been HIV+ for 10 years. In August 1993, his T4 count fell to 235. He decided to try Bitter Melon retention enemas once a day. Since Stanley is his neighbor, he followed the same protocol Stanley used with raw Bitter Melon retention enemas. He did this for 90 days. His T4 count rose to 403.

Note: Most of the Bitter Melon, in pill form, on the market do not work possibly because of the processing, the use of heat and pasteurization may have destroyed the active ingredients. However, if the Bitter melon is freeze dried and a significant quantity is used, it might work. Also not tried is eating a 1/2 cup of fresh bitter melon daily or drinking the juice of the bitter melon. More research is clearly needed here.

SAN FRANCISCO: Dec. 2002. Michael J told Keep Hope Alive he does an enema of 3/4 cup of raw bitter melon juice daily and has done so for the past 15 years. He has never had a symptom, and his current viral load is under 1000, with a CD4 count of 728. To the bitter melon enema bag he also adds 1/2 cup of his own urine. Each year, he buys large quantities of fresh bitten melons, juices them and places 3/4 of a cup in a plastic bag and freezes it until ready to use. He fills up his freezer each year with an extract of the bitter melon plants.

Note: Several sources have reported that Bitter Melon balances blood sugar levels also.

Searching for a herbal cocktail to treat HIV naturally

In 1996, Chang and Kong of Cornell Medical College in New York presented abstract no Mo.B.303 at the Int. AIDS Conf when nearly all the media attention was focused on the new protease inhibitors and triple drug combination therapy. With the passage of time, the need for effective treatments that do not have serious adverse effects as many of the HIV drugs do remains as important a goal as ever.

Chang and Kong researched all the published literature for the thousands of plant extracts that were tested for anti-HIV activity and found 70 compounds and 76 crude plant extracts inhibited HIV in vitro. The compounds were 29 terpenes, 29 flavinoids, 15 polysaccharides, 8 coumarins, 6 tannins, 4 lectins, 4 quinolones, 2 peptides and 7 other alkaloids. The mode or viral inhibition includes reverse transcriptase inhibition, protease inhibition, and interference of infection at the viral cell entry. They reported only a handful of these herbs were studied in uncontrolled studies and (these include ganoderma, momordica, Curcumin, Acemannan, glycyrrhizin, lentinan, hypericin, GLQ233 and PCK-4). The authors concluded that plants and herbs offered an excellent source for discovering low cost treatments for HIV that do not have serious side effects.

A search of the literature finds a variety of anti-HIV botanicals that may work on different angles to stop the viral cycle. These include

Reserve Transcriptase inhibitors:

Prunella Vulgaris (HealAll): Extract of Prunella vulgaris inhibits HIV replication at reverse transcription in vitro and can be absorbed from intestine in vivo. Antivir Chem Chemother. 2000 Mar;11(2):157-64.
by Kageyama S. et al

Abstract: It has been reported that extracts of the spike of Prunella vulgaris (PS) exhibit anti-HIV activity at the adsorption and reverse transcription stages. In this study, the actual activity of PS in cells, kinetic analysis of the inhibitory activity of PS against HIV reverse transcriptase and the feasibility of oral administration were examined. First, to clarify whether this extract shows anti-HIV activity in cells in vitro, the number of copies of proviral DNA in HIV-exposed cells was calculated. The number of copies was significantly decreased in cells cultured in the presence of PS extract, but not in the presence of dextran sulphate.

The activity of PS extract in the cells was also assessed by the drug addition test, during and after HIV adsorption. PS extract and dextran sulphate suppressed HIV production to similar levels when added after HIV adsorption. However, only PS extract suppressed HIV production at the same concentration when the drugs were added during HIV adsorption. Presumably, the penetration of the PS extract into the cells was required for this activity. Secondly, fractionated PS inhibited HIV reverse transcription in a non-competitive manner. This fractionated PS kept anti-HIV activity, but inhibited HIV replication and adsorption to a lesser extent compared to dextran sulphate. Lastly, an active component(s) was detected in plasma in vivo, after injection into the intestine, which demonstrates the feasibility of oral administration dosing.

Other Reverse Transcriptase inhibitors:

Oleuropein from green olives and/or olive leaves. It takes about 200 mg of pure oleuropein 2 or 3 times daily to see results. No known adverse effect but viral resistance has developed in about 8 weeks when used as monotherapy in 2 cases I followed. In one case when it was combined with Epivir, the viral load reached non-detectable levels. This latter case was lost to followup. Green Tea contains tannins that also inhibits HIV.

Integrase inhibitors:

Red Sage Root (Salvia miltiorrhiza) aka Danshen; **Tumeric** (Curcumin) and **Green Coffee Beans**. Salvia miltiorrhiza was studied by Abd-Elazem, Chen, Bates and Huang at John Hopkins Univ. in Baltimore (1). Two integrase inhibitors were isolated from the roots of the plant that "exhibited potent effect against HIV-1 integrase activity in vitro and viral replication in vivo" according to the researchers who identified the two compounds at lithospermic acid and lithospermic acid B. They also stated "These two structurally related compounds are potent anti-HIV inhibitors and showed no cytotoxicity to H9 cell at high concentrations."

The two characteristics of these compounds that are critically important is that the product is a potent inhibitor of HIV and is not toxic to other cells. This means that Red Sage Root also known as Danshen or by its botanical name "salvia miltiorrhiza" is a herb worth considering in the search for a safe a effective herbal cocktail to treat HIV.
1. Isolation of non-toxic inhibitors of HIV-1 integrase from Salvia miltiorrhiza; Abd-elazem, Chen, Bates and Huang; Antiviral Res. 2002 Jul;55(1):91-106

Fusion inhibitors and synctia formation:

Hyssop officinalis. "Mar 10" has been isolated from Hyssop and is a potent inhibitor of HIV as reported by Gollapudi S et al at the Univ. of CA in Irvine (2) Also significant is a lack of toxic effects on healthy cells. Hyssop was first looked at as a treatment for HIV in 1990 by Kreis w et al at North Shore Univ in Manhasset, NY. They reported good antiviral activity in a RT assay and inhibiting syncytia formation. In 2002, researchers in Spain, Bedoya et al tested 15 common herbals and found that Hyssop and Dittrichia viscosa both inhibited HIV at low concentrations and showed no cytotoxicity.

Interleukin 6 (IL-6) inhibitors:

IL-6 is a cytokine or chemical messenger and is one of many found in the body. It is a TH2 type cytokine. IL-6 is to HIV and cancer what gasoline is to fire. Stress is a primary cause of elevated IL-6 levels as is candidiasis and insomnia. Stress reduction appears to be one key to reducing Interleukin 6 levels. The most effective IL-6 inhibitor is low-dose hydrocortisone. See the chapter on the Adrenals for a list of IL-6 inhibitors and how to use them.

Mary Enig Ph.D. on natural coconut oil

On July 19, 1995, Enig was quoted in an article published in "The HINDU," India's National Newspaper as stating that coconut oil is converted by the body into "Monolaurin" a fatty acid with anti-viral properties that might be useful in the treatment of AIDS. The staff reporter for The HINDU wrote about Enig's presentation at a press conference in Kochi and stated:

"There was an instance in the US in which an infant tested HIV positive had become HIV negative. That it was fed with an infant formula with a high coconut oil content gains significance in this context and at present an effort was on to find out how the "viral load" of an HIV-infected baby came down, when fed a diet that helped in the generation of Monolaurin in the body."

The reporter commented on Enig's observations that "Monolaurin helped in inactivating other viruses, such as measles, herpes, vesicular stomatitis and Cytomegalovirus (CMV), and that research undertaken so far on coconut oil also indicated that it offered a certain measure of protection against cancer-inducing substances.

In another article published in the Indian Coconut Journal, Sept., 1995, Dr. Enig stated:

"Recognition of the antimicrobial activity of the monoglyceride of lauric acid (Monolaurin) has been reported since 1966. The seminal work can be credited to Jon Kabara. This early research was directed at the virucidal effects, because of possible problems related to food preservation. Some of the early work by Hierholzer and Kabara (1982), that showed virucidal effects of Monolaurin on enveloped RNA and DNA viruses, was done in conjunction with the Center for Disease Control of the US Public Health Service, with selected prototypes or recognized strains of enveloped viruses. The envelope of these viruses is a lipid membrane."

Enig stated in her article that Monolaurin, of which the precursor is lauric acid, disrupted the lipid membranes of envelope viruses and also inactivated bacteria, yeast and fungi. She wrote: "Of the saturated fatty acids, lauric acid has greater antiviral activity than either caprylic acid (C-10) or myristic acid (C-14). The action attributed to Monolaurin is that of solubilizing the lipids in the envelope of the virus, causing the disintegration of the virus envelope." In India, coconut oil is fed to calves to treat Cryptosporidium, as reported by Lark Lands Ph.D., in her upcoming book "Positively Well" (1).

While HHV-6A was not mentioned by Enig, HHV-6A is an enveloped virus and would be expected to disintegrate in the presence of lauric acid and/or Monolaurin. Some of the pathogens reported by Enig to be inactivated by Monolaurin include HIV, measles, vascular stomatitis virus (VSV), herpes simplex virus (HSV-1), visna, cytomegalovirus (CMV), Influenza virus, Pneumonovirus, Syncytial virus and Rubeola. Some bacteria inactivated by Monolaurin include listeria, Staphylococcus aureus, Streptococcus agalactiae, Groups A, B, F and G streptococci, Gram-positive organisms; and gram-negative organisms, if treated with chelator.

Enig reported that only one infant formula "Impact" contains lauric acid while the more widely promoted formulas like "Ensure" do not contain lauric acid and often contain some hydrogenated fats (trans fatty acids). A modified ester of lauric acid, Monolaurin (available in capsules), is sold in health food stores.

Enig on a therapeutic dose

Based on her calculations on the amount of lauric acid found in human Mother's milk, Dr. Enig suggests a rich lauric acid diet would contain about 24 grams of lauric acid daily for the average adult. This amount could be found in about 3.5 tablespoons of coconut oil or 10 ounces of "Pure Coconut Milk." Coconut Milk is made in Sri Lanka and imported into the United States. It can be found in health food stores and in local grocery stores in the International Foods section or in specialty grocery stores that sell products imported from Thailand, the Philippines or East India. About 7 ounces of raw coconut daily would contain 24 grams of lauric acid. 24 grams of lauric acid is the therapeutic daily dose for adults suggested by Mary Enig based on her research of the lauric acid content of mother's milk. (1)

1. Positively Well, by Lark Lands Ph.D. Her new book discusses lauric acid and suggests many treatment options for persons with AIDS or CFIDS and may be ordered by calling 905-672-7470 or 800-542-8102

Scientific research on the anti-viral effects of monolaurin

Mary Enig cites 24 references in her 7 page article on "Lauric Acid for HIV-infected Individuals," a few of which are as follows:

1. Issacs, C.E. et al. Inactivation of enveloped viruses in human bodily fluids by purified lipids. Annals of the New York Academy of Sciences 1994;724:457-464.
2. Kabara, J.J. Antimicrobial agents derived from fatty acids. Journal of the American Oil Chemists Society 1984;61:397-403.
3. Hierholzer, J.C. and Kabara J.J. In vitro effects on Monolaurin compounds on enveloped RNA and DNA viruses. Journal of Food Safety 1982;4:1-12.
4. Wang, L.L. and Johnson, E.A. Inhibition of Listeria monocytogenes by fatty acids and monoglycerides. Appli Environ Microbiol 1992; 58:624-629.
5. Issacs, C.E. et al. Membrane-disruptive effect of human milk: inactivation of enveloped viruses. Journal of Infectious Diseases 1986;154:966-971.
6. Anti-viral effects of monolaurin. JAQA 1987;2:4-6
7. Issacs C.E. et al. Antiviral and antibacterial lipids in human milk and infant formula feeds. Archives of Disease in Childhood 1990;65:861-864.

Note: Enig's article in the Indian Coconut Journal has 41 reference cites. To obtain a complete set of both articles she wrote, go to our website and search "Enig."

Adult Dosages: Coconut oil - 3 tablespoons daily or 1 cup of coconut milk daily. Mix with pancakes or breakfast cereal or mix with a cup of hot tea with honey. Coconut milk is not recommended to be used more than 3 days per week because it contains arabinogalactins that could throw a TH2 response in the CD4s and drive up CD4 counts too rapidly. A similar effect can happen from the daily use of Echinacea or by drinking too much carrot juice, another source of arabinogalactin polysaccharides. Suggestion: Use coconut milk 3 days per week and coconut oil the other 4 days. Coconut milk may be used on breakfast cereal or mixed with fruit juice.

The most effective form of lauric acid is a patented modified form called "lauricidin." It is very cost effective (about $20 a month) and is available in pellet form from Med Chem, PO Box 339, Galena, IL 61036 at www.lauricidin.com. Monolaurin and Lauricidin are the same product. Lauricidin is a registered name for Monolaurin. For adults – one or two grams 3 times daily is suggested. Recently, one person with EBV, CMV, herpes 1 and 2 and HHV-6 told me "this product has given me my life back." (Monolaurin in capsules is available from Ecological Formulas but the price is 4 fold higher than the bulk pellets.)

The Olive leaf

One of the active ingredients in olive leaves has been identified as "oleuropein." Fredrickson writes: "It is believed that olive leaf extract exerts its main influence by in vivo hydrolysis of oleuropein to (+)-2-epielenolic acid. ...In addition to being antiretroviral, (+)-epielenolic acid is also thought to be immunostimulatory. Finally, it should be mentioned that the other components in the leaf of the olive work synergistically with oleuropein to enhance its natural activity." Wm. Fredrickson told Keep Hope Alive that (+)-2-epielenolic acid was effective against both RNA and DNA viruses. Note: Practical experience using Olive leaf has shown that as a monotherapy, HIV viral resistance develops quickly. If olive leaf is to have a sustained antiviral effect, it needs to be used in combination with at least two other antivirals. One anecdotal report concerned a person who combined olive leaf extract in capsule form with Epivir (3TC) and claimed to have reached non-detectable levels with just these two medicines. Other persons, who have used prescribed drugs to treat HIV, have added olive leaf extract and report better lab results - particularly lower triglycerides and cholesterol levels.

Medical References on the Olive Leaf (Olea Europaea)
1. Cruess WV, and Alsberg CL, The bitter glucoside of the olive. J. Amer. Chem. Soc. 1934; 56:2115-7.
2. Samuelsson G, The blood pressure lowering factor in leaves of Olea Europaea. Farmacevtisk Revy, 1951; 15: 229-39.
3. Juven B et al, Studies on the mechanism of the antimicrobial action of oleuropein. J. Appi. Bad., 1972; 35:559-67.
4. Renis HE, In vitro antiviral activity of calcium elenolate. Antimicrob. Agents Chemother., 1970; 167-72.
5. Soret MG, Antiviral activity of calcium elenolate on parainfluenza infection of hamsters. Antimicrob. Agents Chemother., 1970:160-66.
6. Hirschman SZ, Inactivation of DNA polymerases of Murine Leukaemia viruses by calcium elenolate. Nature New Biology, 1972; 238:277-79.

How to make Olive leaf tea

Place 8 ounces (half of a one pound bag) of dried olive leaves (use olea europaea species only) in a 5 or 6 quart Crock-Pot (i.e. Rival brand K-Mart). Add one gallon of filtered or distilled water. Turn heat on low. 6 hours later, check the temperature with a candy thermometer (from your hardware store). When the temperature falls between a range of 175_ to 185_, move cover off center about 1/4 inch so some heat escapes. This should stabilize the temperature for the next 5 hours. The ideal temperature range to make the tea is at least 175_, but not more than 185_ Fahrenheit. After the temperature reaches the desired level, place the cover off center slightly so some heat escapes. At the 11th hour, add water lost through evaporation until it returns to its original level. Center cover so no more heat escapes and leave on low for one more hour. Total time to make the tea is 12 hours.

Let it cool for 2 to 4 hours, then strain and store in glass bottles in a refrigerator until used. Discard what is not used within two weeks. Also, discard sooner, if a film of mold appears in the jar. A lab test by Irvine Labs using the HPLC method showed 213 mg of oleuropein per 1/2 cup of this home made formula.

The usual adult dose is 1/2 cup twice a day. It tastes better if you mix it with 2 parts ginger ale and add ice. If using a capsule, avoid ground olive leaves with 5% oleuropein in it. Use a powdered extract with 20% or more oleuropein in it (i.e. Ameriden brand is good).

Colloidal Silver

I first heard about Colloidal Silver on the Tony Brown Journal, a national syndicated TV program. Dr. Scott Gregory said it was effective against over 500 kinds of infections. In December, 1993, I talked to "Gary" from Toledo, OH. He said that early in 1993, his T4 count was down to 3 and he was diagnosed with Toxoplasmosis and had lesions on the brain. A local health food store told him about "Colloidal Silver," a solution containing electrically charged finely ground silver. He has used 2 teaspoons daily for the past 6 months. He is convinced that he would not be alive today if it were not for this product. He has also taken PCM-4 for several months. On Jan 25, 1994, I talked to him and he told me the results of an MRI brain scan. He said: "The doctor told me the 3 brain lesions I had have completely disappeared." He is certain that the Colloidal Silver brought about the remission.

Colloidal silver was first used in the 1930's as a wide spectrum infection fighter. It is reported to be effective for Toxoplasmosis, Gonorrhea, Impetigo, Ringworm, Shingles, Thyphoid, Warts and Staph infections but there is no information to indicate it is effective against parasites or protozoa's. I have been told by another source that it is not effective against Cryptosporidium and did not prevent the development of Lymphoma in one case.

I have had no feedback on its use for CMV or MAI, so it is possible benefits here are unknown at this time. A researcher at Brigham Young University sent Colloidal Silver to two different labs, including the UCLA Medical Center, which tested it in vitro and said: "It killed not only the HIV virus but every virus that was tested in the lab." Still, with these impressive results, anecdotal reports of persons taking oral colloidal silver in high doses for HIV showed only a modest reduction in viral loads. The manufacturer claims it is completely safe, there are no known side effects and that it may be used in conjunction with any medication. Note: I would advise taking it 30 minutes before or after taking any prescribed drugs. I would not use colloidal silver on a continuous basis as a prophylaxis, but only when needed to help treat an O.I.

An experiment I followed in the early 1990's tried to cure HIV with very high doses of colloidal silver. After 3 months, the viral load dropped about 50% in the cases I followed. However, the CD4 counts continued to decline with these cases and the experiment was discontinued in favor of more effective conventional treatments.

Colloidal silver or Ozonated oil for genital warts

One of our readers with genital warts told us that he first wiped them off with 3%

Hydrogen Peroxide solution. Then, he placed Colloidal Silver directly on them. He says: "The warts are disappearing." NOTE: In my opinion, ozonated olive oil should work very effectively as well. In fact, if you ozonate 1 ounce of olive oil (about 2 tablespoons) for 20 minutes, you can actually bleach a colored cloth. Making it fresh each time you use it will give you the best results. Ozonated olive oil can be used for ear and mouth infections, on the eyelid, in the nostrils, in the mouth, anus and vagina and anyplace topically where you have a problem except I wouldn't place it directly in the eye. Massage it into tumors and watch them shrink. Ozonated water can be used as an eyewash and for an enema. Just ozonate 8 ounces of distilled water for 2 minutes and use it immediately.

A review of Hulda Clarks's book

"The Cure for HIV/AIDS", by Hulda Clark, Ph.D. N.D. arrived in early October, 1994. I skimmed through it and initially placed it aside, due to its length and the unusual theories of its author. Hulda Clark blames the chemical benzene and an intestinal fluke - Fasciolipis buskii, as the cause of AIDS. She claims the HIV virus grows inside the fluke. She recommends the use of 3 herbs to kill the fluke - green-black walnut extract, wormwood and cloves.

It is my view that many of the author's theories are supported more by her opinions than by good science. She cites 53 cases where persons following her protocol to purge the intestinal fluke have converted to HIV P24 antigen negative. However, only one lab test result is published - that of Roy Ferguson. An unanswered question is whether the other 52 cases reported were tested with her unconventional testing methods or confirmed by independent labs. I highly doubt a fluke is the cause of AIDS. However, if the herbal combination neutralized HHV-6A, parasites mycoplasmas and fungal infections, it would be very beneficial, but not a cure. Black walnut is listed in several herbal books as effective against herpes and may have an effect against HHV-6.

Based on the evidence presented in the book, I would say the title - THE CURE FOR HIV/AIDS is premature. The reason is that there were no PCR tests that were given for the 53 cases cited and no immune function tests. Unless you restore normal immune function, you have not cured AIDS.

However, as unusual as her theories are, H. Clark's belief that flukes, parasites and worms play a role in AIDS is credible. For the sake of discussion, let us give her the benefit of the doubt that she has successfully converted 53 persons with AIDS from P24 antigen reactive to P24 antigen negative. P24 antigen testing is very old technology. For several years now, it has been replaced by PCR.

The three herbs she uses to eradicate the F.B. fluke and the HIV virus are black walnut tincture, wormwood and ground cloves. She advises patients to remain on her program for 6 weeks before being tested for the P24 antigen.

Artemesia anua, black walnut and cloves for treating parasites, worms and mycoplasma

While there is no laboratory evidence that these three herbs are effective against HHV-6, black walnut is effective against herpes. Clark does not mention the other species of wormwood, artemesia annua, that is known to be effective against many types of viruses, the parasite malaria and cancer, and about which there is published research. The type of wormwood used in most of these 3 herb formulas on the market is artemesia absinthium, rather than artemesia annua, although a few products have used both types of wormwood. In my opinion, the 3 herbs could be used for 2 weeks every 6 months just for preventive maintenance to eliminate parasites. Cloves are well-known as an antibiotic.

When using the 3-herb combination in an alcohol tincture form, search for one with artemesia annua added. Dose: take 20 to 40 drops 3 times a day. Various brands have different potencies and tasting the tincture can tell you how concentrated is the extract.

St. Johns Wort

St Johns Wort has been reported in leading magazines on AIDS research for some time. It has some benefit in controlling HIV and other viral infections. Persons taking St. Johns Wort may find their skin sensitized to sunlight. Yerba Prima makes a low cost product. Persons using St. Johns Wort should monitor liver enzymes levels. Recently, it has been discovered that St John's Wort interferes with the effectiveness of protease inhibitors (P.I.s). Persons using P.I.s should not use St John's Wort.

The Venus fly-trap plant (dionaea muscipula) (for normal body temperature and macrophage function)

The Venus Fly Trap is a tropical plant with small jaws that catches and digests insects. It is a carnivorous plant and a German firm that manufactures the extract calls it "Carnivora." It is being used in Germany for treating Cancer, AIDS and Crohn's disease. An article appearing in the May, 1992 issue of The Townsend Letter for Doctors by Morton Walker, D.P.M. tells of a man with AIDS, who received injectable Carnivora for 10 weeks, increased his T4 count from 350 to 915. (A copy of the May, 1992 issue of The Townsend Letter can be obtained by sending $8.00 to: Townsend Letter for Doctors, 911 Tyler St, Port Townsend, WA 98368). Addresses where you can import injectable and oral Carnivora are contained in the article.

The author, Morton Walker, claims that Carnivora has been successfully used for the treatment of "most forms of Cancer, Neurodermitis, Ulcerative Colitis, Crohn's disease, Multiple Sclerosis, Herpes, Polyarthritis, and most any immune deficiency state."

The article concludes with the story of a man from California who had AIDS and who heard a speech by Dr. Keller before the Cancer Control Society convention in Pasadena, California in September 1990. Shortly after, he went to West Germany for the treatment. His T4 Helper cell count started out at 350. After 8 weeks into the treatment, he began to cough up much phlegm. Mucus came out of his nostrils like he had a cold, and various skin eruptions occurred. After 8 weeks, his T4 count began to rise. It climbed to 1700. Within 4 months, he returned to the United States. His blood tests showed no signs of the HIV-1 antigen. Update: A person phoned us to tell us the PWA discontinued using Carnivora after returning to the United States and that his CD4 counts have fallen.

Note: A physician told me that Venus Flytrap Extract is good to kill off candida albicans without causing the die-off effect. It also is good to treat herpes infections. Several reports claim that a low dose, using 20 drops 2 or 3 times daily normalizes body temperature in a few months.

Grapefruit seed - a natural antibiotic

Grapefruit seeds contain factors that, under laboratory conditions, kill over 20 kinds of pathogens. Grapefruit seed extract is marketed under the name "Nutribiotic Liquid Concentrate" (Nutrition Resource). Here is a partial listing of pathogens that grapefruit seed extract has destroyed under laboratory conditions:

Candida albicans, Staphylococcus aureus, Staphylococcus pyogenes, Staphylococcus sp., Streptococcus faecalis, Salmonella cholerasuis, Salmonella typhi, Echerichia coli, Proteus vulgaris, Pseudomonas aeruginosa, Lactobacillus pentoaceticus, Klebsiellus pneumonia, Aspergillus niger, Aspergillus oryzae, Aspergillus parasiticus, Aspergillus terreus, Aspergillus flavus, Fusarium oxysporum, Fusarium oxy. F. sp. tuberosi, Fusarium sambucinum, Penicillium funiculosum, Penicillium sp., Penicillium roqueforti, Pullularia pullulans, Trichophyton interdigital, Scerotinia laxa, Chaetonium globosum, Entamoeba histolytica, Giardia lamblia, Herpes simplex Virus, Type 1, Influenza A2 virus.

Dosage: As an infection fighter, add 5 to 10 drops to a glass of water and take every 2 to 4 hours. May be used as a mouthwash for thrush. Effective for athlete's feet and cold sores. Grapefruit seed extract is sold under various trade names.

Note: Grapefruit seed extract can drive saliva pH in an acid direction, therefore should only be used on a short term-basis - 3 to 10 days.

New books on the benefits of natural sunlight

Many Cancer and AIDS organizations have for years advised their clients to avoid sunlight, as it might stimulate HIV replication in the skin. However, it is the lymphatic system, not the skin, where most HIV replication occurs. U.V. light kills the HIV virus and stimulates the growth of White Blood Cells, the foundation of our immune system. (See "Into the Light" by Dr. William C Douglass M.D.800-728-2288 Fax 404-399-0815). Dr. Douglass, in his book, "Into The Light" shows great success in treating AIDS with full spectrum light containing ultraviolet wavelengths.

Cutting Edge Catalog lists several other books on the health benefits of sunlight. They include:
Health and Light, by Dr. John Ott $9.95
Sunlight, by Dr. Zane Kime. An in depth study on the health benefits of sunlight in general and U.V. light in particular. $14.95
Daylight Robbery, by Dr. Damien Downing, an English Physician. $12.95
Sunbathing Today, by Friedrich Wolff. $9.95. To order, call, 800-497-9516.

Ultraviolet light kills viruses

An article by A Canals (1) discusses an in-vivo test where ASFV was inactivated by UV light. UVA, with a longer wavelength, inactivates viruses and other pathogens. Canals found that active ASFV caused an increase in CD8+ subsets when added to cell cultures of blood cells, whereas ASFV inactivated by UV light caused an increase in both CD4+ and CD8+ subsets.

In one experiment, G. Miolo et al found that "total inactivation of the HIV-1 (200SFU) was obtained in the presence of 1 microgram ml-1of TMP and 20 kJ m-2 of UVA light." (3) Tmp is "8-trimethylpsoralen." In another experiment on cell cultures, MM Saucier found that "heat inactivation, or UV-light treatment of viruses before assays almost completely ablates its ability to induce proliferation." (4).

Note: The latest research published in Positive Health News, Report 18, indicates that UVA light promotes Th1 cytokines, while UVB promotes Th2 cytokines and increased susceptibility to cancer. Readers are advised to use sun tanning salons that use exclusively UVA light and avoid UVB light.

1. A. Canals et al, Vet Microbiol., 1992, Nov: 33 (1-4): 117-27.
2. L.E. Benade et al, Transfusion. Aug, 1994; 34 (8):680-4
3. G. Miolo, J Photochem Photobiol b., 1994 Dec: 26(3):241-7
M.M. Saucier, Symp Nonhum Primate Models AIDS, 1993, Sept 19-23, Abstract No 93. Atlanta, GA.

Radio frequency machines – too dangerous to use. Safety of Rife technology questioned.

In September 1990, Keep Hope Alive began experimenting with radio frequency machines to try to kill the HIV virus, using a BK 3011-B model. My original interest was based on Barry Lynes book – "The Cancer Cure That Worked." After 6 months of experimentation with the machines, I was convinced that they were only partially effective against the virus and other infections and had the potential of causing chromosomal damage in host cells. The radio frequency machines, based on the research of Royal Rife, are dangerous to use, if the control buttons are turned up too high.

While viruses and bacteria are obviously being killed, normal cells may also be torn apart. The misuse of these machines could do permanent damage to the immune system. Because the frequencies were electromagnetic in origin, I distrusted them and have discontinued recommending their use. Electromagnetic fields from high power lines, radio and TV stations, and microwave ovens are all potentially dangerous to your body and are known causes of cancer. The danger of radio frequencies is that they may split chromosomes and damage the membranes of cells. On the other hand, low gauss permanent magnetic fields are gentle and stimulating to the life process. Experiments have shown that low gauss permanent magnets have nearly doubled the life span of laboratory mice, whereas a generator that produces alternating current, when placed in the vicinity of mice, shortened their life span. (Healing by Magnets, by Davis and Bhattacharya; and Magneto Therapy, by Dr. H.L. Bansal).

Bob Becks machine increases HIV viral load

Three persons using the Beck machine to electrocute the HIV virus have told me that they had substantial increases in HIV viral load after 2 or 3 months use. One person's viral load tripled. Could the Bob Beck machine and other similar machines be making cell membranes more porous and vulnerable to viral infection? Could the electrical frequencies that are used to kill viruses and other pathogens be contributing to a weakened cell membrane? Has anyone tested the cortisol levels before and after using these machines?

Note: if the electrical frequencies are damaging cell membranes, as I suspect many of them are, I would expect to see increases in cortisol levels, a response that would weaken cell-mediated immunity. As of this time, I am unconvinced of the safety and effectiveness of the Rife technology and equipment built based on this technology.

Cancell not effective for KS or AIDS

"Cancell," a product with a unique combination of chemicals, has been completely ineffective in one case of KS and in another HIV-related case, as reported to us. However, the product made in Michigan has apparently helped some persons with cancer.

Magnetic fields – for pain relief/anti-inflammatory

Although a north pole seeking side of a magnet can reduce swollen lymph nodes in persons with HIV, it apparently has no effect on the viral load from several case reports I have followed, including one where the persons slept on a strong magnetic mattress every night for several weeks. In localized small cancers, a magnet placed directly over the tumor has caused some to stop growing and even recede. However, a single magnet has not worked, when the cancer was more advanced.

The most practical use of a magnet is for its anti-inflammatory effects and for pain relief, and also to help induce deeper sleep, when used for up to 60 minutes before bedtime. For the purpose of killing viral infections, you can accomplish in 20 minutes with ozone what it would take 6 hours to do on a magnetic mattress. Magnetic therapy has amazing power as a pain reliever. From several years of experience working with magnets, I find they are very effective as pain relievers and have minimal effectiveness as infection fighters. Magnets are widely credited with helping some insomniacs get a good nights sleep and with relieving pain from arthritis.

North pole vs. South pole effects

Every magnet has two poles – one north (_) and the other south (+). Opinions on the use of magnets and their polarity for human conditions vary almost as widely as their authors. Most authors, whose works I have read on the subject of magnets, recommend north pole magnetic energy for infections of all kinds. Several authors have said that south pole magnetic energy will increase infections and stimulate the growth of bacteria. These include Dr. H.L. Bansal, who wrote the book "Magnetotherapy," Dr. Bansal explains the use of magnets in treating over 150 common diseases.

Dr. William Philpott M.D., who wrote the "Biomagnetic Handbook," and who has worked with magnets for over 20 years in the United States, says that north pole magnetic

energy will do the following:
1. Increases cellular oxygen - moves saliva PH in an alkaline direction.
2. Reduces fluid retention
3. Encourages deep restful sleep
4. Fights Infections
5. Reduces Inflammation
6. Stops pain
7. Supports healing

South pole magnetic energy, according to Dr. Philpott, has the opposite effect of north pole energy on the human body. North pole magnetic energy has stopped the growth of cancer in a number of experiments. In addition to stopping the growth of tumors and malignancies, magnets increased the life span of mice by 45% in one experiment. Davis and Bhattacharya report the damaging effects of a high gauss electro-magnetic field generated by an electromagnet that killed a mouse in another experiment. Electro-magnetic pollution, caused by computers, television sets, heaters in water beds, florescent lights and electric blankets, have all demonstrated harmful effects on the body's immune system and cause increased susceptibility to cancer.

Permanent vs electro magnets

There are several problems with electromagnets. The problems start with alternating current, which changes polarity 60 times per second. This causes a magnetic field to alternate, from north pole to south pole (negative to positive), 60 times a second. Since the poles have opposite effects on the body, this creates tremendous stress on the cells. High Gauss electromagnetic fields may even damage cell membranes or possibly split chromosomes. You don't have to do much more than that to cause cancer and suppress the immune system. The suppression of the immune system, caused by electric blankets, has been tested under laboratory conditions. The same stress comes from electric heaters in waterbeds. On the other hand, permanent magnets of low gauss strength mimic the natural magnetic field of the earth and have a positive and gentle healing effect on the body. This has been demonstrated several times in controlled experiments (1).

References:
1. Biomagnetic Handbook, by Philpott M.D. Published
by Enviro-Tech, 17171 S.E. 29th St, Choctaw, OK 73020.
Ceramic Magnets - 4"x 6" x 1/2" can be purchased by calling 405-390-3499. Apply green side (north pole) against the body or place under pillow - green side up.

Cayenne stops internal bleeding

Two Spanish persons from Chicago, with HIV, who ate a lot of Cayenne and Jalepeno peppers daily, reported no progression from HIV to AIDS over a period of 4 years. In 1998, two local persons in West Allis, living with HIV, had bleeding problems that were stopped with the use of cayenne capsules. Dan had bleeding from the gums that would not stop. I offered him 2 cayenne capsules that he took with a glass of water. Within half an hour the bleeding completely stopped. A second PWA, Steve, was coughing up blood from the lungs, a serious problem. I offered to take him to the hospital and he refused, saying "what good will it do?" I then offered him cayenne capsules and he took 2 twice a day. Within 2 days, the bleeding stopped completely and has not returned. Does cayenne have a role in AIDS? Did the bleeding stop because the cayenne inactivated the HHV6A, or did it stop the bleeding through some other unknown mode of action?

Summary of Complementary anti-viral treatments for HIV

1. Neem – 6 capsules daily or Didi's protocol with "Hot Stuff" used in Africa.
2. African herbal remedies (Didi Amanda Rucera's protocol)
3. Manganese – 30 mg once a day or once every other day.
4. Green black walnut plus cloves and wormwood (artemesia annua) - 40 drops 3 times a day
5. Bitter Melon – 1/2 to 3/4 cup of raw juice used as a retention enema daily.
6. Monolaurin (lauricidin) - 2 grams twice daily. Best buy is at www.lauricidin.com or use -
   a. Coconut milk (1/2 cup twice daily or the equivalent in raw or cooked coconut - macaroons) or coconut oil - Coconut oil - One tablespoon eaten three times daily. At the same time take a vegetarian digestive enzyme capsule that has Lipase added (i.e. Absorbaid). The lipase should help convert the lauric acid in the coconut oil to Monolaurin or take Monolaurin capsules – 6 capsules 2 times daily.
7. Curcumin 95 (Jarrow Formulas) 2 caps twice daily along with Red Clover blossoms – three capsules twice daily.
8. Essiac or Ojibwa tea (1/4 cup twice daily)
9. Aged Kyolic Garlic Formula 100 – 5000 mg daily plus 2 or 3 cloves of raw garlic daily.
10. Olive leaf extract with 20% or more Oleuropein (Ameriden) - 2 capsules twice daily.

Designing a treatment protocol.

Immune-based therapies like low-dose hydrocortisone, Naltrexone and many others can be combined with antiviral therapies to maximize results. Immune-based therapies have the advantage of bening non-toxic, low cost and can be used off and on without any conern for viral resistance developing. The downside in advanced disease conditions (full-blown AIDS) is that immune-based therapies alone are not likely to reverse a deteriorating condition. This is why when the CD4's are below 200, it is imperative that the patient use both antiviral drugs plus immune based therapies for optimal results. When pharmaceutical drugs to treat HIV are not affordable or available, consider a combination of options discussed here including some like Neem or Didi's protocol used in Africa that are both antiviral and immune-based.

No one except God knows all the answers. Pray for guidance and direction to open unseen doors on life's path. Consult with an herbal or holistic health care professional in designing a herbal/nutritional treatment protocol and consult with your physician, when combining complementary therapies with prescription pharmaceuticals to avoid unnecessary conflicts and contraindications. Known problems – grapefruit and licorice root interfere with p450 liver enzyme detox pathway and should not be used with protease inhibitors.

Immune-based therapies like Naltrexone can be used continuously with or without prescription antivirals for HIV. Immune-based therapies and over-the-counter alternative antivirals can be tested alone or in combination when on a structured drug treatment holiday. These "drug holidays" can last from a week to 30 days or longer depending on lab tests that would indicate you are doing well enough to stay off the drugs for an extended period of time and thus avoid their unwanted side effects. I know several persons who no longer have AIDS but remain HIV+ and who have stayed off drug cocktails for a year or longer while doing little more than follow a healthy diet along with regular exercise. When the viral load goes over 5000, they go back on a drug cocktail for a minimum of 30 days and then depending on how they feel and their next lab results, plan for their next drug holiday.

Note: It appears at this juncture than the long feared problem of viral resistance develops only when patients are not compliant and reduce and miss doses of drugs one or more times a week. It is better to quit taking a drug cocktail completely than to take it on a hot or miss basis and not regularly as prescribed. The same problem occurs with antibiotics when the prescribed dose is not completely taken or are taken at a reduced dose. In HIV/AIDS, the use of plant-based selenium may help prevent viral mutations and increase the effectiveness of HIV antivirals as well as immune-based treatments.

15

Immune-based therapies

Balancing the TH1/TH2 arms of the immune system is critical to restoring homeostasis in HIV, cancer, candidiasis, CFIDS and many other conditions where interleukin-6 is extremely elevated and, in wasting conditions, tumor necrosis factor (TNF) is as well. Low-dose hydrocortisone and other supplements that lower or normalize IL-6 nad TNF-a have critical therapeutic value in the treatment of AIDS, cancer and many other conditons. The use of hydrocortisone is covered serparately in the chapter on the Adrenals.

Immune-based therapies are intended to restore the ability of the body's natural defenses, usually the white blood cells, to neutralize infections (viral, bacterial and fungal), as well as to destroy cancers. There are over 130 subsets of white blood cells that are specialized components of the immune system with both separate and overlapping functions. Apart from the white blood cells, the lymph nodes, spleen, the skin, gastrointestinal tract and mucus membranes are necessary and critical components of the immune systems primary and filtering defenses against invading organisms.

Interleukin II, alpha interferon and Immunoglobulin inoculations are used by the medical professionals to increase T cells, fight viral hepatitis and bacterial infections, yet many promising over-the counter immune modulators, like transfer factor, Naltrexone and polysaccharides are not as widely known, understood and utilized.

Restoring normal thyroid and adrenal function along with normal body temperature and glutathione levels are some of the most important initial steps that can be taken on the road to immune restoration. From a wholistic perspective, restoring healthy cells and to nourish and detoxify major organs and glands through good diet, nutrition and exercise are the basis of not only immune health but also total health.

Factors in immune function include immunoglobulins, T cell memory, B cell, antibodies, antigen presentation, phagocytosis, Delayed Cutaneous Hypersensitivity (DCH) or DTH, Natural Killer Cell Function and CD8 Cytotoxic Lymphocytes (Killer T cells) and in immune dysfunction include autoantibodies and Anergy – a lack of immune cell memory and response, when challenged. Since we discussed thyroid and adrenal function earlier, we will first examine the role of Glutathione in immune response and detoxification pathways.

Glutathione levels are quickly exhausted, where there is long-term chronic infection(s). The lack of intracellular glutathione causes a shift in the immune response from the more effective TH1 cytokine response to the less effective TH2 (Interleukin 4, 5, 6 and 10 but especially 6), with a deficiency of IgA that is needed for mucosal immunity. A lack of glutathione causes a failure of neutrophils to clear fungal infections and impaired function for monocytes, macrophages and other white blood cells.

Hepatitis viral load correlates to glutathione levels

Several scientific articles I have reviewed found that there was a direct correlation between Glutathione levels and viral activity for hepatitis B and C. As the viral load increases, Glutathione levels decrease. Researchers from Germany reported that adding NAC (N-acetyl cysteine) to HBV producing cells lines reduced hepatitis viral DNA 50 fold. One article reported that alpha lipoic acid, NAC and the amino acid L-Glutamine, when used together, reduced hepatitis B viral load by 60% or more. A search, linking the words "Glutathione" and 'hepatitis," turned up over 40 published scientific articles. Glutathione is needed by the liver to help break down toxins. Glutathione is also needed by infected cells in order to process viral antigen. The processing and presentation of viral antigen on the cell's membrane is the first event that must occur, before an effective immune response from CD8 cytotoxic lymphocytes will occur.

Antigen presentation is the first event that must occur, before the immune system can actually "see" which cells are infected, and then mount an effective attack against the infected cells. The cure for AIDS, CFIDS and hepatitis will only happen when every infected cell in your body can process and present viral antigen on the cells surface. Two major factors play a big role in antigen processing and presentation. They are the antioxidant, L-Glutathione, and Adenosine Tri-Phosphate (ATP), the energy currency of the cell. If you have had any chronic infection for more than 90 days, you need to ask your physician to test your intracellular Glutathione levels. Ask for a "Glutathione Peroxidase Assay" - available from ImmunoSciences Labs (310-657-1077).

CD8 CTL's and the Natural Killer (NK) cells

Natural Killer cells are non-specific effector cells that attack virus infected cells and cancer cells independent of interaction with the CD4 helper cells. A Natural Killer Cell Function test measures the ability of this type of white blood cell to kill cancer cells in a laboratory. NK function tests are measured in lytic units. When the lytic units are less than 20, there is little or no immune resistance to cancer. For minimal resistance to cancer, NK lytic units should be above 50 and ideally above 100. The CD8 Cytotoxic Lymphocytes (CTL's) attack infections inside the cells along with

Naltrexone, low-dose Hydrocortisone, 4-Life Transfer Factor Plus, Maitake mushrooms, IP6 and Garlic are choices to activate Cytotoxic Lymphocytes and NK function, along with some extra help from food high in Beta-Carotene. Improving NK function and CD8 CTL's is an important priority for persons with AIDS, CFIDS, Candidiasis and Cancer. Some treatment options improve more than one type of immune response simultaneously.

Naltrexone and low-dose hydrocortisone are the only ones mentioned here that requires a prescription. Some over-the-counter (OTC) supplements to improve NK and CD8 CTL's include 4-Life Transfer Factor Plus, Maitake or IP6 and aged Kyolic garlic.

Transfer Factor + increased NK function 269%

An in-vitro study of over 200 compounds by Dr. Darryl See, MD, found that Transfer Factor Plus was the most effective (248%) in increasing Natural Killer cell function of all products tested. Of individual products and botanicals tested, IP6 (inositol hexaphosphate) was the highest at 49%. This study was followed by an in-vivo study by Dr. Rob Robertson MD (Paducah, KY) in 10 patients who used 2 capsules daily for 3 weeks of Transfer Factor Plus. Dr. Robertson found an average 269% increase in NK function in these patients. TF

Plus appears to have an even more rapid effect than Naltrexone in improving NK function where the increase occurs slowly over a period of several months.

Transfer Factor Plus from (4-Life Products) contains per 2 capsules - 300 mg transfer factor plus 580 mg of the following: IP6, Cordyceps, Beta glucan, Mannans from Aloe, 10 mg zinc, Maitake D fraction and Shiitake extract. This mix of ingredients supports NK function, macrophage function and CD8 Killer T cells. Several persons I have talked to who have used the product report a significant difference in how they feel in just a few days. One person told me a stubborn sinus infection cleared up in 3 days. I tried TF Plus and broke out with a major cold (a detox effect) that lasted about 5 days but noticed a significant increase in energy and well being beginning in the fifth day. Individuals are reporting benefits in all the following conditions:

Allergies, asthma, autoimmune conditions, respiratory conditions, candida, fibromyalgia, fatigue, hepatitis, infections, psoriasis, shingles, low thyroid and cancer.

Persons with lymphoma or cancer have used 2 or 3 capsules of TF+ 3 times a day between meals. Do not use the product, if you are allergic to any of its ingredients, such as the mushrooms. Start off with 1 capsule 3X and increase to a therapeutic dosage level over a period of 5 to 7 days. Note: The bovine derived ingredients in TF+ are all derived from US sources and are processed in a way so as to be completely sterile.

For more information on Transfer Factor Plus or to order, Call Dr Patricia Salvato MD in Houston, Texas at 713-961-7100. Dr. Salvato has used TF+ extensively in her practice for patients with chronic fatigue syndrome and many other conditions for the past 2 years. Jim Mayhew has used TF+ for his own chronic fatigue condition with good results. He can be reached at 561-805-5787. Internet www.4-life.com. Jan 20, 2003: The current cost for TF+ is $53.95 for 60 capsules.

Five readers with HIV, who used only 2 TF+ capsules daily in combination with 2 or 3 antiviral prescription drugs, have all reported significant increases in CD4 counts and viral loads reaching non-detectable levels in 4 to 6 weeks. Only one of the 5 used a protease inhibitor. The other 4 used Viramune, Zerit and Epivir. These results have been sustained over a period of 3 to 7 months. One of the 5, Jim H, who was on a failing regimen of only Zerit and Epivir, reached non-detectable levels in 4 weeks.

However, two readers with CD4 counts below 150, who used 6 to 9 TF+ capsules daily as a monotherapy, failed to either reduce their viral load or to increase their CD4 counts over a period of 2 to 4 months. From these initial reports, it appears that there is some unique synergism between TF+ and the prescription antivirals for HIV. The use of TF+ alone failed to jump-start the immune system, although both persons on this monotherapy reported feeling better and one gained weight.

TF+ for CFIDS. Persons with chronic fatigue syndrome report less fatigue with TF+, than with plain transfer factor and in improvement in body temperature that moves closer to normal.

Naltrexone stops AIDS progression

Feb. 17, 1995
by Dr. Bernard Bihari M.D.

I am a New York City Physician, specializing in HIV/AIDS. Recently, a patient showed me an article by Craig Horowitz ["Has AIDS Won?"], which had terrified him. Saying that if protease inhibitors "fail, there are no other drugs in the pipeline" is both frightening and inaccurate.

There are several other types of promising anti-viral drugs in early development. There is an immune-stabilizing drug, Naltrexone, which is already FDA approved for the treatment of heroin and alcohol addiction and is in use by several thousand people.

In two studies I have led, my findings have been that Naltrexone, when taken in the 3 mg dose, has completely stopped the progression of the disease and the decline in the immune system in 85 percent of the patients who take it consistently. It has no side effects.

More importantly, development of resistance to Naltrexone does not occur. Some patients in my private practice have had stable immune systems (with regard to T4 numbers) for as long as seven to eight years. This inexpensive, currently available treatment, used in conjunction with good medical care and appropriate drugs to prevent opportunistic infections can keep most people with HIV alive and well until more effective, anti-viral drugs provide the basis for a cure.

1985-86 trial with Naltrexone by Bernard Bihari, MD

The trial was based on a large body of research in basic immunology that demonstrated that endorphins are the key hormones involved in the body's regulation of the immune system and in communications between the brain and the immune system. A survey of serum beta-endorphin levels in 10 AIDS patients showed that they were one-third normal. Naltrexone was chosen for its ability to induce increased production of two endorphins, beta-endorphin and metenkephalin. A 3 mg dose of Naltrexone was chosen to be taken at bedtime. Higher doses were not given, due to concern that they might block endorphin production.

Naltrexone prevents opportunistic infections

The 12-week trial showed a significant difference in the incidence of opportunistic infections. Five out of 16 patients in the placebo group got O.I.s while none of the 22 patients on Naltrexone got opportunistic infections. In the placebo group, lymphocyte mitogen responses declined, but there was no decline for those taking Naltrexone. Finally, pathologically elevated levels of acid labile alpha interferon declined for those taking the drug, but no decline was noted for those on the placebo.

After the trial, Dr. Bihari began to use Naltrexone in his HIV/AIDS practice. He and other physicians were able to do so since the drug is FDA approved for another use - the treatment of heroin addiction at 50 mg/daily.

Naltrexone stabilizes T cells when CD4 counts are above 300

Recently, Dr. Bihari evaluated the use of Naltrexone in 158 patients. The results were stunning. Those patients who had taken the drug regularly as prescribed showed no drop in CD4 cell counts. The average CD4 count in the group taking Naltrexone regularly was 358 in the beginning and after 18 months was 368. The 55 patients who had taken the drug sporadically showed a drop in CD4 count from an average of 297 in the beginning to 176 after 18 months. In the group of 103 using Naltrexone consistently, there was no drop in CD4 levels. The stabilization of the CD4s arrested the disease progression.

The 55 noncompliant patients had 25 opportunistic infections while the 103 compliant patients had a total of 8 O.I.s. Survival was also significantly different between the two groups. There were 13 deaths among the noncompliant group and only one in the 103 compliant patients. Dr. Bihari found that in PWAs starting with fewer than 200 CD4 counts that the CD4 counts would often decline even while taking Naltrexone. However, these patients have far fewer opportunistic infections and most are long-term survivors. In spite of low CD4 counts, patients taking Naltrexone live longer due to the activated Natural Killer cells that prevent O.I.s.

Some patients in this study have been on Naltrexone for as long as 8 years, with no disease progression or CD4 declines. Also, there is no evidence of viral resistance to the drug. None of the patients experienced side effects. In addition, 9 patients on Naltrexone for more than 6 months have had plasma viral titers, as measured by PCR, with extremely low levels of the HIV RNA plate counts. In 3 cases, patients became PCR negative.

Low dose Naltrexone is readily available with a Physicians prescription. Dr. Bernard Bihari M.D. can be reached at 29 West 15th St., New York, NY 10011. Ph. 212-929-4196 Fax 212-229-9371. Your local Physician can prescribe Naltrexone for you. It is available in liquid or capsule form. The daily dose is 3 mgs taken anytime after 8 pm..

End of Press Release

Update: In 2002, Dr. Bihari increased the average Naltrexone dose to 4.5 mg daily. More information can be found at www.lowdosenaltrexone.org.

An interview with Dr. Bernard Bihari

Nov. 10, 1995: This interview should answer a number of frequently asked questions about the immune modulator - Naltrexone.

Mark: What is Naltrexone doing for persons with AIDS over a long period of time?

Bihari: I have a large number of patients who have been on Naltrexone for the past 4 or 5 years with CD4 counts that fluctuate, and yet are as high now as when they started on Naltrexone. I have patients that have been using Naltrexone for as long as 7 years with no decline in immune function and virtually no drop in CD4 levels. I have several patients with very low T cells counts, less than 10, who feel healthy enough to hold full time jobs and have done so for several years. I am not seeing the types or frequency of opportunistic infections that would usually be expected of someone with full-blown AIDS.

Mark: How does Naltrexone work?

Bihari: Naltrexone stimulates the production of the endorphins, beta and Metenkephalin. In a lab, when endorphins are added to cell cultures, macrophage activity is significantly stimulated, as is CD4 and CD8 activity. I have found that CD8 cells increase when infections occur and this helps them fight the infections. When I studied the endorphin Metenkephalin in a controlled study on 20 people, it tripled Natural Killer Cell activity. In the body, endorphins are produced by the adrenal glands. However, people with AIDS, cancer and other immune related diseases have low endorphin production.

Mark: Is there a connection between exercise and endorphin production?

Bihari: Aerobic exercise increases both types of endorphins.

Mark: In your Press Release of Feb. 1995, you stated that three patients became PCR negative. Are any more of your patients PCR negative for HIV?

Bihari: I have tested over 70 of my patients by PCR. Presently, I have 7 patients whose test results by PCR are not measurable, meaning the viral plate count is below 10. The virus may be there, but it is in too small a quantity to be measured by PCR. These 7 patients have used Naltrexone for 2 years or longer. Recently, I tested 6 new patients, who started on Naltrexone, every 90 days for 6 months and they had an average 80% decrease in HIV viral load as measured by PCR. However, this is a very small number and I wouldn't want to hang my hat on it - scientifically. What is interesting is that the acid interferon levels also drop, but very gradually. It takes about 6 months for a significant drop in interferon levels to occur.

Mark: How many of your patients are using AZT, DDI, D4T, DDC and other nucleoside analogs along with Naltrexone?

Bihari: Very few, almost none.

Mark: Some people have said Naltrexone is the same thing as Antabuse, a drug used for the treatment of alcoholism. Is this true?

Bihari: No, it is not. Antabuse and Naltrexone are completely different. Antabuse makes people who drink alcohol feel very sick. Naltrexone in a 3 mg dose has no side effects when alcohol is consumed. However, Naltrexone interferes with narcotic pain killers like Morphine or Codeine and other similar drugs. If narcotic pain killers are used along with Naltrexone, they won't work as Naltrexone interferes with their activity.

Mark: Does Naltrexone decrease Tumor Necrosis Factor (TNF) levels like it lowers acid labile alpha interferon levels?

Bihari: I have not tested for TNF levels. However, the same gene is responsible for making acid interferon as for making TNF. In theory, what lowers acid interferon should also lower TNF levels.

Mark: Does Naltrexone have any effect on Lymphoma?

Bihari: I have had about 1 case out of 100 who develop lymphoma every year. The average is about 4 out of 100. I used Naltrexone on a patient HIV- who had lymphoma. She had 3 golf-size lymph nodes in her groin. She took Naltrexone in 3 mg dose, and in 3 months, the lymphoma completely disappeared.

Mark: What about Naltrexone for cancer?

Bihari: I used Naltrexone on 3 patients with pancreatic cancer. In 3 or 4 months, the pain and jaundice disappeared, and they went back to work. One of the patients has remained stable for the past 4 years and continues to take the Naltrexone. I've also used Naltrexone on patients with colon cancer and non-Hodgkin's lymphoma. One HIV+ patient with lymphoma was successfully treated with a combination of chemotherapy and Naltrexone.

Mark: What effect does Naltrexone have on fatigue, poor appetite and insomnia?

Bihari: Usually fatigue and poor appetite are caused not by HIV, but some opportunistic infection. When you treat the infection, the fatigue disappears and appetite returns.

Mark: What effect has Naltrexone had on swollen lymph nodes?

Bihari; There is a gradual reduction in swollen lymph nodes after 2 or 3 months, although they don't completely disappear.

Mark: What about KS?

Bihari: Most of my patients with KS had it when they came to me. However, I have had a few develop KS, 5 or 6, after being on Naltrexone.
Mark: Was the KS benign or aggressive?
Bihari: Only in one case was it aggressive. In the others it was benign.
Mark: In stabilizing CD4 counts, was there any difference in PWAs with high CD4 counts versus low?
Bihari: In persons with over 300 CD4 cells, Naltrexone is 95% effective in stopping CD4 decline. In persons with CD4 counts between 200 and 300, it is 85% effective and in persons under 100, it is about 60% effective in stopping CD4 count decline. This does not mean that Naltrexone is not doing them any good because their CD4 counts drop.
Mark: Could the higher percentage of patients with low CD4 count continue to drop, because of the immuno-suppressive effects of drugs used as prophylaxis to prevent PCP and other infections?
Bihari: I don't know. I am not aware of alternatives to the current drugs being used as a prophylaxis. I use drugs as prophylaxis to prevent PCP because they are effective.
Mark: Have you found any drugs to prevent PCP that do not have the side effects of Bactrim, Septra or Dapsone?
Bihari: Recently I learned about Mepron (Burroughs Welcome). It has few side effects, when used in a moderate dose, but is very expensive. It was originally developed to treat malaria, but was found to be effective for treating PCP.
Mark: Does Naltrexone reduce the incidence of CMV Retinitis?
Bihari: I have almost no cases of CMV. I have had one case of CMV in 5 years. From the number of patients I have had, I should have had 100 cases. In persons with CD4 counts below 150, I place them on Acyclovir to prevent CMV. The dose I usually prescribe is 800 mg 6 times a day.
Mark: I know of one person who took much higher doses of Acyclovir and developed CMV Retinitis. However, they were not on Naltrexone.
Bihari: All my patients who take Acyclovir are on Naltrexone.
Mark: It looks like the combination therapy is more effective than using Acyclovir alone. Are there any side effects to using Acyclovir?
Bihari: Astoundingly, none, with the exception of one patient who gets fatigue, if he takes over 1600 mg daily.
Mark: What other drugs do you use that have few side effects?
Bihari: Diflucan is effective to prevent and treat thrush and cryptococcal meningitis. There are no side effects. I have had patients on Diflucan, 100 mg daily, Acyclovir and Naltrexone continuously, for several years. I have several patients on these combinations that have CD4 counts below 10 and have been going to work for the past several years. I have one patient who came to me with 4 CD4 cells 4 years ago and he still feels well enough to continue working a full time job. He still has 4 CD4 cells. However, he has more of other immune cells that are very important in AIDS, mainly the Natural Killer cells and macrophages.
Mark: Is Naltrexone the chemical name or the brand name?
Bihari: Naltrexone is the chemical name. Dupont sells it under the brand name "Revia."
Mark: Where do pharmacies get Naltrexone?
Bihari: Any pharmacy can order it from Dupont. Dupont has renamed Naltrexone "Revia". The old name was "Trexon." The tablets come 50 mg each. The pharmacy has to grind the capsules and fill them in 3 mg capsules, as the patient takes just one 3 mg capsule daily. Two

50 mg capsules makes a months supply. Some pharmacies won't bother to do this for one patient, as they won't make money on it, since they have to buy a bottle of 50 mg tablets that costs over $200.00.

Note: Dr. Bernard Bihari can be reached in New York City at 212-929-4196 Fax 212-229-9371.

Adjusting dosages for children

It might be more suitable to use Naltrexone dissolved in a liquid for children with AIDS. The dose should be 1 mg per day per 50 lbs of body weight. A child weighing 25 lbs would receive 1/2 mg daily whereas a child weighing 100 lbs. would use 2 mg daily. Bigelow can compound Naltrexone in any dose prescribed in capsules or place it in a liquid medium. In a liquid, 3 mg per 3 ML would make it easy to measure, when smaller doses are needed. Always keep the liquid Naltrexone in a refrigerator, when not in use. Do not order more than a one-month's supply at a time to maintain potency.

Editor's Note: A friend of mine from Milwaukee recently told me of an end stage PWA he knew 5 years ago in Houston, TX, who did very well, while he was on Naltrexone. At the time he started on the drug, his Physician estimated that he would die within two weeks. When he stopped using the Naltrexone 13 months later, his health rapidly deteriorated and he died one month later. This very impressive record of life extension suggests that no one should rule out using this drug, because they have little or no CD4 cells. The very impressive record of Dr. Bernard Bihari strongly suggests that Naltrexone should be on the top of the list of any protocol being considered by persons living with HIV.

Naltrexone triples Natural Killer (NK) cell activity

Update 12/1/95: In an interview on Nov. 10, 1995, published in Positive Health News, Report No. 10, Dr. Bihari said that Naltrexone increases the production of the endorphin, metenkephalin, which triples Natural Killer Cell activity in AIDS patients. Bihari said that Naltrexone is 95% effective in stopping HIV progression to AIDS in PWA's with CD4 counts over 300. Bihari reported that in PWAs with CD4 counts between 200 and 300, Naltrexone was 85% effective in stopping further declines in the CD4's and was 50% effective in stopping CD4 declines when CD4's were between 0 and 200. Naltrexone stops declines in CD4 counts and brings HIV viral load to very low levels. Naltrexone also enables PWA's with low CD4 counts to become long term survivors. He cites some of his patients with CD4 counts as low as 4 who feel so well that they work full time jobs. One patient of his, who has had a CD4 count of less than 10 for the past 4 years, has used Naltrexone during this entire period and feels so well he continues to work a full time job. This suggests that having Natural Killer cell activity can give you a functional immune system, even with very low CD4s.

Bihari also said that, out of 70 patients who have used Naltrexone for 2 years or longer and have had PCR tests for viral load, 7 are now PCR negative! Bihari said that the viral plate load is less than 10 and can no longer be measured by PCR. He said a significant number of his patients on Naltrexone do not use nucleosides like AZT. Naltrexone provides its benefits alone as a monotherapy. (Note: since this interview, the use of nucleosides or protease inhibitors with Naltrexone has been shown to be compatible).

Robert J, a PWA from California, told me recently that he used Naltrexone in 3 mg daily doses from 1991 through 1994 and that his CD4 count stayed in the 350 range for those 3 years. He used no other drug or medication during this period. He reported having no opportunistic infections during this time and always felt fine. Early in 1995, he got lax and stopped using it for over 8 months. He found out in a recent test that his CD4s had dropped to 150. He also was experiencing thrush. He has since resumed using the Naltrexone.

A PWA from Cloverdale, IN, with a CD4 count of 10 has been on Naltrexone since Sept. 1995. In Dec., 1995, he faxed his lab results. They showed his Absolute NK count at 130 cells/UL (per cubic millimeter of blood). Naltrexone did not increase his CD8, which were already very low. However, his physician said his "sedimentation rate" had dropped significantly indicating a decrease in the rate of cell destruction.

In Milwaukee, WI, a PWA with a CD4 count of 25, noticed an immediate improvement in how he felt, when he started on Naltrexone. When, after 4 weeks, he ran out of the product for two weeks, he felt an immediate decline in well-being. He has since resumed taking Naltrexone and says he now "sleeps like a baby."

Naltrexone treats pancreatic cancer and lymphoma

Bihari told me on Nov. 10th, 1995, that three patients of his with pancreatic cancer, who had used Naltrexone daily in 3 mg doses, were in stable condition with no spread of the cancer, and were in no pain. One patient with pancreatic cancer has been on Naltrexone for 4 years and feels fine. A small indentation in the pancreas is all that remains. Bihari also discussed how Naltrexone had helped some patients overcome pancreatic cancer. In one case, Naltrexone was used along with chemotherapy, and the lymphoma was successfully remitted. Published abstracts I recently reviewed indicate that in Breast Cancer, NK activity can be reduced by as much as 75%. A PWA from Rio Rancho, NM with KS reported that after 3 weeks of using a combination of Naltrexone orally and DNCB topically ,along with the daily Whole Lemon drink, that his KS lesions are drying up.

The endorphin "methionine-enkephalin" (MEK) significantly increases Natural Killer cell activity

A decline in methionine-enkephalin (MEK) levels reduces the production of NK cells. Research done by S. Jody et al (J. Canadian Med Assn. Jan, 1985) shows a decline of up to 91% of NK cells in the lymph nodes of PWAs. Other researchers have also reported NK cell decline that occurs on a parallel track with CD4 T-cell decline. (DL Evans et al in Am J. Psychiatry 1995 Apr.). MEK is also produced by the Adrenal Medulla (Bihari). The amino acid, L-Methionine, is used for the production of methionine enkephalin. Published scientific reports indicate that persons with AIDS are low in L-Methionine. In March, 1998, three HIV+ persons, two of whom had full-blown AIDS, told me that they restored deep restful sleep, by taking 500 to 1000 mg of L-Methionine just before bedtime.

The endorphin, MEK, is a critical pathway for increasing NK cells and regulating CD4's. A trial done on 60 HIV+ patients by Dr. Bernard Bihari (New York City) shows that administration of MEK to PWAs increases NK cell counts threefold and stops further CD4 decline.

HN Bhargava (NIDA Res Monogr. 1990) reports that MEK "enhances the activity of NK cells and induces the production of IL-2, which, in turn, may activate other T-cell subsets like CD4." Several researchers have found that high doses of Interleukin-2 (IL-2) rapidly increase CD4 counts. However, they found the same PWAs with high CD4 counts, obtained through cytokine stimulation with IL-2, were getting PCP, indicating the CD4's were not functional. However, low dose IL-2 does stimulate NK cell activity. VR Bonagura et al (J. Pediatr, 1992 Aug) found that in HIV+ children with PCP and high CD4 counts lacked NK cell activity.

Dr. Bihari has observed that in AIDS, endorphin MEK levels are always low. MEK production is stimulated by the use of small oral doses of the drug Naltrexone. In the body, MEK is produced in the Adrenal Medulla and by Lymphocytes. When using Naltrexone, a critical component of the immune system, the NK cell activity is restored. To date, research shows that one or more subsets of NK cells can destroy cells infected with HHV-6A. CD8 Killer T cells can do likewise. This is indicated by many reports of long term survivors, who have had high CD8 counts.

One of Naltrexone's greatest values is to prevent lymphomas and other forms of cancer, that frequently occur in AIDS, as well as helping to restore DCH (Delayed Cutaneous Hypersensitivity), which indicates improved immune function. Naltrexone helps prevent many opportunistic infections.

Where to buy Naltrexone

A good source that will compound Naltrexone in 3 or 4.5 mg. capsules is Apothecure Pharmacy in Dallas, TX 800-969-6601. The price for 30 capsules is about $20.00 (a months supply).

Another source is Bigelow Pharmacy, 414 6th Ave, New York, NY 10011. 212-533-2700. They compound it in 3 or 4.5 mg capsules. Current cost is $24.00 for 30 capsules. Add $3.00 per order for postage and include your prescription. Also, your physician can phone in an order and you can place it on a credit card.

Other sources: Parnasus Heights Pharmacy in San Francisco at 415-564-9191. Smith Pharmacy in Center Ossipee, NH Ph No 603-539-2020. Motel Pharmacy, No. Miami, FL 305-947-6381.

Local pharmacies may prefer to compound it in a solution. Bihari prefers the capsules, as the product remains more stable. If you use a liquid, keep it refrigerated and do not order more than a one month's supply at a time.

Morphine / Codeine not compatible with Naltrexone

Drug inter-reactions: Persons on morphine or codeine will need to stop using these products for at least 7 days before starting on Naltrexone. Naltrexone will stop the pain killing effects of these opiates almost immediately, which could cause shock in a person addicted to these drugs. The same applies to the street drug - heroin. Check with your physician if you are using heroin, morphine or codeine. No other drug inter-reactions are known.

Where to obtain an NK function test and a prescription for Naltrexone

For an NK function test contact ImmunoSciences Labs - 310-657-1077 or Specialty Labs - 800-421-4449 Fax 310-453-9161 or contact www.specialtylabs.com

For a prescription, show your physician a copy of this article and ask him for a prescription. If your physician is not convinced, and you still want a prescription for Naltrexone, you may phone Dr. Bihari at 212-929-4196 for a telephone conference to receive a prescription for Naltrexone.

Note: Dr. Bihari charges $350 for one hour of telephone consultation. The most cost effective way to get a prescription for Naltrexone is to make reprints of the interview with Dr. Bihari published in this book and give it to your local physician. If your physician won't give you a prescription, you will find more listings of other physicians in your phone directory. You can also write to us for a listing of physicians who purchased this book, and who will be more receptive to giving you a prescription for Naltrexone.

Bihari has reported a gradual reduction in swollen lymph nodes in persons using Naltrexone over a period of several weeks. Activated NK cells are effective against most of the pathogens (viruses, parasites, fungus, bacteria, cancer cells etc.) that cause opportunistic infections in AIDS and other conditions where persons are immune compromised.

There are three subsets of NK cells: CD56+, CD16+ and CD3-. The Absolute NK lab test counts all three together. Reference ranges are from 40 to 380 cells/UL.

Transfer Factor – antigen specific

Transfer factors are protein immunomodulators that transfer ability to express cell-mediated immunity from the immunized donors to nonimmune recipients. The effects are antigen-specific (1) Transfer Factors are molecules that "educate" recipients to express cell-mediated immunity. (2)

A patient with acquired chronic oral and vaginal candidiasis was found to have impaired cell mediated immunity to Candida antigen, and loss of skin test response to tuberculin (Mantous). Treatment with Candida-active transfer factor produced clinical remission lasting 1 year and restitution of in vitro and in vivo immune parameters. (3)

A four-year-old boy, ill for 2 years, was found to have a combined Epstein-Barr virus and cytomegalovirus (CMV) infection. After treatment with an oral form of transfer factor, clinical symptoms and viremia disappeared and specific immunity to CMV developed. (4)

In AIDS, 3 PWAs were treated with anti-HIV murine Transfer Factor (TF). All patients showed a marked improvement in their clinical condition. (5)

The functional activity of CD8 cells (as well as CD4s) will vary in patients. The function of CD8 cells is enhanced by "transfer factor." Transfer Factor is a substance obtained from the leukocytes of a person with a delayed-type sensitivity that can transfer that sensitivity to another person (Stedman's Medical Dictionary). Transfer Factor can restore delayed-type hypersensitivity and improve T-cell mediated immunity. Transfer Factor is found in Colostrum, blood and in the lymph nodes.

1. Kirkpatrick CH, Cell Immunol, 164:2 1995 Sep, 203-6
2. Kirkpatrick; Annals of the New York Academy of Sciences. 685:362-8, 1993.
3. Benz, Thomas, Mandl, Morgan. British Journal of Dermatology. 97(1):87-91, 1977.
4. Jones et al, Treatment of Childhood Combined EBV and CMV infection with Oral Bovine Transfer Factor. Lancet 2 (8238):122-4, 1981.
5. Viza eta l, A Preliminary Report on Three AIDS Patients Treated with Anti-HIV Specific Transfer Factor. Journal of Experimental Pathology, Vol 3, Number 4, pp 653-659, 1987.
Additional Reference: Kirkpatrick CH, Transfer of Cellular Immunity with Transfer Factor (Editorial). Journal of Allergy and Clinical Immunology. 63(2):71-3, 1979.

Transfer Factor for CFIDS or FM - Lyme disease may have a role

March 10th, 1999: Michelle Dopson, of Chisolm Biological Labs, told me a few days ago that they are getting good results with a new transfer factor for persons with CFIDS or Fibromyalgia (FM). The new CFIDS and FM transfer factor was made with blood drawn from 7 persons with FM and 7 with CFIDS. The DS (Disease State) grade of transfer factor for CFIDS is producing good results at one capsule daily. In a surprise development, a person diagnosed with Lou Gehrigs disease, which is crippling and often fatal, actually had late stages of Lyme disease. There are several reports I am now receiving of persons with CFIDS or FM, who are testing positive for Lyme. Anyone who is not responding to immune-based therapies, and has CFIDS, FM or Lou Gehrigs disease, should have a test for Lyme. For many persons, Lyme disease may turn out to be a surprise factor in these conditions. For more info, contact Chisolm Biological Labs, Aiken SC 803-663-9618.

IP6 - boosts NK function, oxygenates the blood, reduce triglycerides, dissolve arterial plaque, kidney stones and reduces lipid peroxidation

Three good choices for boosting Natural Killer cell function are 4-Life Transfer Factor Plus, Naltrexone, and Inositol hexaphosphate (IP6). IP6 is derived from rice bran and has been shown in several studies to significantly increase Natural Killer cell function. Therapeutic doses of IP6 for persons with AIDS, CFIDS, Candidiasis, MS, GWS or cancer is about 1000 mg per 25 pounds of body weight on a daily basis. Example: a person weighing 175 lbs. Divide 175 by 25 which = 7. You would use 7 grams (7000 mg) daily of IP6.

Dr. Shamsuddin MD, who wrote a book on IP6, reports that from extensive animal research with IP6, that it prevents cancer at 1000 to 2000 mg daily and at therapeutic doses of 5 to 8 grams daily, can help shrink tumors and malignancies. Dr. Shamsuddin also reports that IP6 is a powerful antioxidant, prevents platelet sticking, removes calcium deposits (plaque) from the arteries, dissolves kidney stones, reduces triglycerides up to 65% and cholesterol by 19%. In addition, IP6 increases the oxygen carrying power of the blood.

There are no reported adverse effects from IP6 in any published studies or from anecdotal reports. IP6 will do many things to improve your health and well-being. IP6 is best absorbed when taken between meals. The book on IP6 is published by Kensington Books, New York, NY. It can be found in health food stores and bookstores.

When Enzymatic Therapy first introduced IP6, it cost about $125 a month to sustain a therapeutic dose. However, competition has driven prices down. Recently Jarrow Formulas have introduced IP6 in powder form at 100 grams for about $15.00. At 7 grams a day, this is about a two-week supply. This reduces IP6 to the low-cost category of Naltrexone.

I have received several anecdotal reports from readers with either HIV or CFIDS, who are all reporting a significant improvement in how they feel, since using IP6. In April 1999, one lady from Canada, who had had severe symptoms from CFIDS for 10 years, took 1 teaspoon of IP6 powder (Jarrow Formulas) and noticed a reduction in her symptoms 3 hours later. One teaspoon of IP6 powder has about 3000 mg.

Inositol hexaphosphate or IP6 is found naturally in rice bran and in whole kernel corn.

Silica blocks IgG suppression of NK cell activity

An interesting study by Fuji Y et al at the Nagoya Univ. School of Medicine, found that IgG antibodies in-vivo (in a live host) diminished the NK cell activity of nude mouse spleen cells and that preadministration with silica or carrageenan blocked the effects of IgG in suppressing NK cell activity. (1).

This suggests that silica (bioactive silicon), by suppressing TH2 antibody activity, might help promote NK and CTL immune responses that would be beneficial in conditions like AIDS, CFIDS and even cancer. Oatmeal is the single food that is very high in silica. The herb "horsetail" or "shavegrass" is a natural source high in silicon. Other herbs that contain silicon are black walnut, burdock, cornsilk, gentian, ginseng, nettle, oatstraw, peppermint, rosehips and stevia, a natural sweetener. The use of these herbs, as a natural source of silica, might benefit persons affected by AIDS, CFIDS, Gulf War Syndrome and other conditions, if they ultimately are proven to help shift the cytokine profile from TH2 to TH1, thus improving the CD8 cytotoxic lymphocyte and NK cell activity. A daily breakfast of cooked whole oatmeal is an excellent natural source of silica.

Boosting your CD8s with DNCB (DiNitroChloroBenzene)

DNCB is a chemical used in photography labs. The drug has been in use for a long time as an antiviral agent and is considered safe in small doses. From the Mega-Pharmaceutical industry's point of view, its chief drawback is that it is unpatentable and low cost - about $2.00 a month. You can see why no private source is spending money to test its effectiveness. Besides stimulating Natural Killer cell activity, DNCB has been reported to increase CD8 cell counts and to be helpful in reducing KS lesions. DNCB has been used by an estimated 7000 PWAs since 1984. Persistent users show a remarkable record for longevity with few opportunistic infections.

DNCB

No one should use DNCB without first reading all these instructions.

This article was preceded by an interview with Billi Goldberg, who is an expert on the subject of using DNCB. DNCB is a sensitizing agent used in photography. Several decades ago, it was discovered that once a week topical applications would activate cell-mediated immunity and DTH (Delayed Type Hypersensitivity). DNCB has been found to increase total CD8 cell counts and, in particular, CD8 cytotoxic cells, as well as enhance Natural Killer (NK) activity. Some articles published in medical journals about DNCB are listed as follows:

1. "Stimulation of T-cellular immunity by cutaneous application of Dinitrochlorobenzene," by Mills LB, 1986.; J. Acad Dermatol 14:1089-1090.
2. "Dendritic cells and DNCB; a new treatment approach to AIDS," by Stricker RB, Elswood BF, Abrams DI, 1991; Immunol Letters, 29:191-196
3. "Clinical and Immunologic Evaluation of HIV infected patients treated with Dinitrochlorobenzene," by Stricker RD, Elswood BF, Goldberg B et al, 1994. J. Am Acad Dermat 31:462-466.
4. "Safety of topical Dinitrochlorobenzene," by Stricker RB, Goldberg B, 1995 Lancet 346:1293.
5. "Improved results of delayed-type hypersensitivity skin testing in HIV-infected patients treated with topical Dinitrochlorobenzene," by Stricker RB, Goldberg B, Mills LB, Epstein WL, 1995 J. Am Acad Dermatol 33:608-11.

Fred Shaw L.Ac. told me that DNCB topical applications are no different than if someone went into the woods and came in contact with poison ivy or poison oak and developed a skin reaction. The skin reaction that develops is an immune response that sets off a cell-mediated cascade, activating both CD8 CTLs and NK cells. This cell-mediated cascade is also believed to shift the CD4s from the TH2 response to the TH1 response, which makes them more effective in attacking the AIDS virus and other infections inside the cells. Generally, TH2 type CD4s circulate in the blood, while the TH1 type go to the lymph nodes and other sites of active infection. Normally, 90% of the CD4s are in the lymph system. Dr. Jay Levy MD has reported that big increases in CD4 counts in the blood often reflect only a movement of CD4 cells from the lymph system to the blood, and the increase of CD4s in the blood do not reflect newly created CD4 cells.

You can easily tell if the increases in CD4s are of the TH2 type, if you break out with thrush and other opportunistic infections, after your CD4 cells have significantly increased. If the increases in the CD4s were of the TH1 type, this would not be happening. CD4s, of the TH1 type, signal CD8 cytotoxic lymphocytes to clear infections inside the cells or to destroy virus-infected cells, while the TH2 type signal B cells to produce antibodies that are not effective against intracellular infections. The TH2 type of CD4s also increases the percentage of CD8 suppressor cells and decreases the number of CD8 cytotoxic lymphocytes.

DNCB: sensitization and challenge

The first experience one has with DNCB will be the strongest reaction one will ever encounter. This initial reaction is called "sensitization." Initial sensitization is done by using a Q-tip and applying 2 applications of a 10% DNCB solution to an area, ranging in size from 1 inch by 1 inch to as large as 2 inches by 2 inches. The initial application should be applied to the inner left or right forearm. DO NOT APPLY IT ANYWHERE ELSE. As a general rule, DNCB applications should be applied on the upper part of the body, not the legs and thighs. No showers are taken for at least 12 hours after the initial application, or the original area of contact will spread. A large gauze should be placed over the area and adhesive bandage applied, making sure that the adhesive does not touch the area where the DNCB was applied. The person waits 2 weeks minimum before using DNCB again. The initial sensitization reaction usually occurs within 10 to 14 days.

A systemic sensitization reaction, which is the desired reaction, must have all of the following characteristics: Redness, severe itching and raised skin at the application site. If you develop all 3 reactions, you are sensitized. In addition, some swelling of the skin in and around the application site and a feeling of heat being generated, will accompany these reactions. If no reaction occurs, or the only reaction that occurs is that the skin turns red and there is no itching and no raised skin, you are not sensitized. If you are not sensitized to the first application of DNCB, the weekly application of DNCB will do you no good. If you are not sensitized after 2 weeks, administer one application of 10% DNCB solution weekly, each treatment being in a different location on the body, until a sensitization reaction occurs.

A new area of the body needs to be used each time it is applied. When sensitization finally occurs, every area to which you applied DNCB will flare up at once. When that happens, you are sensitized! The first sensitization reaction will take the longest to disappear. The average time is 4 months. Many persons, because of fear of the first reaction, never try DNCB again. Several persons have told me "I got burned the first time I used DNCB; I'll never use that stuff again." Some persons have reported reactions lasting 8 months and even longer. Strangely, no one with an ongoing DNCB reaction, including those that last several months, has ever reported coming down with a major opportunistic infection. Billi Goldberg told me "persons with the strongest initial reaction to DNCB are the long term AIDS survivors."

Dave Pasquerelli, a member of ACT-UP SF, told me "the more you use DNCB, the faster these skin reactions disappear." In Milwaukee, WI, a local PWA, who has used DNCB for the past 3 years, told me his usual skin reactions come and go in 4 days. DNCB solutions are made available in 4 different concentrations: 10%, 2%, .2% and .02%. A DNCB Starter Kit contains all 4 strengths. After sensitization has occurred and if there is a strong reaction, persons usually try the weakest solution, (.02%); to see if they get a reaction called a "challenge" to the immune system. If the reaction was not very strong, use the 2% solution.

Challenge: After sensitization occurs, the immune system is challenged with a weaker concentration of DNCB solution, applied in an area from as small as 1 inch square to a 2 by 2 inch area. At the minimum, the reaction should include a reddening of the skin and itching, some slight swelling and heat generated in the immediate area. If the reaction is too weak, a stronger solution (.2%) is used in the third application. If the reaction is still not strong enough, then the 2% solution is used. The immune reaction increases total CD8 counts, with primary stimulation of the cytotoxic subsets and increased Natural Killer cell activity. The activated CD8 CTLs, and NK cells, provide a significant degree of protection against opportunistic infections.

My own experience with DNCB

In May 1996, I decided to try DNCB to see what reaction would occur. After applying a 10% solution twice to an area about 2 x 2 inches just above my left knee, I waited about two weeks and nothing happened. I thought to myself "Mark Konlee does not have any cell-mediated immunity, isn't that interesting?" I decided to go to a local salon and get a suntan. The very next day the area began to itch, and I began to scratch it (something you are not supposed to do). Within a few days a severe reaction set in, with redness, severe itching, swelling of the skin in the immediate area and raised skin. I was sensitized. Fearing another reaction of this intensity, I decided not to try it again, until this reaction was completely gone. No one told me at the time that the longer you use DNCB, the faster these reactions go away. In a phone call to Dave Pasquerelli, he advised me to apply calamine lotion. I did, and it helped reduce the itching and swelling. Between daily application of Bactine (to prevent infections), aloe vera gel and calamine lotion, it took 4 months before the reaction was completely gone. Recently, I found that coconut oil applied over the DNCB patch helped relieve itching in one local case.

The next time I tried DNCB was in April 1997. Being cautious, I tried the weakest solution - .02%. Within a few hours, it began to itch and turned slightly red, a weak reaction. Within 5 days it was gone. A week later, I decided to try the stronger solution - .2%. Within an hour, a strong reaction set in with red, slightly raised skin and significant itching. Within 5 days it was gone. Two days later, I began taking one Beta 1, 3 Glucan capsule daily. Within two days, the patch that was gone reappeared and began to itch severely. Beta 1, 3 Glucan is known to enhance cell-mediated responses, so it's no surprise that it caused a reactivation of the DNCB patch. I continued taking the Beta 1, 3 Glucan, and after 5 more days observed that the skin reaction was not going away. Apparently, the Beta 1, 3 Glucan was priming the DTH response. I stopped taking the Beta Glucan, and within a week the skin reaction was gone. I have since learned that Thymus and thymic factors will also prime the DTH response. Since an over-reaction can be uncomfortable, I would suggest anyone planning to use DNCB for the first time to stop using Thymus and Thymic factors and Beta 1, 3 Glucan for 2 weeks before using the first application of DNCB. On the other hand, if someone waits two weeks and gets no reaction to the initial double dose of 10% DNCB solution, they might want to take Thymic factors and/or Beta 1, 3 Glucan for a few days, to turn on the sensitization reaction before trying a second application.

In a variation to my experience, a person with less than 10 CD4 cells told me he gets good skin responses to DNCB and he still takes Beta 1, 3 Glucan and Complete Thymic Formula daily. He reports the DTH skin reactions still go away in 5 days. Since his cell-mediated immunity (CMI) is weak, he can use the extra priming of the CMI responses by taking Thymic factors and Beta Glucan. It is important to listen to your body and to observe how you react to DNCB, or any other treatment, and to make changes in your protocol as needed.

Questions and Answers about DNCB

In an interview with Billi Goldberg, an expert on DNCB, I asked several questions.

Mark: Several of our readers have told me that they used DNCB once, got a very strong reaction that took several months to go away and are afraid to use it again. If these persons want to try DNCB again, do they have to re-sensitize with the double dose of 10% DNCB?

Billi: Probably not. Once you are sensitized to DNCB, the T cell memory should last for several years. They could start with weekly applications of the .2% or .02%. If you started with the weakest dose of .02% and do not get a reaction, you can move up to a stronger dose until you get a good reaction.

Mark: I know one person whose doctor told him that if he did not use the drug cocktails, he would be dead in 6 months. He did not like the way the drugs made him feel and refuses to take them. I told him about DNCB and he applied a 10% solution twice to a 2 x 2 inch area on his leg. Note: He should have applied it initially to the left forearm. Even so, about 10 days later, he got a very powerful reaction. It burned and itched severely. He began scratching it with a hairbrush and it spread to an area 4 times its original size. It took daily applications of "Ivarest," a cream for treating poison ivy, plus Calamine lotion to reduce the area of reaction back to its original size. My question is: to achieve initial sensitization, do we need to always start with an area 2 X 2 inches, or could we do it with a smaller area - say one inch square?

Billi: Yes, you could try obtaining sensitization with DNCB, using a smaller area such as one inch square. However, if you do not get a sensitization reaction in 10 to 14 days, you will need to use a weekly application of the 10% solution in a different location, until sensitization occurs. Once sensitization occurs, every other area you applied DNCB to will react at the same time.

Mark: What advice would you have for CFIDS patients trying DNCB?

Billi: For persons with CFIDS, start off with double applications of the 2% solution rather than the 10%. If a sensitization reaction does not occur with 14 days, you can try the 10% solution.

Mark: Does DNCB have to be applied every week for someone with high CD8s and very good DTH responses?

Billi: For someone with high CD8s and good DTH, who is asymptomatic, they could use it less often, such as once every 2 weeks. For some persons, once a month may be sufficient to keep the cell-mediated responses primed.

Mark; Who should not use DNCB?

Billi: Persons with organ transplants, persons with active hepatitis, jaundice, pancreatitis, damaged livers, sarcoidosis, multiple sclerosis and parkinsons disease.

Mark: Who should use DNCB?

Billi: Persons with HIV, CFIDS and other conditions, who have a lack of cell-mediated immunity. They can also check with their physician to find if they have any condition that would be adversely impacted by using DNCB and improving cell-mediated immune responses.

Mark: Thank you for this information. Billi can be reached at 415-826-4928 or e-mail at BiGoldberg@aol.com.

Where to obtain DNCB

By credit card, you can order a DNCB Starter Kit ($50) current price from Dr. Stricker at 415-283-1911 or at this website: www.usmamed.com (Goto HIV link) or write to
Union Square Medical Associates
450 Sutter Street, Suite 1504
San Francisco, CA 94108

Persons planning to use DNCB should stop using all supplements containing "Thymus" for 2 weeks prior to sensitizing with DNCB. This is because thymus fractions may cause an over-reaction to DNCB. Persons with no reaction to DNCB should take thymus supplements to stimulate the DTH response. Other products that enhance DTH responses are Beta 1, 3 Glucan and DHEA.

Beta 1, 3 Glucan – improves macrophage, DTH

Beta 1, 3 Glucan is a polysaccharide derived from the membranes of a common yeast and a known activator of macrophage activity. It is a pure isolate and does not contain any yeast proteins, so persons allergic to yeast should not have a reaction. Beta 1, 3 Glucan is also found in rye sprouts, oat sprouts, lentinan and in kamut, wheat and barley grass. These sprouts also contain Beta 1, 6 Glucan. Beta 1, 3 Glucan and Beta 1, 6 Glucan are also found in over the counter products like Oralmat. There are no known adverse effects from using Beta 1, 3 Glucan and no known drug inter-reactions.

Macrophages are white blood cells that capture foreign invaders (viruses, fungus, bacteria and parasites) and present the invader (antigen) to CD4 cells. If the CD4 cells signal the macrophage that it is an alien, the macrophage destroys the antigen; if not an alien, the macrophage releases it. This antigen presentation from macrophages, monocytes, dendritic cells and CD8 cytotoxic lymphocytes occurs primarily in the lymph nodes. Contributing factors to the failure of antigen presentation and cell-mediated immunity include damage to the germinal centers of the lymph nodes caused by HHV-6A, lack of CD8 cytotoxic lymphocytes, lack of TH1 type CD4s and/or activated macrophages and monocytes, as well as low Glutathione levels.

The scientific community on Beta 1, 3 Glucan

M.L. Patchen, Ph.D., Dept of Experimental Hematology and Radiation Sciences, Armed Forces Radiobiology Research Institute states: "Glucan (Beta 1, 3) has been shown to enhance macrophage function dramatically, and to increase nonspecific host resistance to a variety of bacterial, viral, fungal and parasitic infections."

William Browder MD, Dept of Surgery and Physiology, Tulane University School of Medicine states: "Beta 1, 3 Glucan is a potent macrophage stimulant and is beneficial in the therapy of experimental bacterial, viral and fungal diseases."

Two groups of symptomatic patients were treated with antifungal agents. The first group received Beta 1, 3 polyglucose and the antifungal agent, while the second group only received the antifungal agent. In the first group, 10% had a relapse of fungal infection, while the group treated with the antifungal agent alone had a 62% relapse. The authors, Meira DA et al wrote: "The present results indicate that the patients who received glucan, in spite of being more seriously ill, had a stronger and more favorable response to therapy." (1)

Donald Carrow on Beta 1, 3 Glucan

In the June 1996 edition of The Townsend Letter for Doctors, is found an article by Donald Carrow MD on B-1,3 Glucan as a Primary Immune Activator. Dr Carrow observes "Long before the advent of the germ theory our forefathers had observed that recovery from illnesses could be accomplished by host resistance. You could say that immunology preceded our discovery of microbiology and bacteriology."

Beta 1, 3 Glucan is a polysaccharide molecule, consisting of purified glucose with a unique molecular structure that specifically bonds to receptor sites on macrophages. Research at Harvard University found that there are receptor sites for 7 different sugars (polysaccharides) on the macrophage membranes (3). Unlike pure glucose (white sugar), that suppresses the phagocytic activity of immune cells (1, 2), Beta 1, 3 Glucan activates macrophage activity and sets off a cascade of events, which stimulates immune function in several areas (3).

These include increases in complement production (4), serum cytokines, Interleukin I, Interleukin II and interferon (3). By this cascade of events, Beta 1, 3 Glucan increases non-specific immunity against all infectious diseases (6) including cancer. Peter , resolved within a few days (3).

In his article, Dr. Carrow reports on research done at the Armed Forces Radiobiology Research Institute in Bethesda, MD in 1989 that shows that oral ingestion of Beta 1, 3 Glucan protects against the adverse effects of radiation. An article published by Patchen ML et al, also reports on the beneficial effects of Glucan in radiation exposure (5).

Beta 1, 3 Glucan is isolated from the membranes of Baker's Yeast (Saccharomyces cerevisiae). Brewer's Yeast, used in making beer and wine, also is derived from the same strain of yeast - Saccharomyces cerevisiae (8)

Summary of benefits from using Beta Glucan from Dr. Carrow's article

1. Activation of macrophage and monocyte activity increasing phagocytic activity, of immune cells to destroy virus, fungal and bacterial infections.
2. Increased production of complement, Interleukin I and II. Complement is a sticky substance that coats viruses and makes it easier for the immune system to see them. Complement also punctures holes in the membranes of viruses and weakens their structure.
3. Increased immunity against fungal infections.
4. Protects against damage to normal body cells during radiation therapy.
5. Helps prevent plaque build-up in the arteries and stimulates macrophage activity to

remove plaque build-up.
6. Anti-oxidant activity - scavenges free radicals
7. Releases colony stimulating factor and increases bone marrow production. The bone marrow is the origin for the production of all our white and red blood cells.

References:
1. Sanchez, A, et al. Role of sugars in human neutrophilic phagocytosis. Am J. Clin Nutr., 1973; 26:180-187
2. Bertstein, J, et al, Depression of lymphocyte transformation following oral glucose ingestion. Am J. Clin Nutr., 1977; 30: 613.
3. Carrow, Donald;. B-1,3 Glucan as a Primary Immune Activator; Townsend Letter for Doctors, June, 1996.
4. Jacques PJ, et al. Triggering of Phagocytic Cells, pgs 201-4, 1979.
5. Patchen ML, et al: "Glucan: Mechanisms Involved in its Radioprotective Effect," J. Leuc. Biol, 42:95-105, 1987.
6. Di Luzio NF, "Immunopharmacology of Glucan: A Broad spectrum Enhancer of Host Defense Mechanisms"; Trends in Pharmacological Sciences; 4:344-47; 1983
7. Nutrition Supply Corporation, 2553 North Carson St, #2384, Carson City, NV 89706 Ph No. 800-773-7034.
8. Encyclopedia of Chemical Technology, 3rd Ed, Volume 3. Wiley-Interscience Publication

Benefits of sulfated beta glucan from Lentinan

In an article on Lentinan, a mushroom in its earliest formative stages, contains beta 1, 3 glucan and beta 1, 6 glucan, G Chihara wrote, after observing that Lentinan prevents "cancer recurrence or metastasis after surgery,": "These polysaccharides also increase host resistance to various kinds of bacterial, viral and parasitic infections, including AIDS." (2

Editor's Note: One abstract by K. Hatanaka et al suggested that the sulfated form of beta 1, 3 glucan prevented cytopathic effects of HIV in vitro while a low sulfate form did not. Hatanaka wrote: "Lentinian sulfate, with a sulfur content of more than 13.9%, effectively prevented HIV-induced cytopathic effects at concentrations of more than 3.3 micrograms/ml." (3) However, HIV alone is not known to be cytopathic, which leads to a primary question of cell culture contamination with HHV-6A and a secondary question, whether the sulfated form of beta glucan inhibited HHV-6A along with HIV.

A sulfated form of beta 1, 6 glucan "suppressed the giant cell formation of HIV-infected Molt-4 cells....and inhibited HIV-plaque formation completely at 250 mcg/ml in MT4 cells" (4) The two abstracts which observed that sulfated forms of beta glucan had antiviral properties, raises the possibility that combining a natural source of sulfur rich foods with beta glucan may give it an anti-viral effect. Yeast derived Beta 1, 3 Glucan is not known to have a direct antiviral effect against HIV or other viruses. Beta glucan's action is known to directly stimulate macrophage activity; hence its activity is considered an immune activator, not a direct anti-viral agent. However, the research indicates that the sulfated beta glucan may do both, have a direct anti-viral effect, as well as stimulate macrophage and neutrophil function.

Several of our readers have told me that their T cell counts (CD4 and CD8) have increased since adding the yeast derived beta 1, 3 glucan to their protocols. Two readers thought that lentinan (Shi-Lem), a Source Naturals product, was even more effective than the yeast derived glucan. These results have not been confirmed by scientific studies. A few readers thought they had better results taking Oralmat along with beta 1, 3 glucan in capsule form, than taking either one alone.

1. Meira DA et al ; AM J Trop Med Hyg. 1996 Nov;55(5):496-503.
2. G Chihara;)Dev Biol Stand. 1992;77:191-7.
3. Hatanaka K, et al, Japan J Cancer Res. 1989 Feb;80(2):95-8.
4. Hirabayashi k, et al, Chem Pharm Bull. 1989 Sep; 37(9):2410-2.
5. Neenyah Ostrom, The New York Native, Oct 10, 1994.

Beta glucan - adult dosage

Beta 1, 3 Glucan is available in capsule form in 100 mg or 500 doses. Suggested dose for yeast derived beta glucan: Take 200 mg once daily in the morning or one 500 mg once daily in the morning. Do not take yeast-derived beta glucan several times a day, just once. Another source is oats, raw oatmeal or oatmeal water. For sulfated beta glucan, eat mushrooms - fresh or dried - cooking is thought to destroy the beta glucans (shiitake, maitake are especially well studied).

Beta 1. 3 glucan is also found in rye sprouts, kamut, barley grass and wheat grass sprouts. You won't find it in rye crisp or wheat bread. It is destroyed at temperatures over 140 degrees Fahrenheit. Beta 1,3 Glucan derived from the common baker's yeast is sold in high-concentration 100 mg or 500 mg capsules from Chisolm Labs (800-664-1333 or Fax 803-663-6019).

Lentinan as a source of sulfated beta glucan is sold by Planetary Formulas (Full Spectrum Shiitake) and by Source Naturals in a product called Shi-Lem. Suggested dose: take one or two tablet in the morning and one in the evening. I have heard good reports from persons using both types of beta glucan. My opinion is that the sulfated beta glucan found in lentinan may be more effective than the yeast derived form. Other manufacturers of lentinan products may be found in health food stores. One reader with CFIDS said he had significant relief of symptoms eating rye sprouts that he grew at home.

Proboost (THYMIC PROTEIN A) A sublingual thymic factor boosts platelets, WBC and T cells

Other than injectible IL-2, this sublingual thymus product is, in my opinion, the most under-rated immune modulator on the market. Recently, I have followed two cases, one on a drug cocktail and one on alternative therapies for HIV where this product brought about stunning increases in platelet and CD4 counts in just 10 days.

This product from Longevity Science is made from thymus cells cultured in a lab that were taken from a single healthy calf in the late 1980's. PROBOOST Thymic Protein A (Longevity Science) is a sublingual form of thymic proteins absorbed in the mouth. In cancer patients, it can maintain normal white blood cell counts and other lymphocyte values, even while the patients are on chemotherapy. I have had several reports where Bio-

Pro Thymic Protein A significantly increased Lymphocytes, Platelet, White Blood Cell and T cells counts. Dissolving one packet of granules daily under the tongue. Thymic Protein A increases DTH (delayed type hypersensitivity).

Note: This product is completely sterile as the thymus cells are grown in a laboratory. The original cells were derived from a healthy calf in the US about 10 years ago.

Beta carotene increases NK cells

Dr. Gregg Coodley, MD, speaking at the Third Int'l Conference on Nutrition and AIDS in Philadelphia, PA, Oct, 1994: "Vitamin B-12 deficiency is a causative factor in Neuropathy, Anemia, Encephalatrophy and cognitive dysfunction...intrinsic factor is needed to absorb B-12... Vitamin A deficiency increases the rate of infection...In a study in Africa on 300 pregnant mothers deficient in Vitamin A, the rate of transmission of HIV to their babies was 32%....in a group supplemented with Vitamin A, the rate of transmission was 7%....Vitamin A more favorably reduced HIV transmission than AZT....deficiencies of selenium have been linked to lower T cell counts....Beta-carotene, in one study on 21 patients, boosted CD4 (T4) counts, WBC counts and increased NK cells, compared to a control group...the dosage used was 50 mg twice a day....beta-carotene is one of 600 carotenoids that exist in highly pigmented (colored) vegetables and fruits....breakdown of skin blamed on a deficiency of Vitamin A and C."

DHEA - the "youth" hormone

5/1/97: DHEA, a master hormone, affects many bodily functions. DHEA is safe to use and has no known side effects in small doses in persons with normal immune systems. DHEA makes your skin and hair look younger. It has been called the youth hormone. Users have reported an increase in their sex drive.

A local PWA, who uses DNCB in weekly skin patches to stimulate Delayed Type Hypersensitivity (DTH) reactions, reports that DHEA enhances the DTH responses. He used 50 mg daily. One of the most documented articles on the scientific benefits of DHEA ever published was brought to my attention by a local AIDS activist. After reading over 150 articles published in medical journals, he selected one written by William Regelson, Roger Loria and Mohammed Kalimi that was published in the Annals, New York Academy of Sciences (May 31, 1994, Vol 719). Here is part of what they wrote:

"DHEA has been likened to an "anti-hormone," which cannot serve to excite in the true classical sense of hormone action, but de-excites metabolic processes which overproduce when DHEA is in short supply....Recent broad reviews of DHEA and more specific presentations on immunity, cardiovascular diseases, obesity, carcinogenesis, hepatic function, mitochondrial metabolism, insulin action and receptor availability have been published....Pregnenolone, derived from cholesterol, is a major precursor for all three major groups of adrenal steroids...

In stress, or serious illness, there is a shift in pregnenolone metabolism away from DHEA and its sulfate production to that of the glucocorticoids. Studies have demonstrated that DHEA, at pharmacologic dosage, given subcutaneously, acts to enhance immune resistance to viral and bacterial infection...DHEA has been shown to stimulate T cell proliferation and IL-2 production...according to Daynes' group, the primary immunologic target of DHEA is the TH-1 subclass of the CD4+ T cell population, leading to increased lymphokine IL-2 production, with enhanced cytotoxic activity and reduced lymphokine IL4 levels....The maintenance of IFN-gamma production by DHEA may explain some of its in vivo antiviral activity...The presence of an infection, as a stress, is necessary for DHEA to show its immuno-stimulating action."

The article just quoted contains 79 scientific references. It documents that in chronic illnesses, such as AIDS, Lupus, burn injuries and many others, DHEA levels are suppressed. DHEA levels peak at age 24 and then decline about 20% every 10 years. DHEA is available on prescription and is also sold over the counter in pharmacies and health food stores.

Update 1/19/03: Alfred Plechner told me that if a person is under stress or is estrogen dominant, that taking extra DHEA (pill form) will increase the production of estrogen, further dysregulating the immune system. Wild yam extract is interesting, as it was used in World War II in the manufacture of cortisol. A plant sterol that mimics DHEA is found in Wild Yams. A comparable dose is unknown to me at this time. It is known to contain progesterone precursors. Are the sterols in wild yam more beneficial than the synthetic manufactured forms of DHEA available in pill form? What about the sterols in yucca and tumeric? The use of plant sources of hormone precursors needs further investigation.

16

Chronic Fatigue Syndrome and Fibromyalgia
Does HHV-6A cause Chronic Fatigue Syndrome or CFIDS?

Interview with
Ginny Kloth
(From Positive Health News, Report No 11)

Ginny has traced the origin of her Chronic Fatigue condition of the past 19 years to Sept. 1976, when she had a vaccination for the Swine Flu. The vaccine, which was given to millions of Americans, had live virus in it, and may have been contaminated with HHV-6A. Ginny Kloth, who has direct contacts with several hundred CFIDS patients via the INTERNET, sent out a message on this possible connection, and received 70 replies from CFIDS patients who traced the origin of their illness to the Swine Flu Vaccinations of 1976. This confirmed her worst suspicions, that this vaccination was the origin of many cases of CFIDS and of her own long ordeal with this debilitating disease.

Ginny Kloth had been married most of her adult life and has 3 children. This interview provides a strong case that CFIDS is caused by an infectious agent and may be a transmittable disease.

March 20, 1996:

Mark Konlee: When did you receive the Swine Flu Vaccine?

Ginny: In September of 1976. I first noticed symptoms about one month later.

Mark: What symptoms did you notice?

Ginny: My lymph nodes became sore and enlarged. I found myself becoming tired early in the day. I had extreme fatigue and a rash that would come and go. I had a low-grade fever. I had pain in my joints.

Mark: What did the doctor diagnosis?

Ginny: The doctor diagnosed me as having panic attacks. My sleep patterns became disturbed. I began to develop chemical sensitivities, allergies and asthma. Sometimes, I would wake up feeling paralyzed and unable to move. As a respiratory therapist, I knew three persons who developed Guillain-Barre Syndrome, after they received the Swine Flu vaccine. This happened about 3 weeks after they received the shot.

Mark: What are the symptoms of Guillain-Barre Syndrome?

Ginny: Paralysis, sometimes it affects the whole body. I've read a report of 3 persons who died shortly after receiving the Swine Flu vaccine.

Mark: How long did you continue to work?

Ginny: I worked most of the time until 1989 when I became too weak and tired to continue.

Mark: Do you wake up feeling tired?

Ginny: Yes, this has been going on since the late 1970's. I sometimes only sleep one hour at night and then suddenly wake up. I also have bouts with periodic paralysis, when I cannot move. Sometimes, I cannot even pick up a cup of coffee. During the day, I often have difficulty waking up?

Mark: Have you had burning sensations in your feet? Yeast infections?
Ginny: Yes, I have had burning sensations in my feet. I also have lost all feeling in my mouth. I have had recurring yeast infections and white patches in my mouth.
Mark: Have you had eye floaters?
Ginny: Yes, I have had lots of floaters. Sometimes, my whole field of vision is filled with swarms of floaters. I also had white sparks in my left eye on occasion.
Mark: What was your worst experience?
Ginny: Back in 1991, I was so sick I told my husband I thought I was going to die. I could no longer drive a car. I could not walk without assistance.
Mark: Was your memory affected?
Ginny: By 1991, my memory was gone.
Mark: Do you get frequent colds and flu?
Ginny: Rarely do I get a cold or the flu.
Mark: Persons with AIDS also rarely get colds or the flu. This occurs, when humoral immunity is over-active. Did you turn to Jesus Christ during this period of time?
Ginny: Yes, I have kept my faith in God. I came to know the Lord as my personal Savior in the 1970's. Through this time-period, it was difficult to keep up with my Bible studies.
Mark: Was your husband affected?
Ginny: Yes, he has developed extreme fatigue, but has managed to continue to work. He has lost his libido. The doctor said his body has stopped producing testosterone.
Mark: When did you first contact Keep Hope Alive?
Ginny: Last May, my lymph nodes went wild. My voice went. I could not talk. The doctor placed me on Prednisone. The Prednisone did not help my condition. It actually elevated my blood sugar and I became diabetic. I could barely walk. I had to use a walker. In October, I did a search on the INTERNET and placed the search word "lymph nodes" and found your article on the Whole Lemon drink.
Mark: Did you try the whole lemon/olive oil drink, and what did it do for you?
Ginny: Yes, I started on it right away. I used cold pressed olive oil I bought at a health food store. The article said that I should see results in 5 to 7 days. I started on a Saturday, and after 5 days I did not notice any changes. I told my husband: "This is not working and I began to cry." My husband said to give it a few more days. I did, and two days later, I woke up and noticed the swollen lymph nodes under my chin had gone. I felt the one on my collarbone going down and the one on my neck was gone. I was excited, but I thought, this is too easy. I told my dentist what I had done, and he said he could see that my lymph nodes had gone down.
Mark: How long have you been on the whole lemon drink?
Ginny: Since October 1995
Mark: In February, you called me and obtained a copy of How To Reverse Immune Dysfunction. What information from the book have you incorporated into your treatment program?
Ginny: I am now a vegetarian and eat lots of raw vegetables. I got a prescription for Naltrexone and started on it about March 13th.
Mark: Have you noticed any changes?
Ginny: I don't know how to put this in words. I feel more of inner peace. I am feeling better. Before starting on Naltrexone, I used to have twitches and involuntary spasms and a feeling of things crawling on my skin. These symptoms are subsiding.

Mark: Has Naltrexone affected your sleep patterns?

Ginny: I am no longer waking up with my jaw clenched. Before Naltrexone, I would only sleep one or two hours a night. Now I am sleeping 5 hours and I am waking up feeling more rested.

Mark: What did your lab test show?

Ginny: My CD4's are 1100, CD8's are 220 and CD26+ are 726. The CD26+ are three times above normal.

Mark: Your profile shows hyper CD4 activation and very low CD8s. Your very high CD4's indicates that you have an overactive humoral immunity (antibody mediated immunity), while you have very low CD8's, suggesting that your cell mediated immunity is severely depressed and unable to effectively neutralize the virus or pathogen causing your illness. Since your Natural Killer cells are stimulated into activity by Naltrexone, it is improving your cell-mediated immunity. The result is that some of your symptoms are now subsiding.

End of first interview. Ginny tried a bottle of olive leaf extract capsules. One week later I phoned her.

Mark: Since you have been on olive leaf capsules for one week, what have you experienced?

Ginny: Well, I have always had low body temperature, about 1 to 2 degrees below normal. Right now, I am running a fever, about 100 degrees F. Yet, I do not feel any chills.

Mark: That is wonderful news. It means your immune system is being activated. A low-grade fever can heal a sick body faster than toxic drugs. What else have you noticed?

Ginny: I am sleeping longer now without waking up. I slept a full 7 hours last night. My aching joints are gone. At first, after I started on Eden, my lymph nodes got sore for a few days, then this has subsided and they are now going down. My mental function has improved significantly. I actually feel awake during the day. I have a lot more energy. I don't need the walker anymore. My jaw joints are less sore. I am not having involuntary muscle jerks anymore. I don't feel like there are spiders crawling on my skin. I notice symptoms slowly subsiding each day. I used to feel like my balance was off, that is gone. My kids are surprised at how long I can keep going. I feel like things are settling down inside my body.

Ginny Kloth, 1260 Chase MTN RD, Blue Ridge, GA 30513

Note: Two weeks after being on olive leaf extract, and while still using the whole lemon/olive oil drink, Ginny told me that her "body temperature is now back to normal." Ginny started her recovery with the Whole Lemon/Olive drink, her condition improved further, when she added Naltrexone and the olive leaf extract.

April 26th, 1996 CD4/CD8 ratios reverses

Ginny had just received a new set of lab results and called to tell me her CD4 count fell from 1100 to 237 and her CD8 increased from 220 to 1270. She said: "My CD4s and CD8s have done a flip-flop. My doctor does not understand what is going on. I told my doctor that April has been the first month I have felt normal in 6 years."

I told Ginny that the profile she had now - highly activated CD8s and NK cells is exactly the profile she needed to rapidly reduce viral load of (HHV-6A) and possibly effect a slow cure for her CFIDS condition. Ginny has been tested several times for HIV and has always been negative. I said: "after the HHV-6A is completely eradicated by the CD8 Cytotoxic

Killer Cells and the NK cells, your CD4s will rise, her CD8s will fall and the ratio will most likely return to a normal reference range of 1.0 to 2.5. You don't want the ratio to return to normal until the last virus is gone."

She also said her latest lab result showed platelet counts just above the normal reference range. I suggested she add one tablespoon of cold pressed flax oil to her daily diet to thin the blood and to add it to a salad or mix it with cottage cheese or yogurt and to consider taking one cayenne capsule with each meal.

Ginny also told me that the last swollen lymph node on her collarbone is almost gone. She was so excited she sent me an e-mail message and wrote: I had to share the good news! I have been calling all my family members! Praise the Lord! I spent all the day working...am feeling so good! She said she no longer has sensitive reactions to perfumes and paint like she used to.

A second CFIDS case

Cambridge, MA: Holly, who has CFIDS and Lyme disease and suffers from impaired mental function and systemic yeast infections, found immediate relief using a combination of the Whole lemon drink and olive leaf capsules with 20% oleuropein, the active ingredient, taking a total of about 400 mg of oleuropein daily. After just 10 days, she told me a wide range of symptoms simply vanished and that her mental clarity improved 300%. "The only thing I could compare it to was getting 120 cc of intravenous ozone and then going into an hyper baric chamber." She actually did this. She told me she was going to use DNCB and get a prescription for Naltrexone, as she wants to restore her cell mediated immunity and make a complete recovery.

Hyper CD4 activation in CFIDS

Many people, like Ginny, who have CFIDS, have hyper CD4 activation (over stimulated humoral immunity). In this phase, CD4 counts are high and NK and cytotoxic CD8 activity are suppressed. This is a profile, where people are very sick, often for several months in AIDS, but several years in CFIDS patients. In CFIDS, when the CD4's decrease and the CD8's increase, symptoms subside and the patients feel better.

Full-blown AIDS occurs when both the humoral and cell mediated arms of the immune system stop functioning. The greatest threat to survival in AIDS is not just the loss of CD4 cells, but the loss of CD8 Killer T cells, also known as Cytotoxic T cells, and the loss of NK cell activity. Note: CD8 cells are of two types - suppressor and cytotoxic. The subset of CD8 cells that helps to restore cell-mediated immunity is known as CD57+. CD57+ is known as the Killer T cells or Cytotoxic Killer cells. In a lab test, it would be expressed as: CD8 CD57+, after which the number of cells would be indicated.

The three subsets of Absolute Natural Killer Cells are CD3-, CD16+ and CD56+. The latter two are believed to be the most important. The loss of NK/CD8 function in AIDS leaves them subject to a whole range of infections that spread cell to cell - toxoplasmosis/MAC/MAI etc.

When the CD8's and NK activity increase, cell mediated immunity improves and symptoms subside. When viral load, either HHV-6A and/or HIV is high, it is a treatment error to try to increase CD4 counts and B cells without first bringing down the viral load. Once the viral load reaches zero, CD4s will increase without any special stimulation, CD8's will decrease and the ratio will return to normal. Ginny's CD4/CD8 ratio was 5.0 (CD4's - 1100/ CD8 - 220). At this ratio, she was very ill. This is why simply increasing CD4 counts in AIDS, CFIDS and probably Gulf War Syndrome is a mistake, as it will make the patient more ill while viral load is still high. The antibody-mediated immunity (humoral) is not very effective against the viruses involved in AIDS and CFIDS or the mycoplasmas involved in Gulf War Syndrome (GWS).

Ginny told me of a Gulf War Veteran with GWS and swollen lymph nodes. After doing the Whole Lemon/Olive oil drink for 3 days, he sent her an e-mail message that the swelling in his lymph nodes had substantially decreased.

HHV-6A – antiviral treatment options

Foscarnet has been known for some time to inhibit ASFV, CMV and HHV-6A, while Ganciclovir is a standard treatment for CMV and is also known to inhibit HHV-6A. Both drugs have serious side effects. Anecdotal reports indicate that Butylated Hydroxy Toluene or BHT is very effective against CMV Retinitis. BHT is an over-the-counter antioxidant sold by Twinlabs and comes in 250 mg capsules. For years, it has been widely used to prevent outbreaks of herpes. In doses of 1000 to 2000 mg daily, it can elevate liver enzymes. However, in lower 250 to 500 mg daily doses, it usually does not increase the liver enzymes.

As Konstance Knox has reported in several published scientific journals, HHV-6A causes nearly all the destruction in body tissues and organs in persons who have died from AIDS. In consideration of the success of the Marc Correa protocol, where BHT was used in doses of 1000 mg or more daily, as part of an extensive protocol that reversed full blown AIDS; the recently published interview with Michael Zielinski who used BHT in 250 mg daily doses for the past 15 years and stopped HIV progression to AIDS and in one case, where a CFIDS patient who was using BHT and then thinking it was not helping her, stopped it, only to find that her symptoms suddenly worsened, the use of BHT in the treatment of AIDS and CFIDS needs serious revaluation.

Monolaurin or BHT may help reverse symptoms related to CFIDS & MS

Monolaurin: Recently two persons with multiple viral problems, including HHV-6, CMV, EBV, and in one case HCV, reported a very significant reduction in symptoms using 4 to 6 grams daily of Monolaurin pellets from Med Chem Labs www.lauricidin.com. The pellets are placed on the tongue and swallowed with water or fruit juice. Do not chew them, as they taste like soap. Published scientific research on Monolaurin finds that it dissolves the outer envelope of lipid-enveloped viruses like HHV-6, HIV, CMV and EBV, many kinds of fungal infections and the entire family of herpes viruses. No side effects have been reported.

BHT (antioxidant): In both HIV and CFIDS, the use of at least one 250 mg capsule of

BHT daily could be very helpful in reducing HHV-A replication. Persons who know they already have elevated liver enzymes should have their physician monitor enzyme levels to see if this low a dose has any effect.

To absorb BHT, it needs to be taken with some fat or oil. Opening up the capsule and adding the powder to the whole lemon/olive oil drink would be one very effective way to use it. Another way is to take the capsule with a meal high in fat, at least 2 tablespoons of butter, coconut oil, olive oil or hazelnut oil or any other high quality oil, or take it with a fatty fish like salmon or sardines. If you take BHT on an empty stomach or a meal that does not have any fat, you will absorb very little and it will not give you as much benefit as using it with a high fat meal or predissolved in olive oil.

BHT can be pre-dissolved in a pint of olive oil, almond oil or butter. If you add 16 capsules to one pint, then 2 tablespoons of the oil will provide 250 mg of BHT, or your could add 8 capsules to one cup of melted butter or coconut oil to give you the same potency. BHT may turn out to be a long-term low-cost effective treatment to help prevent or stop AIDS, CFIDS and Multiple Sclerosis (MS) progression.

Using BHT in the lemon olive oil drink

BHT and Co-enzyme Q10 are best absorbed when blended with oils. BHT can raise liver enzymes in the 1000 to 2000 mg daily dose but is not known to do so at a lower 250 mg daily dose. St John's Wort and protease inhibitors also are known to raise liver enzymes. Your physician can monitor your liver enzyme levels for you, before you use BHT, to see if any changes occur.

It is quite unlikely increases in liver enzymes will occur if BHT is added to the whole lemon olive oil drink, as this drink detoxifies and flushes out the liver and lymphatic system. The drink is made by taking the juice of one lemon, the rind of 1/2 lemon (cut up), 1 cup of water or fruit juice and 1 tablespoon of Extra Virgin Olive Oil and adding it to a blender. If you have problems digesting oils, add a small piece of fresh ginger root. Blend on high speed for about 1 minute. Pour through a strainer and use a spatula or spoon to press the juice out of the pulp. Throw out the pulp and drink this mixture once a day; or, if you removed the seeds from the lemon, drink the pulp and all.

For anyone affected by CFIDS, HIV or MS, this drink is a good starting point for your recovery program. In the event you are a person who finds that olive oil disagrees with your system, substitute hazelnut or almond oil and leave in all the other ingredients. The second most important item to add to your immune enhancement protocol is one or more items that boost Natural Killer cell function.

From case reports on persons with CFIDS, other products that are promising for treating HHV-6A infection are Lomatium Dissectum and Venus Fly-Trap extract and Lentinan. Lomatium Dissectum and Venus Fly-trap extract have been widely reported effective against both candidiasis and herpes viruses and have reduced swollen lymph nodes in both AIDS and CFIDS patients. Lentinan, from embryonic shiitake mushrooms, contains sulfated beta glucan that not only activates macrophage and neutrophil function, but also inhibits HIV and other lipid envelope viruses.

Summary of anti-viral therapies for HHV-6A

1. Low-dose Hydrocortisone and Thyroid (see chapters on Adrenals and Thyroid)
2. Whole Lemon/Olive oil drink - use once a day.
3. BHT - 250 mg daily dissolved in olive oil.
4. Monolaurin pellets – 1.5 grams 2 or 3 times daily. www.lauricidin.com
5. LDM-100 - 40 drops 3X Note: For eye infections, add 2 drops to 1 tablespoon of sterile water and use an eye cup wash the eye. Repeat as often as needed.
6. Venus Fly-trap extract - 1/2 tsp in water 3X
7. Mushrooms (Maitake or Shiitake) or Lentinan - (Shi-Lem from Source Naturals) 1 tablet twice daily. A source of sulfated beta glucan.
8. Olive Leaf extract - (from Ameriden- 2 capsules twice daily). Anti-viral, anti-fungal, antioxidant.
9. Oregano (Oregamax from Northern Spice and Herb - 3 capsules twice daily). This brand is made from wild crafted oregano and has powerful antiviral, antifungal and antibacterial properties.
10. Essentials Oils of Lemon, Lavender, Patchouli and Lemon-Eucalyptus and Oregano are effective against herpes viruses and many other viruses, fungal and bacterial infections. Although not specifically tested for their effects on HHV-6, these are the essential oils most likely to inhibit HHV-6A.

External use: 5 drops of 2 or more of the essential oils may be massaged into the abdomen area twice a day, or directly on swollen lymph nodes or other areas. Do not apply in the eyes, as the oils are too strong. Patchouli and Lemon Eucalyptus are a powerful combination.

Internal: Take 3 drops of each oil with a large glass of water one to three times daily. Both internal and external methods may be used together. It is best to start off with one oil and add on gradually until 2 or more of the essential oils are being used together.

Safety data: All available information indicates these essential oils are safe to use as directed.

11. Pharmaceutical antivirals for HHV-6A are
    a. Valtrex
    a. Ganciclovir
    b. Foscarnet

Valtrex is the best of the lot for treating herpes and HHV-6. Ganciclovir and Foscarnet cannot be used long term, as they have serious side effects. No long-term side effects have been reported in persons using items 1 through 9 listed above, with the possible exception of BHT in a few persons who have a seriously impaired or toxic liver. These persons are unable to tolerate chaparral either.

In a nutshell: Low-dose Hydrocortisone, Selenium, immune based therapies - Naltrexone and or TF+, supplements to support glutathione synthesis (ImmunePro, Immunocal etc), restoring normal thyroid and adrenal function, herbs and Glucaric acid to counter estrogen dominance, probiotics and fiber for intestinal and mucosal immunity, liver detox – whole lemon/olive oil drink, diet plan outlined in this book, antivirals for HHV-6 and other lipid enveloped viruses, exercise and prayer.

Dr. Salvato's Regimen for CFS

Posted by PJ on December 31, 2003 on the Message Board at www.keephopealive.org
Hi Maxdel,

Welcome to the board! There are a lot of kind people here who will tell you about their experiences. I have learned a lot here.

I am also a CFIDS patient for the past 14 years, and I have just recently seen some great progress in my condition. My first piece of advice to you (which Mark Konlee, the originator of this board, would also give to you) is to see an immunologist about your condition and treat him/her as your primary physician.

Whatever may cause this disease; it becomes a disorder of the immune system. The disregulated immune system permits the body to be attacked by various invading organisms without giving a proper immune response. The only doctor who will have the tools to monitor your immune system is an immunologist. If you are close or can travel, I recommend Patricia Salvato in Houston, Texas. An infectious disease specialist will not be able to run the same tests or know what to do about them.

Here is a summary of what Dr. Salvato has used to treat me. Below I will describe why.
Products:
Nitroplex / Immunocal/ ImmunePro whey supplement
Glutathione intramuscular injections
ATP-20 (douglaslaboratories.com)
Transfer Factor Plus (4-Life Products)

Now I will tell you what procedure my doctor follows and has followed with me. She begins by ruling out other causes for symptoms, causes such as heart disease, brain tumor, thyroid disease, EBV, CMV, lupus, Lyme disease, MS, HIV, etc. If all these can be ruled out or brought under control and the patient is still symptomatic, she would run a "cytolytic subset panel". This is a blood test which tells the count of your CD3, CD4, CD8, B cell, and Natural Killer cells. These are components of the immune system that ordinarily exist within normal ranges, and in normal proportions to one another.

Of these, the most important would be the NK cells, which should be above 300. CFS patients typically present with low values for this range of cells.

She may also run a test for cyclic AMP. This is a urine test that measures the amount of adenosine triphosphate in your system. ATP is cellular energy. CFS patients are typically low in this value.

If your values were abnormal, the doc's next goals would be:
1) raise the NK cell count to at least 300
2) raise the ATP
3) modulate the immune system so that the CD4:CD8 ratio would be somewhere close to 1.8.

Doctor Salvato has had success with improving NK cell count by improving glutathione through the use of whey supplementation. Glutathione is a liver anti-oxidant. Taking a glutathione pill will not raise glutathione levels. Taking whey supplements provides the precursors for glutathione, which work. She recommends Nitroplex, but okays the use of Immunocal or ImmunePro also. Please look up these products on the net.

She also uses Transfer Factor Plus made by 4Life (see 4Life.com). This product has been shown in clinical trials to improve NK cell count up to 248%. I have been taking it this year and have seen dramatic improvement. Transfer factors are proteins that provide the immune system information on what it ought to attack. The proteins are ordinarily provided from mother to child in the mother's first milk, colostrum. Transfer Factor Plus is made from bovine colostrum.

Dr. Salvato also uses ATP-20, made by Douglas Laboratories (see their website). ATP not only improves the patient's sense of energy, but also is used in critical metabolic pathways of all kinds. Of its many functions, one of the most significant for CFS patients is antigen presentation, which is dependent on having sufficient ATP. As part of its everyday functions, the immune system must decide which foreign proteins (e.g., viruses) to contain and mark for lysing or killing. These proteins must be "presented" by the cells that contain them, and they must have ATP to do it.

Additionally, Dr. Salvato recommends no aerobic exercise until the NK cell count rises, no sugar, caffeine, or alcohol, and no avoidable stress - adrenaline production lowers NK cell counts, so avoid it, even the adrenaline from watching a suspense story. Take a good multi-vitamin which will provide additional anti-oxidants such as vitamin C. Sleep at least eight hours a night if you are able.

When I raised my NK cells recently, I was also taking the whole lemon/olive oil drink described on keephopealive.org for one month and the following:

IP-6 - 4 capsules per day for 2 weeks
Olive leaf extract - 3 per day for 1 week
Compounded T3 for hypothyroidism
Heavy metal detox (naturopathic drops)
Magnesium - 400 mg. per day
Zinc - 100 mg per day
Evening primrose oil
Beta-carotene
Multi vitamin
Sublingual B12 - 1 per day
Cayenne capsules
Kyolic garlic
HiO Silver oxygenated water - 6 per day, 3 days per week

I took these supplements while eating a Mediterranean diet, 3 meals a day.

Not everyone responds to the protocol Dr. Salvato has used with me. There are two other products that she would try if this combination does not work. But this is where she would start.

Wishing you all the best in this New Year,
PJ
Note: Patricia Salvato MD, Houston TX 713-961-7100

CFS and CFIDS organizations

Chronic Fatigue Immune Dysfunction Syndrome (CFIDS) affects millions of Americans. Symptoms include extreme fatigue, swollen lymph nodes, low-grade fevers, aches and pains, flu-like symptoms and nervous symptom disorders (being in a fog, attention deficit disorder). Persistent candidiasis is often reported. The same protocols that benefit persons with AIDS is also benefiting persons with CFIDS.

Organizations to contact:
1. National CFIDS Foundation, 103 Aletha Road, Needham, MA 02491 Phone No 781-449-3535. This is the first CFIDS organization that is now funding research to find treatments effective against HHV-6A.
2. CFS Foundation, 965 Mission St (425), San Fran, CA 94103- 415-882-9986. CFS Foundation has a complete list of CFS related symptoms.
3. The CFIDS Association, PO Box 220398, Charlotte, NC 28222 Fax - 704-365-9755.
4. CFIDS and FM Healthwatch, 1187 Coast Village Rd, #1-280, Santa Barbara, CA 93108 Ph No 800-366-6056. Publishes a newsletter called "Healthwatch."

Guaifenesin for Fibromyalgia

A search about Guaifenesin on the internet yielded some surprises. I read reports of some people with fibromyalgia (FM) recovering nearly completely by using 600 mg or more of guaifenesin 2 times daily. A lot of information about the use of guaifenesin for treating FM is available at a website called www.guaifenesin.com.

Dr Paul St. Amand recommends persons with fibromyalgia avoid products with salicylates when using guaifenesin to treat fibromyalgia. The need to avoid salicylates appears to affect persons with Fibromyalgia in varying degrees. Salicylates are found in Aspirin, similar products and many topical skin creams as well as some foods and herbs. Other conditions for which guaifenesin may be used might not be affected by the use of salicylates.

Over the counter cough syrups like Robitussin whose active ingredient is guaifenesin do not advise against using salicylates . The absence of the notice to avoid salicylates in cold remedies suggests that in treating health conditions that are not related to Fibromyalgia such as HIV/AIDS, sinusitis, respiratory infections, etc that the use of salicylates may not affect the treatment outcome in the same negative way as with Fibromyalgia.

Some people report that guaifenesin is the most effective treatment found for fibromyalgia to date and report complete recovery. However, some people obtain only partial relief and a few obtain no results at all. Very few treatments exist today for any condition that are 100% effective all of the time. This does not diminish the effectiveness of a treatment when it does work.

Some background facts about "Guaifenesin"

The substance originally came from the bark of a tree called "guaiacum." Immunesuport.com reports that the bark of this tree was used to treat rheumatism in the16th century. About 20 years ago, scientists learned how to synthesize the bitter substance from the guaiacum tree and it became known as guaifenesin. It has been widely used in cold medicines for the past two decades.

The standard dose in cold medicines is about 1200 mg daily of guaifenesin in a 24 hour period. While these OTC cold treatments recommend short-term use, if the condition does not clear up, see a doctor. This advice is usually standard for all OTC drugs. At 1200 mg daily, the best available information is that it could be taken for several years and no toxic effects have been reported even at doses up to 3600 mg daily. However there is no point in pushing this envelope. If 800 to 1200 mg daily solves a health problem, then stay at this level as long as you feel comfortable with it.

Note: www.guaifenesin.comn, there are several links to sites where you can obtain Guaifenesin.

Guaifenesin, an expectorant, may enhance mucosal immunity by increasing mucosal IgA levels

Guaifenesin claim to fame is as an expectorant that loosens and thins mucus. That might suffice to help explain how guaifenesin helps overcome a sinus or respiratory infection as a treatment, but this alone does not adequately explain how quaifenesin can prevent strep and other infections of the sinus and lungs when taken as a preventative. What I have found lacking in the published literature are studies of the effects of guaifenesin on cytokines like IgA, IL-12, antigen presentation, DTH and other immune markers.

RH Buckley writes that "Selective absence of serum and secretory IgA is probably the most common form of human innumodeficiency. High frequencies of recurrent sinusitis, otitis media, pneumonia and atopy were noted among a group of 75 such patients all but 4 of whom were Caucasian." (1)

Numerous studies have linked IgA deficiency with sinusitis, bronchitis, allergies, rheumatoid arthritis, sore and swollen joints, anemia, low platelet count, food allergy and asthma. (2, 3)

Lizeng Q et all found that serum IgA suppressed the replication of HIV-2. Lizeng found 96% of all IgA samples reacted against whole HIV-2 antigen and 100% reacted with gp 36. (4)

Challacombe and Sweet state: "There is a paradox that profound HIV-induced immunodeficiency is present systemically, whereas the majority of infections associated with HIV disease are present or initiated at mucosal surfaces.... Considerable attention has been given to the possibility of mucosal immunization against HIV and there is evidence that secretory IgA antibody is neutralizing to different HIV strains." (5)

1. Clinical and immunologic features of selective IgA deficiency, RH Buckley, birth Defects Orig Artic Ser. 1975;11(1):134-42
2. http://www.primaryimmune.org/pubs/
3. Immunologic defects in patients with chronic recurrent sinusitis, Sethi DS et al, Otolaryngol Head Neck surg. 1995 Feb;112(2):242-7
4. IgA mediated immunity in HIV-2 infection, Virology, 2003 apr 10;308(2):225-32
5. Oral Dis. 2002;8 Suppl 2:55-62

17
Pharmaceutical drugs for treating HIV/AIDS

Pharmaceutical drugs, like Norvir, have strong immune enhancing effects. Norvir increases delayed type hypersensitivity (DTH) and has powerful anticancer effects including the treatment of kaposi sarcoma and lymphoma. There are life-saving advantages for immediate use of many pharmaceutical drug combinations although adverse effects may prevent life-long use as a therapy.

Feb 2004. There are now 19 FDA approved drugs to treat HIV plus the two combos "Combivir" and "Trizivir" or 21 drugs total. A complete and objective report (47 pages in length) on all the HIV drugs and combinations can be found in the Fall 2003/winter 2004 issue of ACRIA or AIDS Community Research Initiative of America in New York. A copy of this report can be obtained by calling 212-924-3934. Information can also be found on their website at www.acria.org.

Some of the new drugs recently approved by the FDA include Fuzeon (T-20), the first fusion inhibitor. The new drug is injected and comes with a steep price tag. The two other new drugs are Emtrivia and Reyataz. Emtrivia has mild side effects like Epivir (3TC) and in one study was more effective than Zerit (D4T) in reducing viral load. Reyataz is a new protease inhibitor but without the adverse lipid side effects of the other protease inhibitors. For those of our readers who use the FDA approved drugs when they are not using immune-based treatments for HIV, the new drugs Emtrivia and Reyataz are worth considering.

Pharmaceutical drug combinations to treat HIV/AIDS (excerpts from PHN, Report 16 - updated on 3/1/03)

Suppressing viral replication directly can be very helpful in immune restoration. It reduces stress on the immune system, allowing for some bounce back of the immune system in many individuals. However, anti-viral therapies alone are not always the whole answer for everyone. In March of 1997, I wrote an evaluation of FDA approved drugs used in the treatment of AIDS and separated those combinations that suppressed cell-mediated immune response from those that promoted them. By selecting combinations that are not only antiviral, but also improve the immune response, you will be less likely to have opportunistic infections. Here are the conclusions of the article.

A summary of my findings on the best vs the worst drug cocktail combinations – updated 3/1/03

Protease Inhibitors: Norvir (ritonavir) is by far the most effective of all the protease inhibitors in preventing and remitting nearly all opportunistic infections including Kaposi sarcoma, lymphomas and cancers. Crixivan (indinavir), Viracept (nelfinavir) and Invirase (saquinavir) also have therapeutic value, but are less effective than Norvir. Norvir significantly increases CD8 cytotoxic lymphocyte activity and improves antigen presentation (DCH and DTH) skin responses, when challenged with an antigen or topical DNCB solution that demonstrates DTH/DCH (antigen presentation) and cell mediated immunity.

A report by A. Carr et al at the 3rd Conf Retro and Oppor Infect. Jan 28-Feb 1, 1996, reported that Norvir (Ritonavir) increased and sustained higher CD8 counts by 892 cells/mm3 over a 40 week period as a monotherapy, whereas AZT, in combination with other nucleosides, initially increased, then decreased, the CD8 counts to baseline by the 24th week. These high CD8 counts, especially with improved DTH responses to DNCB indicates the TH1 branch of the immune system (CD8 cytotoxic lymphocyte and NK activity) is improving. A good drug cocktail combination can mop up the opportunistic infections, as immune function is restored.

Nucleosides: On the 6 nukes, D4T (Zerit) and 3TC (Epivir) are the safest and most effective for preventing or remitting opportunistic infections, when used in combination therapy with protease inhibitors. However, based on a significant number of anecdotal reports, the two nucleosides, AZT and DDI, are linked to nearly all the AIDS-related cancers, lymphomas and wasting syndrome, when used in combination with protease inhibitors. DDC is generally not used in combination therapy and little interest remains in this drug. About 40% of persons using DDC (HIVID) develop peripheral neuropathy (Report from the Medical College of Wisconsin)

Non-nucleoside Reverse Transcriptase Inhibitors (NNRTI's). Rescriptor (delavirdine) increases absorption of protease inhibitors where as the other NNRTI, Viramune (nevirapine) inhibits absorption of all the protease inhibitors. (Data from the Medical College of Wisconsin - CME program). Viramune is effective when used with D4T or Viread, and 3TC. Note: About 1 in 7 people may develop a rash using either delavirdine or nevirapine. If the rash cannot be controlled with antihistamines, you may consider using either Viread or D4T and 3TC.

Note: Norvir must be kept refrigerated, and there are several prescribed medications that should not be used with Norvir. When taking Norvir, you can start with a low dose and take up to two weeks to get up to the full dose. To obtain more information, see your physician and also call Abbott Laboratories at 847-937-7069. Website: www.abbott.com. Information fact sheets on Norvir and other drugs are available from GHMC at 212-367-1455.

The best triple drug combination therapies – without the use of protease inhibitors.

The following 3 drug combinations (in bold lettering) work well together as they each attack a different part of or point of the HIV replication cycle. So far, we have near consistent reports of non-detectable viral loads on these combinations. The belief that you cannot get and sustain a non-detectable viral load without also using protease inhibitors is not supported by the facts.

1. Viread, Viramune and Epivir (3TC) or Zerit (D4T). Viread is a relative newcomer and has brought few complaints. 3TC is well tolerated and Viramune is usually well tolerated

although associated with neuropathy in a few cases. D4T has also been associated with neuropathy and higher triglycerides in some cases.
2. Viread, Sustiva and Epivir (3TC)
3. Rescriptor, Viread and 3TC
4. Viramune or Sustiva or Rescriptor plus D4T and 3TC. Some have also used the Lemon/Olive oil drink daily as well to prevent the D4T or Viramune from causing neuropathy.

Note: Sustiva may cause colorful dreams or nightmares.

The best drug combinations with protease inhibitors.

Experiences in the past few years have convinced us that D4T should not be used with protease inhibitors, as it aggravates the lipodystrophy problem. Also, no one should use any protease inhibitor without also taking Naltrexone (4.5 mg once daily in the evening) that helps to prevent lipodystrophy. However, if the lipid profile worsens, then stop the drug cocktail for a while and consider a drug combination without the use of protease inhibitors.

1. Norvir (use 1/2 dose only – 2 capsules 3 times daily), Viread and 3TC or Rescriptor. Important: Use Norvir, not Kaletra, if cancer or any kind of lymphoma is present. Once the cancer is gone, go to a non-protease combination and use Naltrexone as an immune modulator to maintain the NK function that controls cancer. 12 capsules of Norvir daily as recommended by Abbott causes diarrhea and is too much for most people to handle and is not necessary.
2. Viracept or Agenerase or Kaletra plus Viread and 3TC Note: One of the NNRTIs Sustiva or Rescriptor may be substituted for the 3TC or the Viread but not both at the same time. The use of Viramune is not recommended with any of the protease inhibitors as it inhibits their absorption. Kaletra is not in bold here as we have had many complaints of side effects – high triglycerides and cholesterol although this problem plagues all the protease inhibitors that are used long-term 6 to 18 months or longer. That is why a drug holiday for a couple months or a change to a non-protease combination should be part of the evolving treatment pattern. These breaks do not cause viral resistance. More on this later in this chapter.

Note: The main reason some persons have avoided protease inhibitors is that lipodystrophy and/or elevated cholesterol and triglycerides have lead to heart disease in a number of cases.

Important note: Whether you use a drug combination with or without protease inhibitors, the minimum immune-based therapies that you should use in conjunction with these drugs is Naltrexone once a day in the evening 4.5 mg and selenium (plant-based sources only like Bio-Active Selenium or Selenomax – 800 to 1200 mcg daily).

The worst of the drug combination therapies

1. Crixivan and Combivir (AZT and Epivir) – associated with several cases of lymphomas and cancer.
2. AZT plus DDI when used in combination with any of the protease inhibitors. (Most

dangerous combination)
3. AZT OR DDI or Combivir (AZT +3TC) when used in combination with any of the protease inhibitors.
4. ANY TWO protease inhibitors used together in any person with active hepatitis or who has elevated liver enzymes or impaired kidney function.
5. ZIAGEN (Abacavir) with AZT, DDI, Combivir or Trizivir.
   Note: We have also had several readers report bad side effects from Ziagen (Abacavir).

A bad 6-pack – a summary of the 6 worst HIV drugs

Of the 15 FDA approved drugs to treat HIV, the following six drugs have the worst side effect profiles and should not be used at all or only used short term for salvage therapy or until something better is found. They are 1. Crixivan (indinavir), 2. Videx (DDI), 3. Ziagen (Abacavir), 4. Retrovir (Zidovudine aka AZT) and Glaxo's two combos, 5. Combivir and 6. Trizivir.

These bad drugs when used in combinations have, in several case reports, led to gastrointestinal distress, lymphomas, brain tumors, heart attacks, lung cancer, melanomas, MAC, candidiasis, Retinitis, PML, wasting syndrome, beer bellies, buffalo hump and many other AIDS related opportunistic infections and several deaths. Suppression of ATP production in the mitochondria by AZT and DDI cannot alone explain all these O.I.'s. There must be some toxic drug inter-reaction occurring between AZT or DDI and the protease inhibitors.

Note: regarding the use of Fortovase (Saquinavir), I am concerned that a few cases of leukemia have developed. However, in these cases, AZT was used in combination with Saquinavir. GMHC has published an article in "Treatment Issues," in which they received survey reports from 37 physicians using protease inhibitor drug cocktail combinations and the successes and failures are discussed. For a copy, write to GMHC, The Tisch Bldg, 119 W. 24 St, NYC, NY 10011 and ask for Volume 12, No 1, copy of Treatment Issues.

Anecdotal reports & scientific evidence

The combination of Crixivan, AZT and 3TC has resulted in several cases of lymphomas and cancers among persons I know here in Wisconsin. Two people I know have died of lymphomas on this combination and one non-smoker died of lung cancer. Another person had one lung removed for cancer on this combination and is now being treated with chemotherapy. In yet another case, a PWA who used both AZT and DDI in combination with Crixivan and Invirase now has melanoma, a rare form of skin cancer.

M.W, who used Crixivan, AZT and 3TC, developed both a "crix-belly" and a brain tumor. Not everyone using AZT or DDI with protease inhibitors is developing lymphomas and beer bellies. However, other problems are showing up like an increase in mental confusion and dementia. One of the most striking things about Norvir (ritonavir) is the almost complete absence of reports of lymphomas, cancers, wasting syndrome or other opportunistic infections. I recently became aware of about 12 local persons using Norvir, either in combination with delavirdine (Rescriptor) or Viramune plus D4T or 3TC or D4T plus 3TC, who have had remissions of all opportunistic infections and no adverse side effects from these drug combinations for more than 12 months. The only exceptions when Norvir failed were when DDI or AZT was used in combination with it.

Marc Correa's case is one example. He used Norvir, D4T and DDI. He developed 5 major opportunistic infections including KS and also accumulated a lot of fat in the abdomen area. I am certain from other cases I have followed that the DDI was the cause of his protocol failure, not the Norvir or the D4T. Orlando, who lives in Washington, DC, recently called to tell me that on the combination DDI, Viracept and 3TC, he became very ill and within one month was diagnosed with Non-Hodgkins Lymphoma, after which his physician changed his protocol to Norvir, Invirase, D4T and 3TC, which he tolerates much better. He is currently on chemotherapy for the lymphoma. My own opinion is that he would do better dropping the Invirase and adding 4-Life Transfer Factor Plus, Naltrexone, and raw garlic to his daily regimen, along with the whole lemon/olive oil drink.

HIV antivirals (AZT, DDI and DDC) suppress immune responses and are toxic to the mitochondria of cells

B Tindall et al (AIDS, 1993 Jan, 7(1):127-8) writes: "Primary HIV-1 infection is associated with the development of a predominately CD8+ lymphocytosis (cytotoxic lymphocytes) during the second month following onset of acute illness. This is part of a vigorous host response that is presumably aimed at controlling viral replication during the acute stage of infection. Here we report seven subjects with primary HIV-1 infection who were treated with zidovudine (AZT) and in whom this acute CD8+ response was significantly depressed, compared with an untreated control group."

L. Mecure et al (Immunology, 1994 Jul, 1(4):482-5) reports that "AZT, but not two other nucleosides tested, inhibited the Interleukin-2 dependent proliferation of CD8+ lymphocytes in a dose-dependent manner." Writing in the New England Journal of Medicine (10/30/97). Michael Oldstone MD states: "Cytotoxic T lymphocytes have an important role in controlling HIV infection, and loss of their activity in the end stages of HIV infection leads to an increased viral load...A single peptide molecule, in complex with the correct MHC molecule on the cell's surface, is sufficient to generate a cytotoxic -T- lymphocyte response. In contrast, more than 5×10^6 antibody molecules, as well as complement, are required to lyse a virally infected cell."

Olstone reported on a case of a patient whose CD8 cytotoxic lymphocyte response rallied against the HIV infection, causing viral load to drop from 300,000 to 1000 copies per ml. Despite AZT's success in lowering HIV viral loads, AZT fails to restore the immune response needed to prevent opportunistic infections, because it has been found to suppress CD8 cytotoxic lymphocyte activity. AZT, DDI and DDC have been reported to have a toxic effect on the mitochondria, where Adenosine Tri-Phosphate (ATP) is produced. ATP is needed to help transport antigen to the cell's membrane, where it is bound to MHC molecules. E. Benbrik et al (J Neurol Sci 1997 Jul;149(1):19-25) states: "AZT, DDI and DDC all exert cytotoxic effects...and induce alterations of mitochondria...All 3 compounds can inhibit mitochondrial mtDNA polymerase..." By impairing mitochondria function and ATP production, AZT, DDI and DDC also impair antigen presentation and an effective cell mediated immune response against HIV, HHV-6A and other intracellular infections.

In one study, AZT was used with Norvir and 3TC. In the first two weeks, there were significant increases in both CD4 and CD8 counts, but a 15% decrease in Natural Killer cells. An immunosuppressive drug like AZT can eventually spoil the benefits of a good drugs like Norvir and Epivir, over time. Depressing Natural Killer cell activity leaves you with little or no immunity against cancer and lymphomas. The most important fact to note about drug cocktail combinations is that all drugs in the same class are not created equal and neither are the combinations. There are both good and bad drug cocktail combinations. Only by monitoring immune function on a continuous basis will we ever know which combinations will have long-term benefits in preventing and remitting opportunistic infections.

Ziagen (Abacavir) and Trizivir?

The FDA approved (Ziagen) Abacavir for the treatment of AIDS. A few people have died from strong allergic reactions to the drug. It has been reported in several AIDS publications that if you ever get a rash from Abacavir, you can never use it again. It will kill you. One person from New York who used the drug developed impaired thyroid function. For the time being, I would avoid this one. While DDI has been a disaster when used in combination with AZT and protease inhibitors, DDI and Hydroxyurea has substantially reduced HIV viral load in some persons, while others report they cannot tolerate the side effects. Glaxo Wellcome markets a drug combination called Trizivir that is a combination of Abacavir, AZT and 3TC. In my opinion, two bad drugs (Abacavir and AZT) and one good (Epivir also called 3TC) do add up to a good treatment.

Structured treatment interruptions & self-immunization

Fred Walters experiment with a Pulsed Protocol

Houston, TX. Fred Walters who directs the Houston Buyers Club is open as far as his HIV status is concerned. Recently he shared the results of a 3-month experiment pulsing HIV meds one week on and week off from December 2003 through February 2004.

Mark: What HIV meds did you use during these 3 months?

Fred: I used a simple formula – Viramune and Combivir. I took these two drugs for 7 days, then took 7 days off. This cycle went on for 3 months.

Mark: Combivir is AZT and 3TC. How did you feel while on this combination?

Fred: I felt fine.

Mark: What other supplements did you use?

Fred: I used IP6, Beta Glucan, and a Ginseng product called CM4 and numerous vitamin and mineral supplements.

Mark: What were the results?

Fred: The CD4's increased from 350 to 650. The viral load decreased from 50,000 to 5,000.

Mark: Are you still on this pulsed protocol?

Fred: No, I stopped this month in March. I am satisfied with the results and I am going to be off the drugs for a while. When the CD4's get into the 300 range again, I will resume the use of the HIV meds using either this combo or some other one.

Mark: What products have you found helpful in increasing CD4 counts?

Fred: IP6 and CM4, the ginseng product made by Omega NutriPharm in Birmingham, AL. I have followed 4 cases where CM-4 has increased the CD4 counts.

Mark: Have you found any supplements that lower triglycerides?

Fred: Yes. Fish oil capsules (3 to 6 daily) lowers triglyceride levels.

Mark: What about diarrhea in persons using protease inhibitors?

Fred: About 2000 mgs daily of calcium citrate will stop that in most cases. If there is too much stomach acid already – acid reflux, calcium carbonate or coral calcium works best as it lowers the stomach acid at the same time. If the calcium supplements do not stop the diarrhea, they should ask their physician to check them for parasites.

Note: Fred can be reached during the day in Houston, Texas at 713-520-5288

Long-term immunological control of HIV

Wodarz D, Nowak MA.
Proc Natl Acad Sci U S A. 1999 Dec 7;96(25):14464-9.

Institute for Advanced Study, Olden Lane, Princeton, NJ 08540, USA. wodarz@ias.edu

We used mathematical models to study the relationship between HIV and the immune system during the natural course of infection and in the context of different antiviral treatment regimes. The models suggest that an efficient cytotoxic T lymphocyte (CTL) memory response is required to control the virus.

We define CTL memory as long-term persistence of CTL precursors in the absence of antigen. Infection and depletion of CD4 T helper cells interfere with CTL memory generation, resulting in persistent viral replication and disease progression.

We find that antiviral drug therapy during primary infection can enable the development of CTL memory. In chronically infected patients, specific treatment schedules, either including deliberate drug holidays or antigenic boosts of the immune system, can lead to a re-establishment of CTL memory.

Immune restoration in patients with HIV: HAART and beyond.

Verheggen R.J Assoc Nurses AIDS Care. 2003 Nov;14(6):76-82.

Integrative Medicine Center, Advocate Illinois Masonic Medical Center, Chicago, IL,

Since the introduction of highly active antiretroviral therapy (HAART), there has been a dramatic decrease in HIV-related morbidity and mortality. Suppressing HIV replication by HAART can result in a restoration of the CD4+ T-cell count and, consequently, a diminished risk of opportunistic infections.

However, the degree of immune restoration that can be achieved with HAART varies from patient to patient. It is often incomplete and can be poorest in those patients who, because of their very low CD4+ counts, need it the most. Additional approaches are needed to increase immune restoration still further. Structured treatment interruptions, therapeutic immunization, and recombinant interleukin-2 are three such options that are currently being investigated.

A skin test to measure immune response

Self-Test: A quick way to determine if a drug cocktail combination is improving or depressing immune function, or how the immune system is working during a structured interruption period, is to observe the DTH skin response to a topical application of DNCB. If the DTH response gets stronger, cell mediated immunity (CMI) is improving; if it gets weaker or stops, antigen presentation and CMI are failing.

From readers who have used Norvir in combination with 3TC, we know DTH responses to DNCB improve dramatically and flu-like symptoms often occur, an indication of cell-mediated immune activation. These strong reactions to DNCB can occur in as little as a few hours after taking Norvir. Testing DTH responses to DNCB is a fast screening test to evaluate the potential of a drug cocktail combination to help in immune restoration. Anecdotal reports from readers who have used either AZT or DDI with protease inhibitors indicate that DTH responses to DNCB get weaker or stop completely.

The HIV Drug book

The HIV Drug Book, by Project Inform (www.projinf.org) is published by POCKET BOOKS and is available in most bookstores. The 688-page book lists almost every drug used in the treatment of AIDS, its benefits, side effects and drug interactions. For anyone who uses drugs to treat HIV/AIDS, it is a must reference book. The information in this book can help you self-diagnosis drug-related symptoms that your physician may overlook. Persons taking several drugs may need to consider the side effects of each drug plus the side effects of the various drug combination interactions.

In 1996, a local PWA faithfully took 20 drugs prescribed by his physician and then died. Physicians will not admit that intereactions due to drugs they prescribe can kill a patient. Patients must stop allowing themselves to be used as guinea pigs and educate themselves about the drugs they use. Benefits and side effects of drugs are also found in the Physicians Desk Reference available at your local library. There are several news HIV drugs in the pipeline.You can learn more about these new classes of drugs at www.acria.org or call 212-924-3934 for a copy of the ACRIA publication.

Note: "The HIV Drug Book," is not recommended as a source of information on immune-based therapies.

18

Osteoporosis and Bone Mineral Density

Loss of bone density affects millions of people

The aging population, women with PMS, and millions of people addicted to soda pop especially Coke, Pepsi, Tab and all the other sodas high in phosphoric acid, are developing weaker bone structures by the day. A lack of quality sources of calcium, dark green vegetables, almonds, etc and lack of sunshine that produces Vitamin D all contribute to the national osteoporosis epidemic.

The end result is that more people are getting surgery for damaged spinal vertebrae, knee and hip replacements. Those not getting these drastic measures have lower and upper back pain and/or bone pain in the legs and arms. When you walk into a grocery store and look at the long isles of soda pop, cookies and sweet rolls, you can see why America's health is going to hell in a shopping cart.

Research on the benefits of Black Cohosh and Red Clover

Black Cohosh inhibits HIV and cancer.

Sakurai N et al reports that Actein, a tetracyclic triterpenoid from black cohosh showed potent activity against the HIV virus. (1) Einbond LS et al researchers at Columbia Univ College in NY found growth inhibitory activity of alcohol based extracts of black cohosh on human breast cancer cells. Research continues as to why Actein and other compounds in black cohosh would inhibit breast cancer. (2)

Powles T writing in Breast cancer Research, states: *"Plant extracts such as Red Clover, which contain high levels of isoflavanoids, have been used to reduce menopausal symptoms and have been shown to reduce bone loss in healthy women."* (3)

In her book on "Today's Herbal Health," Louise Tenny M.H. states that Red Clover has been used for bronchitis, as a blood purifier, in treating cancer and for the nerves.

Black Cohosh: In a study published in the Journal of Bone Mineral Metabolism (4), Nisselein T et al reported on the results of an extract of Black Cohosh given to rats who were ovariectomized and placed on a soy-free diet. They were given a Black cohosh product called "Remifemin" that has been marketed in Europe for the treatment of hot flashes in women with PMS. The researchers checked for markers of bone loss in the urine including pyridinoline (PYR) and deoxypyridinoline (DPY) and baseline and weekly intervals. The results indicated that the extract of black cohosh significantly diminished the urinary content of PYR and DPY indicating that bone loss was decreasing.

Nisslein stated: *"Because extracts of black cohosh are already recognized as safe and effective in the treatment of certain gynecological disorders, a longer-term clinical trial of this herbal remedy for the treatment of osteoporosis is warranted."* (4)

Folk medicine uses: Louise Tenny reports Black Cohosh has been used as a tonic for the central nervous system, for hot flashes, for asthma, bronchitis, epilepsy, high blood pressure, hormone balance, menstrual problems, menopause, TB and whooping cough.

Black Cohosh and Red Clover may help prevent and even strengthen bone density as well as be an adjunct treatment for cancer. This is in comparison to low dose estrogen (hormone replacement therapy) that helps prevent bone loss but is also known to be carcinogenic. A search of the literature indicates that black cohosh and red clover are safe choices for both men and women.

Licorice is a herb that taken in small amounts can benefit the adrenal glands of men and women. However, too much may cause high blood pressure.

Holy Basil (Ocimum Sanctum) is used in India as a Cox-2 inhibitor and reduces inflammation in the body. In animal studies, the "Control rats" under noise stress had a decline in cortisol levels while the rats taking Holy Basil and exposed to the same noise stress had cortisol levels that remained the same. This indicates that Holy Basil has anti-stress effects (5).

1. Anti-AIDS agents – Actein from black cohosh, Sakurai et al; Bioorg Med Chem Lett. 2004 Mar 8;14(5):1329-32
2. Black Cohosh on human breast cancer cells, Einbond ES et al; Breast Cancer Res Treat. 2004 Feb;83(3):221-31
3. Isoflavones and women's health, Powles T Breast Cancer Res 2004;6(3):140-2
4. "rat model of osteoporosis" Nisselein T et al, J Bone Miner Metab 2003;21(6):370-6
5. Indian J Physiol Pharma. 1997 Oct;41(4):429-30

Osteoporosis and HIV Meds:

A few months ago, I talked with a 31 year-old man from the Midwest who had recently had hip replacement surgery. I said: "31 years old – you are too young for hip replacement surgery." He said he was HIV+ and mentioned a long list of HIV meds he was taking. He blamed his hip bone deterioration on the HIV. I told him I disagreed as there is no proof that HIV alone can cause this especially in someone this young. Most of the reported cases of osteoporosis now widespread in the HIV community in the US have occurred since 1996 when the use of protease inhibitors and drug cocktails became a treatment standard. I don't recall hearing of any cases of osteoporosis in HIV+ people before 1996. Today the problem of bone deterioration in HIV+ persons on anti-HIV drugs is an epidemic and may be a serious side effect of some HIV medications.

Emerging drug toxicities of highly active antiretroviral therapy

by Heath KV, Montaner JS, Bondy G, Singer J, O'Shaughnessy MV, Hogg RS.
Curr Drug Targets. 2003 Jan;4(1):13-22.
Centre for Excellence in HIV/AIDS, University of British Columbia, Vancouver, Canada.

To provide an overview of the epidemiologic parameters of emerging adverse effects associated with antiretroviral therapy for human immunodeficiency virus (HIV) disease. All available antiretroviral agents are associated with significant adverse drug effects. Of particular interest are newly emerging suspected adverse drug effects which were not generally noted in pre-marketing trials nor captured under current standard clinical care practices. Suspected antiretroviral toxicities meeting these criteria include: HIV-associated lipodystrophy which can include peripheral lipoatrophy, lipohypertrophy and metabolic abnormalities; hyperlactatemia and lactic acidosis; and metabolic bone abnormalities such as decreased bone mineral density, osteoporosis and osteonecrosis.

Results of prospective and observational studies reported to date suggest that these abnormalities, while aetiologically complex, are likely attributable to treatment factors and may be intricately interrelated. The medical management of these symptoms remains unsatisfactory given the unexplored efficacy of traditional approaches in the HIV positive population. While the pathogenic mechanism of these disorders remains obscure, a theory of tissue-specific mitochondrial toxicity has been proposed.

With the continued introduction of novel therapies and standard treatment with combination therapy, new adverse events will continue to emerge among persons being treated for HIV disease. Beyond their immediate clinical implications, these events may contribute to changing patterns of antiretroviral utilization including therapy initiation, adherence and cessation.

Editor's Note: There is disagreement among the experts whether or not HAART for HIV is causing loss of bone density with some studies saying it is and others saying it is not with a few studies finding that the length of time a person is infected is a more predictable factor for osteoporosis. There is a case to be made for both arguments, but suspicions that the protease inhibitors are contributing factors is gaining some traction.

To preserve Bone Mineral Density, consider the following

1. Exercise – Walk 3 to 5 miles a day or find an active hobby like dancing or roller skating. Throw away the remote control for the TV.

2. Diet – AVOID Coca Cola, Pepsi Cola, Tab etc and other sodas that contain phosphoric acid. Phosphoric acid leeches calcium out of your bones and directly destroys vertebrae in the spinal column. I know two people who were one case a day drinkers of Coke for over a decade that have since had back surgery for ruptured discs and are now limited to a wheel chair. Unable to walk normally, they live with constant back pain.

AVOID SALT Sodium Chloride increases bone mineral loss among many other adverse effects. Try to keep sodium intake to 500 mg daily or less, not the 2500 to 5000 mg currently consumed.

Eat whole foods - fruit, vegetables, nuts (almonds) and cultured foods – yogurt, cottage cheese, and no sweets with added corn syrup or white sugar added.

3. Calcium lactate – 4 to 6 capsules once daily in the evening. Note: People with very acid stomachs may do better using Coral Calcium which also neutralizes the stomach acid..

4. Cod liver oil (1 tsp daily) or other natural sources of vitamin D (indoor tanning)

5. Magnesium Citrate or magnesium oxide – about 500 mg daily

6. Boron and trace minerals – Marine Liquid Ionic Minerals from the Great Salt Lake Utah 20 to 40 drops daily. Zinc deficiency has been associated with loss of BMD in men. (Suggestion: eat pumpkin seeds daily for zinc and the prostate).

7. Nutrients: Vitamin B 12 deficiency has been associated with loss of bone density in vegetarians. Daily B12 should be considered.

8. Herbs to help preserve mineral bone density -

a. Black Cohosh – 2 capsules twice daily and/or

b. Red Clover – 2 capsules twice daily.

9. Natural Hormones to help preserve BMD

a. Progesterone cream or consider Wild Yam capsules or extract.

b. DHEA – low dose for men or women over 40 years of age. Dr Brownstein's recommendations: For men over 40 – 25 mg 3 days a week (Mon, Weds, Fri). For women – 10 mg daily for 5 days per week or 25 mg twice a week (e.g. Mon and Fri). Have your physician monitor DHEA levels after 4 to 8 weeks. Brownstein advises against high doses of DHEA (over 25 mg daily) as this can reduce adrenal production of other hormones

Other hormone herbs: For women – Dong Quai, Damiana. For men – Ginseng, Sarsaparilla.

19

Bio-oxidative Therapies

Ozone – the "good" (negatively charged) and the "bad" (positively charged)

Medical ozone has a wide range of health benefits and, for most purposes, should be administered by a trained health care professional, although ozone rectal insufflation, ozone in a sauna bag and ozonated olive oil or glycerin can be safely used at home by an informed patient. In terms of medical opinion, ozone has been both over rated and under rated. Many people have a bad opinion of ozone, based on news reports of "ozone alerts" that occur, when sunlight causes (positively charged) ozone to form in the presence of air pollutants.

This "bad ozone" is produced by sunlight in polluted air and possesses a positive electrical charge and steals electrons, much like a free radical would. This bad ozone can make it difficult for someone to breathe and, when inhaled, slows down the production of energy in the cells and causes fatigue, both mental and physical. Positively charged (i.e. electron-deficient) ozone produced by the Sun's ultraviolet light in the presence of pollutants not only has no medicinal value, it is harmful to the body when inhaled and especially to those with emphysema, asthma or heart conditions.

In contrast, the "good ozone" used for medicinal purposes has a negative electrical charge and is the same as the ozone that is naturally produced in a lightning storm. This good ozone consists of three or more atoms of oxygen attached in groups or chains and possessing extra electrons that can be donated. This "good ozone" invigorates the body and increases the energy output of the cells. Today, ozone produced with electricity is used to disinfect hundreds of municipal water supplies throughout the world, including the City of Milwaukee, that added it after the cryptosporidium outbreak in 1991.

Ozone is a triatomic form of oxygen that is highly unstable. It is the most powerful oxidizer known to man next to fluorine. Ozone is produced naturally in lightning storms, in pine forests and by the action of the sun's ultraviolet light on oxygen. It is also produced in small quantities by ultraviolet light in a sun tanning bed. Negative ionizers produce small amounts of ozone along with negative ions. Ozone in water will kill viruses 3125 faster than chlorine (from Milwaukee Public Library Science Section). Ozone is the most potent anti-viral substance known to man that is safe to use in controlled doses and is effective against viruses, even in low concentrations. However, it is not effective against bacterial and fungal infections in low concentrations.

Ozone is produced commercially and for home use by a machine that passes oxygen through a glass tube subject to high voltage. The cold spark method produces ozone of consistent concentration. The hot spark method of producing ozone is not safe for medical purposes as ozone concentration may start off very high and then drop off suddenly. As the oxygen absorbs electrons, it forms clusters of O_3 and even higher forms of ozone - O_4, O_5 and O_6. In the presence of water, ozone (O_3) breaks down to O_2 plus O_1. In the process of breaking down, ozone releases electrons into the water. The difference between hydrogen peroxide and ozone is electrons. While both are oxidizers, only ozone releases free electrons. Because of this unique quality, ozone (negatively charged) destroys free radicals.

The definition of a free radical is "a substance that steals electrons from healthy cells." In this way, free radicals can damage normal cells. Hydrogen peroxide is a natural part of the life cycle and is produced by granulocytes as a first line, without causing free radical damage. This is due to an enzyme called "catalase," present in normal healthy cells which inactivates hydrogen peroxide. However, if catalase reserves become depleted, hydrogen peroxide in high concentrations can have an aging effect on normal cells, like free radicals. Catalase reserves in cells can be enhanced by a diet high in natural carotenes found in raw vegetables (raw potatoes are high in catalase and alpha lipoic acid) and anti-oxidant supplementation.

Ozone's effect on the immune system

In an article written by Dr. Horst Kief of Germany, he reports on using ozone in HIV+ patients. He claims that B cell function more than doubles during ozone therapy, increasing antibody production. Several sources have told me that, while ozone therapy is underway, about half will have increases in T4 counts and half will have decreases. This source also reported one patient that had excess B cells returned to normal values, after ozone therapy, and that Monocytes, Granulocytes and Lymphocytes moved toward normal values, after several ozone treatments.

Several anecdotal cases, including some written by Dr. John Pittman, appear to confirm this observation of T4 count increases, after ozone therapy is stopped. An example is a case reported by Dr. Pittman of a person who started with a T4 count of 600 in July 1991. After one month of receiving autohemotherapy daily, his T4 count dropped to 400. Then ozone therapy was stopped and in 2 months it rose to 900. Dr. Pittman reports on a second case of a person who underwent 70 autohemotherapy treatments, starting with low doses of ozone that were gradually increased to 10,000 mcg per treatment. He started with a T4 count of 153. He also received 70 infusions of Vitamin C and Herb's. After ozone therapy was stopped, his T4 count rose to 928 in June 1992.

An article published in an Italian Medical Journal - HAEMATOLOGICA, 1990; 75:510-5, by Prof. Velio Bocci of the Instituto di Fisiologia Genrale, Sienna, Italy is titled: "STUDIES ON THE BIOLOGICAL EFFECTS OF OZONE - INDUCTION OF INTERFERON ON HUMAN LEUCOCYTES." reports on several tests that show that after ozone autohemotherapy treatments, using concentration of ozone ranging from 2.2 mcg/ml to 42 mcg/ml, there was in increase in interferon along with an increase in Tumor Necrosis Factor and Interleukin II. Concentrations of ozone in autohemotherapy above 42 mcg/ml produced no interferon and stressed the membranes of red blood cells. The best results were seen at 42 mcg/ml, while a very small amount of IFN production occurred at 2.2 mcg/ml. The report concluded: "The results presented in this paper show that under strictly defined conditions of ozonisation, PBMC, either in whole blood or after isolation, can be induced to produce significant amounts of Interferon."

Ozone stops CMV and hepatitis

In January, 1994, I talked with Dr. Shallenberger, M.D., Minden, NV. He has used IV ozone on over 20 patients with HIV. One patient had been on Ganciclovir for CMV for sometime. Dr. Shallenberger said: "If he stopped using the Ganciclovir for 1 week, he began to lose his eyesight. After receiving 10 treatments of ozone over a two month period and then stopping the treatments, it took 2 and 1/2 months before the CMV became active again." Persons doing Ozone at home will need an aggressive program to reverse active CMV. See protocols for CMV in the chapter on "Symptoms and Remedies." Shallenberger also told me of two patients on ozone autohemotherapy that completely cleared the Hepatitis B virus from the blood in three weeks.

Ozone therapy choices

Major Autohemotherapy (M.A.H.) is the process of removing a pint of blood and adding ozone gas to it and returning it to the patient's body. It was originally developed in Germany. Major autohemotherapy is considered to be safe and effective. Autohemotherapy is the treatment of choice for all conditions affecting the blood. Hundreds of thousands of treatments have been safely used in Germany for the past several decades. Intravenous Ozone, called I.V. infusions, is used by some physicians in the United States, but is not used in Europe. IV ozone treatment requires continuous monitoring to prevent too much ozone gas from entering the blood at one time, which could cause an embolism. In IV, small amounts of ozone gas are directly fed into a vein over a period of time. One problem with I.V. ozone is a hardening of the vein at the site of entry. A new technique is being developed by Renate Viebahn for I.V. ozone, where it first is placed into a solution and then the solution is used in an i.v. drip. If the new technique is successful, it could simplify ozone treatments and lower their cost to patients. Since this new technique is still being developed, I would advise Physicians not to use I.V. ozone at this time, but to use Major Autohemotherapy that has an excellent track record for safety and effectiveness.

Home methods include Rectal Ozone insufflation, where ozone is fed into the colon for about 1 and 1/2 minutes per treatment at concentrations up to 27 mcg/ml. The average adult colon can hold about 750 ml (about 3/4 or a liter). Another home method is the use of a Sauna bag filled with ozone gas. The patient gets into a plastic suit or Sauna Bag, after taking a shower, and fills the suit or bag with ozone gas for absorption through the skin. Concentration of ozone from 20 to 30 mcg/ml is used. The person stays in the Sauna Bag with the ozone flowing continuously at a rate from 1/2 to 1 L.P.M. for 30 to 45 minutes per treatment. The Sauna Bag method is very effective for treating burns and preventing the formation of scar tissue. Other treatments, like bathing in ozonated water, are considered by many people, including myself, to be less effective than the Sauna Bag. However, in one case, drinking 2 glasses of ozonated water each day, along with 30 minutes in the Sauna Bag, produced impressive results in raising white blood counts, normalizing blood pressure and pulse rates in just two weeks.

The effectiveness of various ozone treatments

On a scale of 1 to 10, with 10 being the most effective, I would rate both autohemotherapy and I.V. ozone at a 10, with autohemotherapy being the safest. For autohemotherapy, concentration of ozone should be 30 mcg/ml. 200 ml. of ozone should be mixed with 200 m.l. of blood in a 500 ml bag per treatment for adults. Autohemotherapy is the treatment of choice and should be administered by a Physician. Only medical grade oxygen is to be used for autohemotherapy.

For home use, the Sauna Bag method is very promising, if done 30 to 45 minutes daily. With the Sauna Bag method, there were two cases of swollen lymph nodes completely disappearing. Two cases of complete remission of Herpes were reported. While the overall results were encouraging, in terms of T4 counts, results have been mixed. While the Sauna Bag method was effective for most problems in the skin and in the lymph system, it was totally ineffective for problems of the gastro-intestinal tract, like diarrhea. As compared to Autohemotherapy, I would rate the Sauna bag method at a 4.

On Ozone rectal insufflation, I have 4 confirmed cases of increases in T4 counts and 2 cases of decreases. In all 4 cases of T4 count increases, rectal insufflation was done 3 to 5 times a week with about 750 cc (3/4 of a liter) in the range of 20 to 30 mcg/ml. In both cases of T4 count decreases, ozone rectal insufflation was done only once a week. Rectal insufflation, done daily, has been reported by Dr. Michael Carpendale of San Francisco as effective against all types of diarrhea, except for cryptosporidium. Rectal ozone insufflation should always be done after giving yourself a warm water enema. Concentrations of ozone should be in the range of 20 to 22 mcg/ml. Treatment should be done 5 times a week with 2 days off. For HIV, hepatitis and herpes, I would rate rectal insufflation at a 5.

An excellent protocol would be to do the Sauna Bag method one day and rectal insufflation the next day, and to do this alternating combination 6 days a week, with one day off. A combination of the Sauna Bag alternated with rectal insufflation would probably yiekd a higher rating such as a 6 or 7. In interpreting the data, most failures with ozone therapy are attributable to the failure to deliver enough ozone into the blood supply to attain positive results. A second and equally important cause of failure is to rely on ozone alone to reverse AIDS, and not to change the diet to eliminate junk food and destructive habits like alcohol and tobacco.

Up to a 100% loss of ozone when used with a humidifier

In Sept 1993, several domestic "experts" on ozone advised us to recommend the use of a humidifier with ozone to activate the ozone and to prevent irritation and burning in the colon from high concentrations of ozone. We were also told by several of the same "experts" that the effective concentration of ozone for rectal insufflation was from 27 to 32 mcg/ml. As it now turns out, they were right on one point and wrong on another. Humidified ozone will not burn the colon, as most of the ozone is either absorbed by the water it passes through or inactivated by it.

A test was done by passing ozone gas through a humidifier containing 8 fl. ozs of distilled water. The ozone unit that was used for the test was manufactured by Ozotech (Yreka, CA), Model OZ2PCS. This unit produces ozone by the cold spark method. Ozone output is

17.2 mcg/ml at a flow rate of 1/2 liter per minute. The ozone input into the humidifier was adjusted at 17 mcg/ml, using an Ozone analyzer. The water temperature was 72 degrees F.

Ozone

INPUT	TIME (Minutes)	OZONE OUTPUT (Humidified)
17 mcg/ml	1	0.0 mcg/ml
17 mcg/ml	2	1.3 mcg/ml
17 mcg/ml	3	4.1 mcg/ml
17 mcg/ml	4	7.4 mcg/ml
17 mcg/ml	5	9.0 mcg/ml
17 mcg/ml	6	11.7 mcg/ml
17 mcg/ml	7	13.2 mcg/ml
17 mcg/ml	8	14.4 mcg/ml
17 mcg/ml	9	15.3 mcg/ml
17 mcg/ml	10	15.8 mcg/ml
17 mcg/ml	11	16.2 mcg/ml
17 mcg/ml	12	16.4 mcg/ml

The experiment was stopped after 12 minutes. Even after 12 minutes, the ozone output did not match the input of 17 mcg/ml. It shows that ozone rectal insufflation, done within the first 3 minutes of turning on an ozone machine, would be approximately 90% ineffective. To be 90% effective, ozone would have to be continuously passed through the humidifier for 9 minutes before it is inserted into the colon. It is little wonder that people using humidified ozone immediately after turning on the ozone unit were not getting desired results. In place of the humidifier, we are recommending an enema of purified water before doing rectal insufflation. Second, we are suggesting an ozone concentration output for rectal insufflation range from 17 mcg/ml to 22 mcg/ml or .4 LPM for the OZ2PCS or 1 LPM for the OZ4PC10 (Ozotech). You will need data from the manufacturer on ozone output at various flow rates, when using other models, or rent an analyzer to find out exactly how much ozone the unit produces. In purifying water, complete destruction of germs and bacteria occurs at concentration as low as 1 mcg/ml. We don't buy the argument that you need ozone concentrations of 27 to 32 mcg/ml for rectal insufflation to get effective results. Concentrations in that range will produce a burning sensation in the colon, if done without doing a warm water enema first.

We also ran a test passing ozone through 8 fl ozs. of olive oil at 17 mcg/ml and found a zero ozone output for 20 minutes, at which time we discontinued the experiment. This means that the ozone totally inter-reacts with the olive oil, allowing none to escape. We do not know what types of oxidative byproducts are formed or if ozone is actually stored in the olive oil. Only chemical analysis of the ozonated olive oil will determine if there is any ozone in it and how long it lasts at a given temperature, or if there are oxidative byproducts with germicidal properties that could last for long periods of time. Last fall, we had done an experiment ozonating glycerin and found its disinfectant properties lasted only 7 days, when stored in a refrigerator.

High quantities of low concentrations of ozone believed to be more beneficial that high concentrations of ozone

Viebahn and Rilling's book on The Use of Ozone in Medicine (Haug Publishers, Germany) suggest that small concentrations of ozone are immune stimulating with a range of 10 to 20 mcg/ml for immune stimulation. In autohemotherapy, most of the sources I have spoken with indicate that immune depression starts at ozone concentrations over 35 mcg/ml. Concentrations over 35 mcg/ml may be harmful to red blood cell membranes, particularly in those persons who have been on junk food diets and have not taken antioxidants. At the same time, Viebahn recommends high concentrations up to 70 mcg/ml for their germicidal effect.

This creates a "Catch-22" situation where, if you use high concentrations of ozone or an antibiotic to kill an infection, you will also suppress the immune system. Our own observations are that you don't need high concentrations of ozone to have a germicidal effect, if you increase the total amount of ozone absorbed in a given treatment. In other words, if the protocol is designed right, you can attain both effects simultaneously. That is, you can kill off the infections, while stimulating the immune system at the same time. If you take 10 Vitamin C tablets each containing 100 mg of Vitamin C, you will ingest 1000 mg of Vitamin C. If you apply the logic of the "experts" you would need to take the 1000 mg of Vitamin C in one tablet. Their argument is not logical. 1000 mg of Vitamin C is the same dose, whether you take it in one tablet or in 10 tablets.

At the March, 1994 IBOM conference in Dallas, TX, Dr. Shallenberger recommended 100 ml of blood mixed with 100 ml of ozone at 40 mcg/ml (4,000 mcg total). We would suggest using a higher quantity of blood and ozone and to add ozone at a lower concentration - that is, mix 200 ml of blood with 200 ml of ozone at a concentration of 30 mcg/ml (6,000 mcg total). A higher quantity of ozone at a lower concentration will result in a higher percentage of patients having increases in their CD4 counts, along with more destruction of viruses and other pathogens. This would be the suggested dose for an adult of 140 to 180 lbs. For children, use a proportionally smaller dose.

Warm water enema before ozone insufflation

The use of an enema of warm water before inserting the catheter for rectal insufflation is recommended to clean the colon and remove feces that can obstruct the absorption of the ozone gas. Use one pint to 1 quart of purified warm water. An Enema/Douche Kit sold in drugstores will work fine. Water from the hot water side of the tap is usually safe. You can also use distilled water that is preozonated for 3 minutes with a sandstone bubbler for enemas prior to insufflation.

How to do ozone rectal insufflation

To do direct ozone rectal insufflation, ozone concentration should be set for 15 to 20 mcg/ml. After turning on ozone unit and allowing it to run for 1 minute or until you smell the output of ozone, insert catheter into colon. Allow 500 to 750 M.L. of ozone gas to enter colon, then remove the catheter. At 1/2 LPM, it takes 90 seconds to obtain 750 ML. If you feel excess pressure or pain at any time while doing the insufflation, remove the catheter immediately and redo your enema, or contact a Physician to determine if there is a colon obstruction. Retain ozone gas in colon for 15 minutes after the catheter is removed. While you can do direct ozone rectal insufflation from the ozone unit, a better method is to fill a Teflon bag with a shut off valve with 750 m.l. of ozone and then to squeeze the ozone into the colon quickly, to inflate the colon with the ozone. Ozone resistant bags are available in Germany (Viebahn). I have not located a U.S.source. Check with your Physician and medical supply sources.

Note: Some persons have run ozone continuously into the colon for up to 10 minutes per treatment at 1/2 LPM. By consciously relaxing the muscle, excess ozone gas is released as pressure builds up in the colon. The treatment is stopped early if cramping occurs.

For immune modulation only, ozone rectal insufflation should be done 2 or 3 times a week and not every day.

Side effects: Ozone rectal insufflation causes an initial release of mucus in the colon and sometimes a discharge of mucus and water that subsides after about one hour. Note: if there is any cramping or soreness in the colon area after an insufflation treatment, the ozone concentration should be reduced to 10 mcg/ml in the next treatment.

Ozone in a Sauna bag

Ozone in a Sauna Bag is done after taking a shower. Get into the Sauna bag wet. Ozone output for Sauna Bag is 1/2 to 1 LPM at a concentration of 20 to 30 mcg/ml. Ozone unit should run continuously 30 to 45 minutes per treatment. The exhaust fan should be on, while you are doing it, or you may wrap a wet towel around your neck to prevent breathing in too much ozone. When getting into the Sauna Bag, press the bag against your body to push the air out before turning on the Ozone. Start with your feet and push up toward your neckline. Leaving a lot of air in the bag when you start will dilute the ozone concentration and reduce the effectiveness of the treatment.

A word of caution for persons with gross catheters

Gross Catheters are implanted in the upper part of the chest area and are not ozone resistant and may be damaged during a Sauna Bag ozone treatment. If the Sauna Bag method is used, the upper drawstring should be lowered until it is below the Catheter to prevent high concentrations of ozone from coming into contact with the catheter. Also, no one should ever place anything in the catheter, unless it is prescribed by his or her Physician. GMHC (NY) recently reported one death, when a patient placed a high concentration of hydrogen peroxide in the Catheter. A gas embolism resulted.

Home Ozone protocols

1. Rectal Insufflation twice a week- Tues and Thurs. or Sauna Bag method - 30 to 45 minutes a day 3 days a week.

Do not use ozone within 3 hours after eating a heavy meal. You can be creative in designing your own treatment protocol. We suggest that you be consistent between blood test results. Take note of what makes you feel better and stronger.

Special notes for physicians

In Dr. Frank Shallenberger's presentation at IBOM in Dallas, TX. March, 1994, he recommended 100 ML of Ozone at a concentration of 40 mcg/ml mixed with 100 ml of blood for AHT. We are recommending a variation of his protocol that we believe will have a substantially more positive effect in raising CD4 counts. Specifically, I am suggesting drawing 200 ml of blood and mixing it with 200 ml of ozone at a concentration of 30 mcg/ml. Shallenberger's protocol gives 4000 mcg of ozone while our gives 6,000 mcg of ozone at a lower concentration. Several sources have reported that lower concentrations have a greater effect in immune stimulation. (See Ozone Compendium: IBOM). Very ill patients should be given two treatments daily (6,000 mcg of ozone each), until infections have substantially reduced, then one treatment daily, 5 days a week, is suggested, until the infection being treated has completely cleared from the blood. Monitoring white blood cell counts every 7 days will determine the degree of success in attaining immune stimulation. The goal is to get white blood cell counts into the upper level of the normal reference ranges or even slightly above it.

In Germany, a safety procedure used to prevent a patient from accidentally getting the wrong blood is to place a label with the patients name on it on the plastic bag into which the blood is to be drawn, before any treatment begins. It is a procedure that should be made mandatory for all employees. The day may come when you will be treating two or more patients with ozone at the same time.

Videotape on how to do "Major Autohemotherapy"

Medical doctors wanting to do major autohemotherapy should get the videotape of how to do it, made at the IBOM convention. You can obtain a copy by calling Tree Farm Cassettes at 800-468-0464 and asking for Dr. Frank Shallenberger M.D.'s workshop presentation on how to do major autohemotherapy. They can provide you with a complete list of other audio and videotape presentations available.

Now available – The 2nd English edition of "THE USES OF OZONE IN MEDICINE," by Renate Viebahn, PhD. This book is a must for physicians. It gives technical details for doing Major Autohemotherapy and how to use ozone for various medical applications. 187 pages. Soft cover. $29.95. Order from: Medicina Biologica, 2937 NE Flanders St, Portland, OR 97232. 503-287-6775. Add $4.00 for postage in the U.S. Canadians, add $5.00.

More information is available from The Int'l Ozone Assn., 31 Strawberry Hill Ave, Stamford, CT 06902, which has several publications on the uses of ozone in medicine. You may call them weekdays at 203-348-3542 for more information on the publications and their cost. Physicians should contact International Bio-Oxidative Medicine - call 405-478-4266 for an application form or write to IBOM, PO Box 891954, Okla City, OK 73189 to find out about the latest available video tapes on using medical ozone and seminar courses they offer to train physicians on the latest techniques of using autohemotherapy. Consumers can also contact IBOM to find the names and phone numbers of local physicians trained in the application of bio-oxidative therapies.

An earlier book, "THE THERAPEUTICAL APPLICATIONS OF HYDROZONE AND GLYCOZONE," by Chemist Charles Marchand was published in 1904. It reprints articles appearing in over 100 medical journals on the use of ozonated water and ozonated glycerin in treating infections of all kinds. Hydrozone is ozonated water, and Glycozone is ozonated glycerine. These products have a short shelf life. In spite of this, these ozonated products were used to treat every infectious disease known to man at that time. The articles are a culminative collection of successful anecdotal cases, using this unique form of oxidative therapy. Reprints of this book are available from: ECHO, PO Box 126, Delano, MN 55328. $17.00 a copy ppd.

Distributors of ozone units, Sauna bags and tents

Ozone units: Ozotech, Inc, 2401 Oberlin Rd, Yreka, CA 96097. Ozotech manufactures over a dozen varieties of ozone units for multiple purposes - 530-842-4189. www.ozotech.com. For consumers, a convenient unit with a built in oxygen accumulator and flow meter is model OZ2OEAP. Health care professionals may want to inquire about the suitcase model OZ2PTS-SS, made of stainless steel.

Cleanwater Systems - 800-837-8655. Check with more than one source before making a decision on purchasing an ozone unit. Ask for references and equipment specifications as well as ozone analyzer output data and who did the testing.

Sauna Bags and Ozone tents: Custom made sauna bags, ozone tents and for suits for specific body areas: Healing Arts at 818-992-1353

Regulators with built in Flowmeter (1/8, 1/4. 1/2, 3/4 and 1 LPM adjustable): B and F Medical Products - 419-729-0606 Model 81020 for Yoke type small oxygen tank or Model 83020 for nut type larger tanks. Physician's prescription required to purchase. Ozone resistant tubing can be obtained from the source that distributes Ozone units or from Tygon Tubing (Ozone resistant) - Type R3603 - Cope Plastics, 262-784-6882 Do not use rubber or PVC tubing from a local hardware store as this will release toxic gases. Note: Teflon tubing is hard to bend but is totally ozone resistant.

Dangers of ozone inhalation and antidotes

While inhaling a small amount of ozone is harmless, inhaling high concentrations of ozone for more than 10 minutes will do damage to the mucus membranes of the lungs. No one should set up any ozone unit in their home without having a bathroom exhaust fan or window exhaust fan. Over exposure to ozone can cause headaches and burning lungs and can lead to an asthma-like condition. Ozonating bath water will not work as hot water will not absorb ozone and most of the ozone will end up in the air you breathe. In the event of an ozone overdose, take 5,000 mg of Vitamin C or take oral EDTA to turn off the ozone reactions.

Ozonated Olive oil

The Uses of Ozone in Medicine, by Rilling and Viebahn, recommends the external use of ozonated olive oil for fungal infections, fistulae, anal fissure, decubitus, epidermorophyton, and mycosis. It is our opinion that ozonated olive oil should be effective for any external viral, bacterial of fungal infection and other uses for which ozone gas is also effective. That would include herpes, burns and the stimulation of wound healing. Ozonated olive oil must be stored in a refrigerator, or it will break down into oxygen in a few days. Do not ozonate more olive oil than you will use in 7 days. Ozonated olive oil may be used in conjunction with either rectal insufflation or the ozone body suit method.

You can make your own ozonated olive oil by buying a small sandstone from a pet shop that is used to bubble air in an Aquarium, or you can attach a brass of stainless steel fitting to the end of your hose. Take 4 to 8 ounces of olive oil and place it in a tall glass container. Attach the ozone outlet from the Ozone unit to the inlet of sandstone or brass fitting. Place sandstone or fitting in the bottom of the container and bubble ozone through olive oil for 5 to 10 minutes. Mark your bottle "Ozonated," and place it in your refrigerator until you are ready to use it. Use it within 2 days. To make a smaller quantity of ozonated olive oil for daily use, fill a 1 oz. shot glass with olive oil and hold output hose from ozone unit in bottom of shot glass for 10 minutes. Use immediately for best results. Note: One person said that ozonated olive oil was very effective in getting rid of herpes infections in his facial area.

Rectal insufflation - a case report

Ozone gas should never be bubbled through a Humidifier before using it, as the water in the Humidifier will absorb most of the ozone, rendering the treatment ineffective. One PWA, from St. Louis, MO, recently wrote that he has been doing rectal ozone insufflation since 1989 - about 5 years. He uses about 27 mcg/ml - a half liter three times a week and retains it for 20 minutes. He says his T4 count was in the 600 range 5 years ago and is in the 400 range today. He says he rarely uses prescription drugs and is in good health. Once a year, he does rectal insufflation every day for 21 days, then reduces treatment to 3 times a week.

Hydrogen Peroxide therapy

Two methods of using hydrogen peroxide are described here - bathing in hot water with a pint of 35% H2O2 added or oral H2O2. However, I do not recommend using both the ozone treatment and the hydrogen peroxide treatments in the same day as a regular course of treatment for long-term use. That is simply too much nascent oxygen for your body.

Oral hydrogen peroxide - benefits and side effects

Hydrogen peroxide is H2O2 which is one water molecule (H2O) with one nascent oxygen atom added (O1). While I don't recommend the long-term use of oral hydrogen peroxide, I want to report this story that I heard first hand. An Illinois man, first name

"John" told me he stopped using AZT and tried oral hydrogen peroxide drops. He started with 5 drops in a glass of water three times a day on an empty stomach - about 3 hours after meals. He used 35% H2O2 (food grade). He increased the dosage by one drop a day until he was taking 20 drops three times a day. After two months of using 20 drops 3X a day, he gradually reduced the dosage to 5 drops 3x. At that point, his T4 count was tested and it was over 800.

Updated protocol for using 35% H2O2 for HIV (2/25/95)

When ozone is not available or unaffordable, oral H2O2 may be used in its place for the following purposes: to kill HIV and raise T4 cell counts. Like Ozone, a pulsed therapy is recommended. For persons without symptoms - start with 5 drops of 35% H2O2 (food grade or reagent grade) in a glass of water 3 times a day on an empty stomach. Increase the dosage by 1 drop 3 times per day, until you are doing 20 drops 3 times a day. When you reach 20 drops 3X, continue this for 2 weeks, then reduce dosage by 1 drop 3 times a day until you are down to 5 drops 3 times a day. Then stop using hydrogen peroxide for 2 weeks and ,at the end of the second week, have your blood tested for T4 counts and NK counts (if available). This cycle will take 2 months, after which you repeat it. Do not get a blood test until you have stopped using H2O2 for 2 weeks, and do not wait for more than 4 weeks before getting tested. I believe that the high point in your T4 count will occur between the second and fourth week after you have stopped using the H2O2. After 4 weeks of being off either ozone or H2O2, existing information indicates that T4 counts may start to decline. Many of the infectious diseases that respond to ozone will also respond to H2O2 therapy. However, results from users indicate that Ozone is more effective for most conditions than H2O2. For persons with serious infections, use 10 drops in a glass of distilled water up to 7 times a day, until infection has subsided. Be sure to check body temperature and take supplements to raise it, if necessary.

Hydrogen peroxide and iron (well water) – a combination that produces free radicals

Inflammation of the stomach mucosa has occurred in some case where H2O2 was taken with well water, which is often high in iron. This combination produces Super Oxide Radicals, which can cause rapid breakdown of H2O2 in the stomach and irritate the G.I. tract. However, I have confirmed that, when these same persons switch from well water to distilled water, they had no problems taking H2O2 orally. The enzyme, catalase, which controls H2O2, is in low supply in the stomach area, while plentiful elsewhere in the body. By using distilled water, little H2O2 breaks down in the stomach and most of it is absorbed into the blood

Should an ulcerated condition develop from using H2O2 orally, it can be reversed by stopping the oral use of hydrogen peroxide, eating a bland diet and taking Herb's like whole leaf aloe vera juice and drinking cultured cabbage juice. However, this problem can be avoided by using distilled water, that should not create any problems. Supplements containing iron and blackstrap molasses should not be taken for 1 hr before or after taking

H2O2 orally.

Skin problems? try Oxy-spray

While the baths in warm water with a pint of 35% H2O2 added are an excellent choice in hydrogen peroxide treatment, Oxy-Spray contains Aloe Vera that heals many kinds of skin conditions. To make oxy-spray, mix 1 cup of 3% H2O2 (sold in drug stores) with 1 cup of aloe vera juice and place it in a spray bottle. This product contains 1.5% H2O2. Spray on the skin 2 or 3 times a day, where topical infections exist. A stronger formula is to mix one part 35% H2O2 with 5 parts of aloe vera juice. Place in a spray bottle. This mixture contains 6% H2O2. It can be sprayed on any ache or pain and on swollen lymph nodes.

For more information on Ozone and Hydrogen Peroxide for home and professional use, send for the book called "Hydrogen Peroxide and Ozone," by Conrad LeBeau. $3.95 plus $1 for postage. Send to Vital Health, 8544 W National Ave #21, West Allis, WI 53227 414-329-0648 or www.vhp4.com. Sources of 6% H2O2 solution food-grade are listed in the book.

Safe storage recommendations – Antidote for accidental ingestion

Note: Never store unmarked 35% H2O2 in a refrigerator, where it can be accidentally ingested. A refrigerator is to store food, not chemicals. Never assume that a visitor to your home will not accidentally drink some, when you are not looking. It will do damage to the stomach if accidentally ingested. It will remain liquid up to 35 degrees below zero. 35% H2O2 is too concentrated for direct application on the skin and must be diluted before using. 35% H2O2 may be stored safely and indefinitely in a freezer.

In the event of accidental ingestion of one teaspoon or more, do not attempt to induce vomiting, immediately drink a large amount of fruit juice (up to 1 quart) or a large quantity of water. Then eat one or more raw potatoes. Raw potatoes contain catalase, an enzyme that will break down the H2O2 into oxygen and water, and a lot of gas will be released. Charcoal capsules will need to be given immediately after eating the potato to help absorb the gas. Then, contact a physician or hospital and ask them to pump your stomach. After your stomach is empty, drink another pint of apple or other fruit juice and take 5,000 mg of regular Vitamin C to normalize (lower) the blood pH levels that will be elevated from the H2O2.

Note: There have been three recorded deaths from people drinking 35% H2O2 ,where they mistook it for water stored in a refrigerator and effective antidote procedures listed here were not followed.

20
Nutrition for immunity and weight gain

In Africa, AIDS is commonly called "Slim's Disease", as the infected person loses weight from diarrhea and malnutrition. In an article written in the ANNALS OF INTERNAL MEDICINE, Oct, 1984, by Donald Kotler, MD. et al, he writes: "The potential role of malnutrition in the clinical course of acquired immunodeficiency syndrome has not been emphasized. Protein-calorie malnutrition and deficiencies of specific nutrients, such as zinc, adversely affect cell-mediated immunity. Among other deficits, malnutrition decreases total T-lymphocyte counts, T-helper and suppresser counts, and IgA secretion. Of note, protein-calorie malnutrition has been believed to be an important factor in epidemics of Pneumocystis carinii pneumonia in children."

In another article published in THE AMERICAN JOURNAL OF GASTROENTEROLOGY, Oct, 1985, Dr. Brad Dworkin, MD et al writes: "Severely diminished plasma selenium levels were noted in AIDS patients. This manifestation most likely represents generalized protein-calorie malnutrition, rather than a specific defect in selenium metabolism....Therefore, it is possible that the malnutrition commonly seen in AIDS, including abnormalities of trace minerals, may lead to further impairment of immune function..."

Low-dose hydrocortisone for treating TNF and wasting syndrome

Serious weight loss in AIDS and cancer is almost always due to elevated levels of tumor necrosis factor (TNF). Low-dose hydrocortisone (20 to 30 mg daily) can help normalize the TNF and lower the IL-6 leading to weight gain. Fish oil supplements has also been found to do this in pancreatic cancer patients. See the chapter on the Adrenal glands and low–dose cortisol. Persons with serious loss of muscle mass would be well advised to use both hydrocortisone and fish oil supplements to loer the TNF and reverse the weight loss.

Whole lemon drink

The Whole Lemon drink is the most important drink you can take to return your weight to normal. The success of supplements to gain weight depends on returning your saliva pH to a normal 6.4. The saliva pH factor is indicative of how well you assimilate nutrients, including vitamins, minerals, amino acids, essential fatty acids and carbohydrates. Acidosis, indicated by an acid saliva pH, has always been associated with a failure to gain weight. In several PWA's I have consulted with, weight gain starts when saliva pH reaches 6.2. Once your saliva pH reaches 6.2, weight gain supplements will work effectively to gain lean muscle mass.

Note: If saliva pH does not return to normal in 7 days after starting on the whole lemon/olive oil drink, add lime water to your daily regimen- 1 tsp in a glass of water 3 times a day and/or drink one cup of fig juice daily. You may discontinue these very alkalizing supplements, when pH returns to normal.

A case report: J.C., PWA in Idaho, was using the whole lemon drink for several weeks, yet his saliva pH remained below 5.5 and he continued to lose weight and was 40 lbs underweight. He started using limewater daily (1 tablespoon twice a day) and within one week his saliva pH returned to a normal 6.4. Immediately, he began to gain weight at the rate or 2 to 3 pounds per week. After 3 months, he gained nearly 40 lbs and was back to his normal weight. What is also significant is that most of his weight gain was muscle and not fat. He continued to exercise and also used 30 grams daily of cold processed whey proteins.

ImmunePro - a good choice

Excellent cold processed protein supplements include ImmunePro or Immunocal. It is lactose free, sugar free and is easily digested. It is a cold processed whey product. Several persons have reported 1 to 3 pounds weight gain monthly of lean muscle mass, not fat. Available in health food stores. Others have reported weight gain from Designer Protein or Optimune. One local PWA, Doug, gained 25 lbs on Designer Protein alone, and it was muscle mass, not fat. More information on ImmunoPro can be found at www.wellwisdom.com.

Third international symposium on Nutrition and AIDS

Over 500 health care professionals attended the "Symposium on Nutrition and AIDS," along with a number of PWA's. The event was sponsored by Philadelphia Fight; Physicians Assn for AIDS Care and PA AIDS Education and Training Center on Oct 13-14, 1994. Speakers reported on products to stimulate appetite and weight gain. Pharmaceutical companies provided information on Megace, Testoderm (transdermal source of Testosterone), Marinol and nutritional drinks like Advera (Ross Labs). Advera is actually a good choice for persons with wasting syndrome, as it contains deodorized sardine oil, a source of omega-3 fatty acids (DHA/EPA) that promotes cell mediated immunity.

9/8/97 Update: Based on our successful efforts to increase body mass with cold processed whey proteins like Optimune and Designer Protein and the good results with the whole lemon/olive oil drink, I would advise using these options and to strictly avoid megace, which only adds body fat. Also avoid Testoderm and Testosterone therapy. Avoid Marijuana, as it suppresses DTH skin responses to DNCB. Especially avoid Megace and steroids to gain weight. They suppress cell mediated immunity and adrenal cortisol production. As for herbs, Siberian Ginseng and Sarsaparilla are good choices.

Vitamin and mineral absorption depends on normal saliva pH and calcium

Calcium is the mailman that carries nutrients into the cells, while saliva pH, when taken between meals in a resting mode, is a very important indicator of how well you are absorbing nutrients. A normal healthy person has a Saliva pH reading of 6.4, when taken before meals. When taken during a meal or immediately after a meal it should be around 7.2. The Immune enhancement diet, with its emphasis on alkaline vegetables, and particularly, the Whole Lemon/Olive oil drink, will restore saliva Ph to a normal value faster than anything else known. However, in a few cases, the whole lemon/olive oil drink alone did not restore pH to normal, then the use of lime water (calcium hydroxide) did the job. Use one teaspoon in a glass of water up to three times daily - a very alkaline formula or one tablespoon to a quart of water. Drink 2 or 3 glasses daily and you should see your saliva pH rapidly increase. Stop the limewater, when the saliva pH reaches normal levels. Another powerful alkalizing drink is fig juice or simply eat whole figs.

If you eat only wholesome foods, whole grains, vegetables, easily digested proteins (yogurt, cottage cheese, poached eggs, sprouts, pea soup, boiled meats etc.), and foods high in natural carotenes, like yams and squash, then most of you will not need to take dietary supplements, unless malabsorption of nutrients remains a problem. However, if you drink canned soda (coke, Pepsi etc.), eat white bread, pasta, pizza and other products made from white flour, sweets, pastry, cakes, etc., you certainly need vitamin and mineral supplementation.

I suggest that you avoid all the cheap synthetic vitamins that are often incorrectly marked "natural" and use only 100% whole-food based natural vitamin/mineral supplements like "Vitalerbs" by Dr. Christopher. Vitalerbs contains alfalfa, barley grass and kamut greens, dandelion, kelp, purple dulse, spirulina, irish moss, rose hips, beet, nutritional yeast, cayenne, blue violet, oatstraw, carrot juice and ginger.

Other whole food based vitamins are brewers yeast, desiccated liver, cod liver oil capsules, for vitamin C (Camu, Rose hips or Acerola cherries), for vitamin e (wheat germ oil or raw wheat germ), coral calcium, raw pumpkin seeds for zinc, brazil nuts for selenium, horsetail herb for silica, blackstrap molasses for iron, magnesium and copper and trace minerals plus ionic trace minerals from the Great Salt lake.

I recommend Cod Liver oil capsules only, 3 to 6 daily, and not the liquid as it too often goes rancid. The capsules should be in a brown bottle and preferably also in brown cellulose or gelatin caplets. For free radical scavengers (sic: antioxidants), see the chapter on "Free Radicals." Zinc stimulates the Thymus gland to produce the hormone, Thymulin. The Thymus gland matures the CD4 cells produced in the bone marrow. Suntanning 3 to 5 times weekly is also recommended to build up white blood cell counts.

Vitamin A reduces HIV transmission

Vitamin A: In a study in Africa (Lancet, June 25, 1994, page 1593), pregnant women with the highest serum levels of Vitamin A reduced HIV transmission to their offspring to 7%, compared to those with the lowest blood levels of Vitamin A, who had a HIV transmission rate of 32% to their offspring. The authors of the article, Semba, Miotti, Saah at al, wrote: "The underlying biological mechanisms concerning vitamin A in mother-to-child transmission may include the essential role vitamin A plays in immunity and maintenance of mucosal surfaces...Lack of vitamin A is associated with compromised T-cell and B-cell function which may contribute to higher viral loads..."

In contrast, a study with AZT (Zidovudine), in HIV+ pregnant women showed that the group receiving the AZT reduced the rate of HIV transmission to 8.3%, compared to 25.5% in the control group. Vitamin A certainly was slightly more effective than AZT in reducing the rate of HIV transmission. On a side note, one person I spoke with recently told me that several years ago, when he had low white blood cells, his physician prescribed vitamin A supplementation to build up the white blood cells. He told me his white blood cells returned to normal values.

Beta Carotene

Increases in NK counts have been reported by Dr. Coodley. Modest doses of Beta-Carotene stimulate immune responses (1). Supplementation of diet with beta-carotene increases T4 Helper cell counts. In an experimental study, 180 mg daily of beta-carotene increased the frequency of T4 cells in normal volunteers. After two weeks, it significantly increased the frequency of all T cells. The frequency of T8 cells was unaffected compared to controls. (2) Beta-carotene is found in high concentrations in carrots, squash, pumpkin, dark green leafy vegetables, like parsley, spinach and endive, spirulina and blue-green algae. The body cannot always effectively convert Beta-carotene into Vitamin A. It is important to use both Beta-carotene and Vitamin A in your supplement program. We have received several letters from HIV+ persons who claim to have increased their T4 counts with either Spirulina or Beta-carotene supplements. Beta-carotene promotes growth of friendly flora.
1. Contemporary Nutrition, 11(11), 1986. "Nutrition and Immunity," by R.K. Chandra.
2. Immunology Letters 9:221-24, 1985. "Oral beta-carotene can increase T4 cells..." M. Alexander et al.

Vitamin A and Cod Liver Oil capsules

Dr. Stephen Langer M.D. in "SOLVED: THE RIDDLE OF ILLNESS," reports that Vitamin A is needed for the body to assimilate protein. Deficiency reduces the response of both T and B cells to mitogens and antigens, while modest doses stimulate immune responses. (1) Severe deficiency leads to atrophy of the thymus and spleen and marked decrease in circulating leukocytes and lymphocytes (2). In an experimental study, lymphocytes were counted on the first and seventh day of post-surgery. In the experimental group, which received 300,000 units of Vitamin A for 7 days, there was no change, while lymphocyte counts fell in the control group (3). It should be warned here that such a large dose of Vitamin A (over 100,000 i.u. daily) over a long period of time would cause liver poisoning, which would depress the immune system (2). For adults, 10,000 units of Vitamin A may be taken daily on a continuous basis without fear of harmful side effects.

One good best source is Cod Liver oil. I used to recommend liquid Cod Liver oil, except I am now convinced that sitting on a shelf exposed to light and oxygen, will cause it to turn rancid. Your freshest source of cod liver oil will be capsules, preferably stored in a brown bottle, and even better, if the capsules themselves are brown or black in color. Upon opening a bottle, store it in the refrigerator. Cod liver oil also has essential fatty acids that support the Thyroid. Long-term AIDS survivors have higher serum levels of Vitamin A.
1. Contemporary Nutrition, 11(11), 1986. "Nutrition and immunity," by R.K. Chandra.
2. Basic and Clinical Immunology, 4th Edition, Lange Publications, Los Altos, CA, 1982.

3. Surg. Gynecol Obstet, 149:658-62, 1979. "Reversal of postoperative immunosuppression in man with Vitamin A," B. Cohen et al.

The B vitamins

Deficiencies of B vitamins generally are associated with decreased antibody responses and impaired cellular immunity. B vitamins may be beneficial for the following ailments - insomnia, adrenal exhaustion, swollen glands, fatigue, angina pectoris, celiac disease, indigestion, hepatitis, pneumonia, gastroenteritis, cancer, stress and infection. (1) Denny Smith of AIDS Treatment News reported that several of their readers said that injections of B-12 lessened their neuropathy (2). Many symptoms may be alleviated by supplementation with B vitamins. Low body temperature was reported, by Dr. Langer M.D., to stop Vitamin B-12 assimilation. Other sources have reported that B-12 deficiency can cause neuropathy. Good sources of all the B vitamins are liver, Spirulina and Chlorella, Brewer's yeast, blackstrap molasses, bran and wheat germ. Acidophilus bacteria in the colon produce a wide range of B vitamins. Synthetic B vitamins that you can buy at any drug store or health food store are less expensive, but also less effective than their natural counterparts that occur in whole food or are produced by bifido bacteria in the colon. However, when a high dose of a particular B vitamin is needed for a drug effect, you may have no choice but to use the high potency "manufactured" form.

B1 - Thiamine

Thiamine is probably the most important of all the B vitamins. It is essential in the manufacture of hydrochloric acid, which aids in the digestion of proteins (1). This fact, alone, makes thiamine indispensable for restoring the body's ability to digest proteins. Lack of hydrochloric acid, in turn, is often a cause of growth of parasites and yeast in the colon. Thiamine helps normalize body temperature.

In studies, Thiamine, in doses of 200 to 300 mg daily, has been used to reduce hepatitic B and C viral loads. In some cases, they have reached non-detectable levels. Thiamine used at these levels is like taking a drug. In healthy persons adverse effects might occur at levels this high. For more info on hepatitis and thiamine, go to mercola.com/2001/apr/21/thiamine.htm or askemilyss.com/n&d/thiamine.htm or see "Hepatitis" in the chapter on "Symptoms and Remedies."

B2 - Riboflavin:

Riboflavin is part of a group of enzymes involved in the utilization of proteins, fats and carbohydrates. It is also involved in cell respiration (1). B-2 is needed to produce ATP in cells, which creates both heat and energy. Deficiency of riboflavin in animals is associated with a diminished ability to generate antibodies in response to antigens (2).

1. Nutrition Almanac, 2nd Edition, by John Kirschmann and Lavon J Dunne, 1984. McGraw-Hill Book Co, San Francisco, CA.
2. American Journal of Clinical Nutrition, 35:417-68 Supplement, 1982. "Single Nutrients and Immunity," W.R. Beisel.

B3 - Niacin:

Deficiencies of niacin can cause small ulcers, insomnia and depression. Niacin also stimulates the production of hydrochloric acid and is used to reverse arteriosclerosis. Niacin increases body temperature (1)

1. Nutrition Almanac, 2nd Edition, by John Kirschmann and Lavon J Dunne, 1984. McGraw-Hill Book Co, San Francisco, CA.

B5 - Pantothenic acid:

B-5 is supportive of adrenal gland functions and is helpful to persons with stress and allergies. (1) In experiments on animals, pantothenic acid prevented infections in 44 out of 45 rats in a controlled experiment. (2)

1. American Journal of Clinical Nutrition, 35:417-68 Supplement, 1982. "Single Nutrients and Immunity," W.R. Beisel.
2. Encyclopedia for Healthful Living, J.I. Rodale quoting from Nutrition Review, Feb., 1957.

B6 - Pyridoxine:

Required for the absorption of B-12 and for the production of hydrochloric acid. Maintains the balance between sodium and potassium. Helps produce antibodies and red blood cells (1). A deficiency is associated with a reduction in both T and B cells, reduced thymus cell functions and phagocytic activity of neutrophils. (2) Dose: 100 mg twice daily. B6 and Biotin are important for persons with chronic candidiasis. Biotin helps keep yeast in the single cell state where they are not invasive.

1. Nutrition Almanac, 2nd Edition, by John Kirschmann and Lavon J Dunne, 1984. McGraw-Hill Book Co, San Francisco, CA.
2. Basic and Clinical Immunology, 4th Edition, Lange Publications, Los Altos, CA, 1982. "Nutrition and the Immune System," J.A. Levy.

Vitamin B12:

Vitamin B-12 deficiency is common in persons with AIDS. B-12 deficiency can cause neuropathy. Symptoms of B-12 deficiency include weakness in arms and limbs, diminished reflex response, difficulty in walking and speaking, and jerking of limbs (1). Several readers of AIDS Treatment News reported that injections of B-12 relieved symptoms of neuropathy. (2) Restoring body temperature to normal, 98.6 F., improves assimilation of B-12. B12 with Folic acid also is reported to build up red blood cells. A sublingual form of B12 with Folic acid is sold in health foods stores (Bricker Labs). B12 deficiency is common in CFIDS as well.

1. Nutrition Almanac, 2nd Edition, by John Kirschmann and Lavon J Dunne, 1984. McGraw-Hill Book Co, San Francisco, CA.
2. AIDS Treatment News, Sept. 6, 1991, from an interview with Neil Graham, M.D. Denny Smith. PO Box 411256, San Francisco, CA 94141.

Folic acid:

Folic acid is essential for the production of heme, the iron containing protein used to make hemoglobin. Folic acid works in conjunction with other B vitamins in building red blood cells, which carry oxygen. Folic acid is found in dark green leafy vegetables, brewer's

yeast and blue-green algae.
1. Nutrition Almanac, 2nd Edition, by John Kirschmann and Lavon J Dunne, 1984. McGraw-Hill Book Co, San Francisco, CA.

Dimethylglycine:

Dimethylglycine (DMG) significantly enhanced both humoral and cell-mediated immunity in double-blind experiments. Ten healthy volunteers who took 180 mg of DMG daily had a fourfold increase in antibody response to pneumoccal vaccine after 10 weeks (1). In an in vitro study of diabetic patients, mitogen was increased threefold after addition of DMG (1).

N,N-Dimethylglycine is a natural oxygenator of the blood. Besides improving immune functions, it is used to improve blood circulation, to relieve angina pain, for arteriosclerosis and for asthma. Sublingual DMG is sold in health food stores. Red beets are a very good source of Trimethylglycine that reduces homocysteine* levels and also helps oxygenate the blood. *Homocysteine is widely implicated as a major cause of heart disease.

1. Journal of Infectious Disease 143(1):101-5, 1981. "Immunomodulating properties of DMG in humans," C.D. Graber.

Coenzymated B vitamins (Source Naturals)

In some persons, malabsorption of nutrients from food is a major impediment to recovery and for B vitamins to be utilized by the body; they must first be converted into their active coenzyme forms. When wasting or malabsorption of nutrients is a known factor, a source of Coenzymated B vitamins should be considered. The synthetic formulation that does this is Coenzymated B Vitamin Complex by Source Naturals called "Coenzymate B Complex." If blood tests indicate low levels of B vitamins including B 12, then taking one of these Coenzymated B vitamins daily might be good idea. The Coenzymated B vitamin is dissolved sublingually and some enters the blood stream as an active and bio-available form of B vitamins. Other than plant or animal sources that are the preferred choice, Coenzymate B Complex is the only manufactured (synthetic) form of B vitamins I would consider using. Available in health food stores.

Vitamin C

If you bruise easily, it indicates capillary weakness and may be a sign of Vitamin C deficiency. Vitamin C aids in the destruction of viruses engulfed by WBCs. T cells exposed to Vitamin C containing calcium threonate were able to absorb more Vitamin C than without the calcium additive.

There is some confusion as to how much Vitamin C one should take to be effective. One study on stressed mice shows that large daily doses suppressed immune response by over stimulating the adrenal glands (1). It is my view that a safe level of Vitamin C intake is to gradually increase the daily dosage until you no longer bruise easily. Rose hips tea, a rich natural source of Vitamin C, has unknown co-factors that enhances immune function. Due to the presence of many toxins, persons with AIDS and CFIDS need higher doses of Vitamin C than most persons would normally take. Natural Vitamin C improves Natural

Killer cell function. However, finding natural Vitamin C is very difficult, as nearly 100% of all Vitamin C sold today in health food stores and pharmacies is synthetic (manufactured) from derivatives of corn. Published research shows that synthetic Synthetic Vitamin C in amounts as low as 500 mg daily will cause DNA damage to the cells. This research has been confirmed by retesting. This throws a dark cloud of doubt about the safety of other cheap synthetic vitamins that are being mass marketed today.

There is no research that has discovered any DNA damage from the 100% natural Vitamin C found in oranges, Rose hips and Acerola cherries, gooseberries and other plant sources. The foods with the highest natural Vitamin C content are Camu Camu, Acerola cherries, Indian gooseberries and Rose Hips followed by oranges. Persons who buy these whole foods, including oranges, instead of cheap synthetic vitamin C tablets are making a much wiser choice for their health. Unfortunately, millions of bottles of synthetic vitamin C sold today are often mislabeled as "natural."

1. International J. Vitam. Nutr. Res. 47(3):248-57, 1977.
1. Med. Hypotheses 21(4):383-85, 1986.

Vitamin D

Experimental Controlled Study of 63 elderly men and women showed 30% had both a deficiency of Vitamin D and depressed immune responses. Supplementation with Vitamin D and/or exposure to ultraviolet light (sun tanning) normalized immune responses. Best sources are exposure to sunlight, sun tanning salons and Cod Liver Oil. Suggested dosage: 20 minutes of sun tanning twice a week, plus Cod Liver oil capsules twice daily. Vitamin D3 is the natural form found in Cod Liver Oil and is produced naturally, when the skin is exposed to sunlight or full spectrum light in a sun-tanning salon. The synthetic form, Vitamin D2, commonly added to milk, is not recommended.

Vitamin E

Mega doses of Vitamin E depressed the immune system in one study (1) while vitamin E supplementation in another study enhanced several immune functions (2). In a study on aging animals, high doses of vitamin E caused several immune functions to equal those of younger animals (3). We suggest 400 I.U. daily of mixed tocopherols - a natural Vitamin E derived from wheat germ oil for long-term use. (Synthetic d-alpha tocopherol acetate, while less expensive, should be avoided as it lowers gamma tocopherol levels)

References:
1. Am J. of Clinical Nutr. 33:606-8, 1980. "Effect of vitamin E on leukocyte function," J.S. Prasad.
2. Basic and Clinical Immunology, 4th Ed, Los Altos, CA. Lange Publications, 1982.
3. Med. Tribune, Jan 8, 1986. J. Blumberg.

MINERALS

Calcium

Calcium is necessary for strong teeth and bones and regulates the passage of nutrients in and out of cell walls. It helps in nerve transmission and in stimulating deep restful sleep. Most advanced cases of cancer, CFIDS and AIDS are deficient in calcium for a number of reasons. First is a deficiency of hydrochloric acid in the stomach, which aids in the assimilation of calcium and other minerals along with amino acids. Lack of hydrochloric acid and calcium leads to low blood levels that cause both blood and saliva PH to be on the acid side. This causes food to move quickly through the digestive tract, which further impairs the assimilation of calcium and other minerals.

The second reason for low calcium levels is a lack of bifidobacteria in the large intestines. Bifidobacteria produce a variety of short chain fatty acids that bind with minerals and help in their absorption. Some of these acids are lactic, acetic and butyric. A variety of mineral lactates, acetates and butyrates is the result of a normal digestive process with Bifidobacteria. Minerals also bind to fibers that contain phytic acid. In the presence and activity of Bifidobacteria, the mineral phytates become IP6 or inositol hexaphosphate and increased mineral absorption takes place. In the absence of bifidobacteria, minerals bound to phytic acid are excreted in the stools and not absorbed. In the absence of bifidobacteria, the stools will sink in water and over a long period of time, osteoporosis will develop. In several cases I have followed, when the stools start floating, mineral absorption and bone density increases.

Calcium is also critical to the nourishment of cells, as it is the mailman that transports nutrients across cell walls. When a severe deficiency of calcium exists, nothing else may work. All dark green vegetables are rich in calcium, as are canned sardines and cooked salmon with the fish bones. Other good sources of calcium are blackstrap molasses, almonds, peas and beans, yogurt and cottage cheese. The best form of pure calcium is Calcium Lactate. Coral calcium, with over 60 naturally occurring trace minerals, is usually well absorbed and increases bone density. It helps restore deep restful sleep and should be taken before bedtime. Suggested dose for adults: 1/2 teaspoon in water or 3 capsules (740 mg ea).

Copper

Deficiency of Copper has been associated with increased susceptibility to infections (1). Copper is needed to help hemoglobin carry oxygen throughout the body. Food sources are blackstrap molasses, dark leafy vegetables, seafood and legumes. Too much zinc can cause a copper deficiency. If you take zinc in supplemental form, make certain the formula also contains copper.

Iodine

Lack of iodine can result in a lower level of thyroid activity and lower body temperature. Deficiency is related to reduced microbicidal activity of leukocytes.

Iron

The Dangers of using too much…………..

Iron helps hemoglobin transport oxygen and has no other known function in the body. Too much iron can produce Super Oxide free radicals that can damage the intestinal lining of the stomach and have an aging effect on other cells. In 1992, the CDC reported 11 deaths in children who ate large amounts of iron tablets. Iron is used by viruses for replication. Dietary supplements with iron should be avoided. An all-natural and safe source of iron is Blackstrap molasses which is also high in calcium and most other trace minerals. Spinach, dark green leafy vegetables, fish, oysters organ meats, liver, whole grains and legumes are also high in iron.

Magnesium

Magnesium deficient animals have reduced Immunoglobulin levels (1). Magnesium activates enzymes necessary for the metabolism of carbohydrates and amino acids. Magnesium is needed by the body to help retain potassium. Muscle cramps are often caused by a deficiency of magnesium. Magnesium supplementation is beneficial in all forms of cancer. Persons suffering from fatigue are frequently deficient in both potassium and magnesium. All vegetables and fruits are high in potassium, as are whole grains. Pumpkin seeds and almonds are high in magnesium, as are all dark green leafy vegetables. For supplementation, consider magnesium chloride (Alta Health Products) or magnesium sulfate (Epson Salt) as your best choices for easy absorption. Less impressive are chelated magnesium or magnesium oxide that are poorly absorbed.

Note on Magnesium: Dr. Patricia Salvato published an abstract on the successful use of Magnesium in the treatment of neuropathy.

1. Basic and Clinical Immunology, 4th Ed, Los Altos, CA. Lange Publications, 1982.

Manganese

Deficiencies are related to depressed thyroid functions and can cause increased susceptibility to allergies (1). Manganese is found in kelp, green leafy vegetables, raw egg yolk, beets, peas, blueberries, apricots and wheat germ.

1. How to Get Well, Dr. Paavo Airola, Health Plus Publishers, Phoenix, AZ.

Selenium

Cell-mediated immunity is reduced with Selenium deficiency (1). Selenium increases intracellular Glutathione levels. T cells ability to attack viruses is reduced (2). Sources: Brazil nuts, kelp, garlic, seafoods, brewers yeast and eggs. Sodium Selenite – up to 500 mcg daily may be used safely, although it is not the preferred choice, as is the plant derived sources of selenium that can be safely used in much higher doses. Best choices as dietary supplements are Phytosel (Nucycle) or high selenium yeast. See separate chapter on this mineral elsewhere in this book.

1. J. Am Coll Nutr., 4(1):5-16, 1985.
2. Basic and Clinical Immunology, 4th Ed, Los Altos, CA. Lange Publications, 1982.

Sulfur

Deficiencies of sulfur can cause skin disorders, rashes and blemishes. Sources are onions, cayenne, horseradish, celery, radishes, egg yolk and garlic.

1. Systemic glutathione deficiency in HIV-seropositive individuals, Buhl, Roland et al. The Lancet, 2(8675):1294-8(Dec 2, 1989.

2. Evidence that the intact glutathione molecule is required by the neoplastic tissue to undergo regression of malignancy, Novi, A.M., Florke, R., and Stukenkemper, M. Science, 212:541-2(1981).
3. Amino Acids in Therapy, by Leon Chaitow, D.O., N.D. Healing Arts Press, Rochester, VT.

Zinc and T Cells

Zinc is used along with Vitamin B-6 and Magnesium to produce gamma linolenic acid (GLA) that is used by the body to produce PGE1, an anti-inflammatory prostaglandin (1). Zinc is also used by the thymus to promote the growth of T cells, and in one controlled study, the use of zinc sulfate caused the output of thymus hormone to return to normal in aged persons (2). In another experiment, 150 mgs of elemental zinc taken daily depressed immune system function (3). However, the same amount of zinc taken as zinc sulfate caused T-lymphocytes to proliferate and persistent infections were cured in another study (4). A deficiency of zinc intake has been associated with depression of the immune system, including T cell response.

A considerable amount of research links deficiencies of zinc with progression of HIV infection, as found in NUTRITION AND HIV INFECTION (1). The book clearly establishes that it is not how low your T cell count is that determines how long you live, but rather, your body mass (weight) (1). When your body mass is two-thirds of your ideal weight, you are near death. The primary key to longevity is to maintain normal body weight.

Caselli and Bicocchi (1) reported that serum zinc levels in patients with AIDS were substantially lower than those of normal subjects. Libonore et al, found that zinc levels decreased progressively with the worsening clinical and immunological condition represented in the progression from lymphadenopathy syndrome to AIDS.

The usefulness of zinc salts against HIV was proposed by Sergio in 1988, based on their known antiviral capabilities. The use of zinc gluconate increased T4 and T8 cells, and significantly improved the T4/T8 ratio (1). Zinc is an integral part of Thymulin, a hormone produced by the thymus gland. Zinc deficiency has been noted to cause atrophy of the thymus gland. In one study on aged people, the use of zinc sulfate, 660 mg daily (150 mg of elemental zinc), caused the thymus hormone function to return to normal (2). In our opinion, zinc sulfate is a good choice. 220 mg of zinc sulfate daily provide 50 mg of elemental zinc, although food sources like pumpkin seeds are your most safe and effective choice. When taking up to 50 mg of zinc daily, supplement your copper levels with 1 Tbsp of Blackstrap Molasses daily.

Food sources: pumpkin seeds, garlic, spinach, sunflower seeds, brewer's yeast, wheat germ and bran, brown rice, other whole grains, seafood and especially herring. Too much zinc can depress copper levels.

1. "The Healing Magic of Evening Primrose Oil", by Alan Donald. Bestways Magazine, Sept, 1981.
2. "Zinc Nutrition and cell-mediated Immunity in the Aged." Int. J. Vit. Nutr. Res. 53(1): 94-101, 1983. Also see "Typic hormone deficiency in normal aging and Down's Syndrome", Lancet, 1:983-86, 1983.
3. "Excessive Zinc intake Impairs Immune Response", JAMA, 252:1443-46, 1984.
4. "Fed. Am. Soc. Experiment", Biol. Abst. April, 1979.

Physicians comments at the Third Int'l Conference on Nutrition and AIDS

Philadelphia, PA, 1994:

Dr. Gregg Coodley, MD: "Malabsorption is a small intestinal dysfunction...Vitamin B-12 deficiency is a causative factor in Neuropathy, Anemia, Encephalatrophy and cognitive dysfunction...intrinsic factor is needed to absorb B-12....Vitamin B-6 deficiency decreases NK cell activity....Vitamin A deficiency increases the rate of infection...In a study in Africa on 300 pregnant mothers deficient in Vitamin A, the rate of transmission of HIV to their babies was 32%....in a group supplemented with Vitamin A, the rate of transmission was 7%....Vitamin A more favorably reduced HIV transmission than AZT....deficiencies of selenium have been linked to lower T cell counts....Beta-carotene in one study on 21 patients boosted CD4 (T4) counts, WBC counts and increased NK cells compared to a control group...the dosage used was 50 mg twice a day....beta-carotene is one of 600 carotenoids that exist in highly pigmented (colored) vegetables and fruits....in another study, beta-carotene increased Interleukin II levels....breakdown of skin blamed on a deficiency of Vitamin A and C."

Dr. William Kassler, MD: "Vitamins B1, B2, B6, Niacin and Vitamin C made a difference in malabsorption...especially B-6."

Dr. Donald Kotler MD: "At the intermediate stage of HIV, protein deficiency is noticeable, patients tire easily...gastro-intestinal tract infections may contribute to weight loss...other factors are low appetite, diarrhea, bloating, flatus, fatigue, tachycardia and fever.....low testosterone levels are caused by low protein levels..... we need to use common sense in making prescriptions...I wouldn't give a Testoderm patch to someone who is fighting an active infection, has nausea or who has no appetite....." In an article on "HIV WASTING SYNDROME," published in the Journal of Acquired Immune Deficiency Syndrome 7:681-694, 1994, by Gregg Coodley et al, is listed a number on pathogens that can cause wasting syndrome. They are: Cytomegalovirus, MAI, Cryptosporidia, Isospora belli, Campybacter jejuni, Giardia, Microsporidia, Entamoeba histolytica and Enteric viruses (picobirnavirus, adenoviruses, astrovirus). Other causes: HIV enteropathy, infection with (salmonellae, shigellae or Clostridium difficile), Pancreatic insufficiency, medication-induced diarrhea, and protein calorie malabsorption leading to mucosal atrophy, gluten intolerance and intestinal autonomic neuropathy.

21

Immune enhancement diet

Detecting food allergies

The first thing to consider doing is to obtain an IgG Food Allergy test for 90 food groups, to determine which ones your immune system is attacking with antibodies and to eliminate these foods from your diet. The information from this test will help you custom design a diet that is more compatible with your body chemistry. Your Physician can order this test by calling ImmunoSciences Labs at 800-950-4686 and order this test for you. There are two kinds of tests - immediate and delayed reaction and you should do both. By eliminating foods that your immune system attacks will help you feel better and improve your digestion and the assimilation of nutrients.

The following diet will work well for most people. Persons who are very ill should consider a parasite-cleansing program for 30 days, along with one or more drinks to heal the gastro-intestinal tract. See the chapter on (Detoxification and Colon Cleaning) You should start with the (Rapid Recovery Procedures) in this chapter that emphasizes raw vegetable juices. The Whole Lemon/Olive Oil drink should be used daily and then as needed, to keep your saliva pH at a normal reading of 6.4. This will solve many digestive problems.

In designing your self-treatment program, it is important to have a physician who has an open-mind on the subject matter of this book and who can diagnose specific problems you may have, which are beyond the scope of this book.

The most common food allergies and sensitivities are to milk and ice cream, then cheese, wheat gluten, corn and eggs. However, individual testing is the only sure way of determining food sensitivities.

Rapid recovery procedures

The Liquid Healing Diet
Revised March, 2003

Anyone who is very sick should not be given any solid foods and should be on an all-liquid diet. A PERSON WHO IS VERY ILL WILL NEED A FULL-TIME HELPER, NURSE OR FRIEND TO ASSIST IN MAKING THE JUICES AND HELPING IMPLEMENT THE PROGRAM. Full-time help will be needed, until the patient's strength has returned and they are able to manage the program for themselves. The duration of this program will vary from person to person. When substantial progress is made, the patient may gradually phase in one solid meal a day for several days, then increasing to two solid meals a day. The times set for the drinks in this chapter are arbitrary and may be changed at the discretion of the user and his physician. As a general rule, one meal with solid food may be introduced after 3 days of using the rapid recovery program and should be introduced by day 7.

The most rapid progress in healing can be achieved by a combination of freshly squeezed raw vegetable juices, raw fruit juices, liquid and predigested proteins and liquid nutritional supplementation. All juices should be made in a food juicer. When a juicer is not available, pureed vegetable juice may be made by placing vegetables in a blender, with an equal amount of water, and blending them at high speed for 2 minutes. After this, run pureed vegetables through a screen strainer to remove most of the pulp. Beet tops, carrot tops, parsley, endive and spinach may be juiced or blended for a daily green drink. The pureed mixture may be passed through a strainer to remove the pulp, although this is not necessary.

Stimulating appetite and hunger

The following Rapid Recovery Program should be used until genuine and strong hunger sensations arise in the patient. Then solid foods should be introduced. If by day 4 hunger pangs are not present, give the patient 2 or 3 Cayenne capsules with a glass of water 3 times a day and 1 or two cups of Gentian root tea. Gradually phase in the solid foods, rather than make an abrupt switch from a liquid diet. Liquid diets are the easiest to digest and they create little or no stress on the digestive organs, while nourishing the immune system. The person who has no appetite is too toxic, with major organs having impaired function (liver, pancreas, kidneys, thyroid etc). The high liquid diet helps to detoxify the body and cayenne helps to stimulate all metabolic processes.

Total parenteral nutrition (TPN)

The person who is seriously underweight should be given TPN (intravenous nutrition) for 2 to 4 weeks, until they have gained some weight, appetite returns and they are able to digest solid food. Without TPN, the use of liquid whole food supplements (from the chapter on "Supplements for Weight Gain") will be needed to build up weight. One solid meal per day should be introduced from day 3 to day 7 and 2 solid meals per day by the 10th day. After that, rapid recovery should consist of about one pint of raw vegetable juice daily along with meals from this chapter. Neither fat nor muscle will be lost, but fluids with toxins in them will be washed out of the body. Under Rapid Recovery, eat as much of any foods listed as you desire. Rapid Recovery Procedures will work more effectively, when protocols from the chapter on "Detoxification and Colon Cleansing" are done first or simultaneously.

All protein supplements should be avoided in the first few days, until hunger for protein rich foods occurs naturally.

A suggested rapid recovery program

(modify quantities and times as desired)

Special first day instructions for persons who are very ill: Skip all protein supplements and soy-based supplements, like Advera, until you actually develop an appetite for a protein food. If you do not consume proteins at all the first day, that is OK. Start in gradually the second day. The important thing is to detoxify the body first, which is what the vegetable and fruit juices will do, along with the colon cleansing drinks. Then you add the nutritional drinks, as appetite for protein returns. In other words - listen to what your body is trying to tell you. Last point: When diarrhea occurs, add 1 level teaspoon of psyllium husk powder to each glass of vegetable, fruit juice or liquid replacement meal (i.e. Advera). This will slow down peristaltic movement and help solid stools return. Use a food juicer like the Champion brand to make fresh juice, or mix the vegetables in a blender with water and strain before drinking.

7:30 - Enema - with water, chlorophyll, vinegar and garlic and a bath in warm water. When doing an enema with garlic for the first time, start off with 1/2 clove, or just use plain water with chlorophyll added. Gradually increase to 2 cloves per enema, as your colon heals. See the chapter on "Detoxification of the Liver and Colon."
8am - Whole Lemon/Olive oil drink.
8:30am. Glass of freshly squeezed fruit juice (from lemons, oranges and grapefruit).
10:30am. Glass of fresh vegetable juice (carrot, celery and beet, beet tops, carrot tops).
11am. Cup of red clover or hops tea with honey and lemon.
12 noon: Green juice - 1 cup made from one or more dark green vegetables (endive, kale, parsley, carrot tops, beet tops). Use dark green vegetables like parsley, endive, carrot tops and beet tops to make the green drink. This may be followed by a bowl of Vegetable Soup or a dish of cooked squash.
2pm. 1/2 cup of cultured cabbage juice, Kombuchu or Whole Aloe Juice drink.
3pm: 1 cup of red clover or hops tea with honey and lemon. Relax.
5pm: Green juice - 1 cup made from one or more dark green vegetables (endive, kale, parsley, carrot tops, beet tops). This may be followed by a bowl of Vegetable Soup or pea soup and a dish of cooked squash.
7:30pm. Take a bath in warm water.
9pm. Prior to bedtime, do your Castor Oil pack for 1 hour. Take 1 tsp. or (about 5 capsules) of calcium lactate in water. Drink a cup of Marjoram and Thyme tea. Add no honey. To make the tea, add 1/2 tsp. of Marjoram, and 1/2 tsp. of Thyme to a cup of hot water and steep for 5 minutes or you may make it in an automatic coffee maker. Optional: Insert a small serrated clove of raw garlic dipped in olive oil and insert into colon before bedtime.

After 2 or 3 days, if hunger pangs do not develop, take 2 or 3 Cayenne capsules with a glass of water about 1/2 hour before your normal mealtime, followed by a cup of Gentian tea. Both cayenne and gentian will stimulate appetite.

Hungry for something solid to eat?

When the cayenne and/or gentian stimulate hunger pangs, that is a good sign. Listen to your body's cravings. Easy to digest proteins are cottage cheese with raw pineapple or soft-boiled eggs. Serve these with rye crisp, whole rye bread, brown rice bread or some other whole grain gluten-free bread. Use butter if desired.

Easy to digest foods

The main difference between this section and the one that follows is that most of the vegetables are steamed and the proteins are also easy to digest. The following are suggestions only. When body temperature increases to normal, you may mix meals from this section with the one that follows, which emphasizes raw vegetable salads.

Breakfast: 1/2 grapefruit or a glass of Apricot Nectar and one or two poached eggs served with hot salsa and gluten-free toast (spelt, rye, brown rice etc); or a dish of cream of rice cereal served with applesauce and lactose reduced milk. Green tea.
Lunch: Hot Chili, served over brown rice, or mashed potatoes, along with steamed asparagus or hot pickled beets. Buttered Rye Crisp with slices of raw garlic cloves. Garnish with lemon slices and parsley. Green tea.
Mid-afternoon snacks: a glass of almond milk with peaches, kiwi, pineapple, strawberries or other fruit blended in or a glass of low sodium V8 with Tabasco sauce added and/or a spoonful of Barley Green.
Dinner: Baked squash with a few almonds added with butter and sea salt, cottage cheese with chopped hazelnuts or filberts added or cold pressed flaxseed oil (1 tbsp), Buttered Rye Crisp with fresh garlic clove slices, steamed broccoli or cauliflower and carrots, seasoned with Curry, hot Salsa or Jalapeno peppers. Garnish with Lemon slices and parsley. Green tea.
Sweets (allowed if no yeast or thrush problem exists): A glass of plain almond milk or with some fruit blended in, or a dish of apple sauce or a Fig or Apricot Nectar Gelatin, served with real whipped cream.

Oils for cooking

For frying foods, the best choices are Olive oil (Extra Virgin or Light), hazelnut or filbert oil. You may also use some coconut oil and/or butter. For certain foods (bakery etc), where the strong taste of Extra Virgin Olive is objectionable or for higher temperature cooking, use Light olive oil (the bitter faction is removed) or a special Safflower oil, that, like olive oil, also contains 90% monounsaturated fats. Both coconut oil and butter may be mixed and used together or blended with olive oil.

Do not use hydrogenated coconut oil; use only natural coconut oil that melts at 80_F. Do not cook with margarine, vegetable shortening or hydrogenated vegetable oils, which contain transfatty acids that can cause damage to blood vessels. Do not fry foods with other types of vegetable oil that contain more than 20% polyunsaturated fatty acids, as the heat will form transfatty acids. Cold pressed vegetable oils should be used only on salads and never used in cooking. Due to toxic ingredients, never use Canola or Cottonseed oil. Source: Fats and Oils, by Udo Erasmus.
Note: Soybean oil suppresses the thyroid and should be avoided.

Breakfast choices
Citrus juices and others

This first choice is the best for a person who is not hungry and leads a sedentary life style. Take one grapefruit, two oranges and one lemon and juice them with a hand or electric juicer. Add ice cubes and enjoy it. (A good cleansing drink in the beginning). After drinking this tasty cocktail, wait until you feel real hungry before eating any solid food. A glass of freshly made carrot and celery juice would make a good mid-morning snack.

Gluten-free pancakes

Gluten free (wheat free) pancakes can be made with pancake mixes sold in health food stores. Use almond milk in place of regular milk and Egg Replacer by Ener-G. Add blueberries or other berries. Cook in butter. Top with applesauce or other natural cooked or raw fruit. Enjoy 2 or 3 medium pancakes.

Note: 100% whole Buckwheat pancakes are also gluten-free and should be tolerated by most persons, although I am aware of a few cases where they were not tolerated.

Eggs sunnyside or poached

Do not use if diarrhea is present

One or two eggs poached or cooked at low temperature, leaving the yolk soft. Serve with Spelt, Kamut or other gluten-free breads. You may season with crushed red pepper and/or herbal seasonings. Poached eggs may also be served with gluten-free pancakes, corn bread or hash browns. Serve with hot apple cider.

Apple sauce and cream of rice cereal

Serve rice cereal with coconut milk and unsweetened apple sauce. Add a dash of cinnamon.

Hot corn muffin, butter and honey

For a light snack, try hot corn muffins with butter and apple sauce. Corn is a gluten-free grain.

Gluten-free hot cereal choices

Protein Content: 15 Grams

Choose one - Quinoa (A gluten-free grain imported from South America) or Cream of Rice or millet cereal. Cook cereal according to directions. Top with applesauce and add almond milk or coconut milk.

Note: For cooking Quinoa, add 1/2 cup of quinoa to 1 cup of water. Boil for 10 minutes. This serves one person. For millet and rice combo, add 1/4 cup of whole millet to 1 and 1/2 cups of water and boil at a low temperature for 15 minutes, or until the grains pop. Then add 1/4 cup of cream of rice cereal. Cook an additional one-minute. Enjoy. Portions may be increased as appetite increases.

Almond milk yogurt, fruit and wheat germ (RAW) Protein Content: 20 grams

To two cups of almond milk yogurt, add 1 cup of chopped fresh fruit (pineapple, kiwi, blueberries, blackberries, seedless red grapes etc.) and top with one tablespoon raw embryo wheat germ. (Raw embryo wheat germ is sold in health food stores. Keep refrigerated to maintain freshness and to prevent rancidity).

Lunch choices

Special salad combo/yogurt plus baked squash
The most valuable healing meal in this book

Mix in a bowl or platter - endive, (Kale, Romaine lettuce or spinach), parsley, sliced yellow onions or green onions with tops, carrots, red or ripe bell peppers - any color, 1/2 red beet, one clove of garlic sliced, and hot peppers, Shiitake mushrooms and add one Tbsp of raw sunflower seeds (presoaked in water) and a couple of ripe or green olives. You may add any other vegetable, except do not add broccoli, cabbage or cauliflower, if you have low body temperature. Add fresh lemon juice over the salad and cold pressed Extra Virgin olive oil. Top with Paprika. Dip vegetables in one cup of plain yogurt, with a tablespoon of fresh flax oil added, and topped with paprika. (Do not use iceberg lettuce). Other raw vegetables, such as ripe tomatoes or cucumbers, may be added to the salad. Refrigerate olive oil after opening. If it turns solid, place bottle in warm water to liquefy.

Serve yourself 1/2 to 1 lb of cooked squash. Squash may be baked with brown sugar and butter. Any one or more of the following (baked or boiled) vegetables - potatoes, corn on cob, whole kernel corn, cooked brown rice or rye crisp. Season with a little sea salt and butter.

Dessert: Try applesauce with a gluten-free cookie or a glass of soy milk (plain or with fruit blended in). Green tea or rose hip tea with honey and lemon to taste.

Dry-curd cottage cheese or Baker's cheese may be mixed with flax oil and used in place of the yogurt.

Sunflower/mashed potato/baked onion meal.

Over one cup of mashed potatoes on a plate, add one clove of raw garlic sliced plus 1/3 cup of raw sunflower seeds (presoaked). Add 1/2 cup of plain yogurt plus butter over potatoes. Serve with a baked onion. Garnish plate with parsley. Top with paprika. Serve with a side dish of coleslaw. Green tea or rose hip tea with honey and lemon to taste.

Special yogurt and flax oil vegetable dip

To one cup of Non-Fat Plain Yogurt (or home-made yogurt), add 1 Tbsp of refrigerated flax seed oil plus chives or chopped onions and blend slowly. Top with paprika. This special yogurt dip with raw vegetables is the most powerful healing formula of the Immune Enhancement Diet as the flaxseed oil helps oxygenate the blood.

Have a 1/2 cup of chilled red sockeye salmon, a baked potato, cooked asparagus, plus a small salad made from endive/parsley/spinach, garlic cloves, red cabbage, cucumber, carrots and olives. Season with lemon juice and olive oil. A crunchy, tasty and very nourishing meal. Green tea. Serve butter and sour cream with your baked potato. Sugar Snap Peas - a baked potato and a small cob of boiled corn.

A lot of variations to this meal are possible. Any cooked or raw vegetable may be used. A small salad or coleslaw may be substituted for the cooked vegetable. For tea, try green tea or rose hips tea. Season with honey.

Chili over potatoes or rice plus a salad.

Over a plate of mashed potatoes, add one clove of sliced raw garlic. Pour hot Chili over the potatoes and sprinkle a little Parmesan cheese over the chili. Have a Jalapeno pepper, coleslaw, carrot salad or broccoli in dill dip. Green tea. Ground beef or turkey in Chili should be well tolerated by most people.

Cottage cheese and raw pineapple, potatoes and vegetables

To one-half cup of creamed cottage cheese, add 1 Tbsp of flax oil or pumpkin seed oil and some chopped garlic or chives. Top with paprika. Have some boiled or baked potatoes, onions plus coleslaw or a small salad. Green tea or rose hip tea with honey and lemon to taste. Serve chunks or fresh raw pineapple with the cottage cheese. (Avoid cottage cheese if mucus is an immediate problem). Note: Pineapple contains a protein digestive enzyme called bromelain.

Brown rice or spelt pasta

Gluten-free Spelt macaroni and spaghetti is sold in health food stores. It tastes great too. Try it with a flavored tomato sauce and browned hamburger and a sprinkle of Parmesan or Romano cheese. You can also serve it with broiled fish and coleslaw. Several combinations are possible.

Recipe for great tasting Chili with grass-fed ground beef

Buy a package of Chili seasoning mix, the hotter the better. Brown 1 lb of finely ground organic or grass-fed beef. Brown beef first, then add seasoning mix plus tomato paste and water or tomato sauce.

In a separate pan, add one cup of sliced celery, one cup of chopped onions, 1/2 cup of chopped green pepper and one cup of sliced mushrooms. Put celery, onions, green pepper and mushrooms in a large cooking pot and add just enough water to cover vegetables. Simmer for 20 minutes until cooked. Add the cooked ground beef with Chili seasoning and tomato sauce to the cooked vegetables and one 16 oz can of pinto beans plus one 16 oz can of whole tomatoes (cut up) and two sliced Jalapeno peppers. Simmer for 15 additional minutes. It is delicious. Refrigerate until ready to use.

Recipe for great tasting vegetable soup

Into an 8 qt pot, add the following: Brown 1 lb of grass-fed or organic ground beef or sirloin and add 1 and 1/2 cup of diced celery, 1 cups of diced onions, 1 cup of diced carrots, 1/2 cup of diced green pepper and 1 cup of diced rutabagas. Add 2 pieces of dried seaweed

- Nori or Kombu (sold in health food stores). Add enough water to cover the vegetables, cover pot and simmer for 10 minutes. Add 2 bay leaves, 1/2 cup of chopped parsley, one clove of sliced garlic and 1/2 Teaspoon of herbal (i.e. Spike) seasoning. Add 3 cups of chopped green cabbage, one pint of V8 or tomato juice and one large can of whole canned tomatoes. Cut whole tomatoes into quarters. Cover and simmer for 20 more minutes. Soups done! Serve with rye crisp. Add more herbal seasoning to taste, if desired. Optional: Add Sea salt

Recipe for Cream of Broccoli soup

1 cup of chopped leeks (use stem only)
2 medium size red-skin potatoes - cubed
2 Tablespoons of butter
1/4th cup of water
5 cups of coarsely chopped broccoli
6 cups of chicken broth (To make your own, boil 3 chicken necks or wings in 7 cups of water for 30 minutes with one carrot and one celery stalk added). Remove chicken from broth and proceed with recipe.
1/2 cup of plain yogurt (made from whole milk).

In a frying pan, add butter and water, leeks and red potatoes. Cover and simmer for 5 minutes. Remove and place contents in a larger porcelain, Pyrex or stainless steel pot. Add chicken broth and broccoli. Cover and simmer for 30 minutes. Remove from heat, add yogurt or natural sour cream and blend in. Puree soup in blender or food processor. Serve warm. Add extra sea salt or Spike to taste. Enjoy.

Recipe for raw nut (Almond) milk or pumpkin seed milk

Into a blender add 1/2 cup of raw almonds or pumpkin seeds, presoaked in water for 8 hrs or more. Add one tablespoon of ground flaxseeds. (Optional - Add 1 tsp. of lecithin granules and 1 tsp. of ground slippery elm powder). Add 2 cups of warm water and blend at high speed for 3 minutes. Add 1 more cup of water and blend at high speed with cover on for 2 minutes. Strain to remove pulp. Add 1 Tbsp. of maple syrup or honey, 1/4 tsp vanilla and 1/8 tsp. of sea salt. Shake and pour liquid into a quart glass jar with a funnel. Refrigerate nut milk until you are ready to use it. An almond milk available in health food stores is "Nutquick," by EnerG. You can also use hazelnuts or filberts to make nut milk.

Special Instructions on how to eat

Listen to your body. Relax. Reduce portions to avoid overeating. Chew your food well and eat slowly, mixing saliva with each bite. This is absolutely essential for good digestion. Let your saliva be the liquid to mix the food together. Persons with digestive problems should eat only one kind of food at a time. Avoid mixing. Soak sunflower seeds in water in the refrigerator 8 to 24 hrs. before eating them. Pour off excess liquid and store unused seeds in refrigerator until needed. 1/2 cup of sunflower seeds provides 16 grams of the highest quality protein. Don't stuff yourself. Take a long slow walk after a meal as an aid to digestion.

Snacks that heal

Raw garlic with avocado on rye crisp

On rye crisp, add slices of avocado. Slice a large clove of garlic. Add hot salsa sauce and enjoy. Variations: Cucumber, tomato or other vegetables can be eaten over rye crisp with add garlic slices. Enjoy.

Sweet and sour red beets and onions

Slice two raw or cooked red beets. Slice one small onion and place in a dish with the beets. Add 1/2 cup of apple cider vinegar with 1 tsp. of raw cane sugar to sweeten. Add two cloves and stir. Let soak for 1 hour and enjoy.

Soups

Unless you have a favorite recipe for vegetable soup, I highly recommend a book called Vegetarian Soup Cookbook, by Janice Cook Migliaccio. It contains over 50 enticing recipes for soups. At least 35 recipes are usable on the IED program. Soups are tasty and a very digestible way to consume vegetables. The book is highly recommended. Another book, "Nut Milks," contains 40 recipes for delicious, digestible nut milks, which are free from the lactose and casein in cow's milk.

Raw vegetable juices

A vegetable juicer is a great asset to healing an injured and sick body. A centrifugal juicer will do an adequate job, but I prefer a Champion juicer. Most people quickly and easily digest juices. Drinking a glass of carrot and celery juice, with the juice of a small beet added, will alkalize the blood and stimulate the liver and lymphatic system. Another nutritious juice is a glass of "green" juice. Juice endive, parsley, kale, spinach, beet-tops, romaine lettuce and carrot tops. One glassful a day provides miraculous healing nutrients to the body.

Raw veggie and rice cake snacks

Here is a great snack idea. Place a rice cake on a leaf of green cabbage. Spread plain yogurt on rice cake. Add some raw sunflower seeds and top with slices of garlic, parsley, broccoli, carrots, tomato, cucumber etc. and enjoy. Note: If your body can handle some gluten, try rye crisp topped with raw veggies. Raw green onions and rye crisp are also good.

Late evening snacks

Do not eat raw foods within 3 hours of bedtime. Do not eat popcorn before bedtime, if you get night sweats. Otherwise, enjoy a bowl of popcorn made with coconut oil. Try vegetable soup as a good late evening snack. Other snack ideas: Try marinated Artichoke hearts on rye crisp. Consider cabbage soup or many choices available from the Vegetarian

Soup Cookbook.

Miso, Tempeh and Tofu may be good choices, but what about beans and pea soup?

With the exception of green beans, some persons ,immune-compromised, do not tolerate pea soup or beans very well. They are hard to digest. You know your own body. If you can tolerate pea soup and bean soup, it is OK to use these in moderation. Tofu and Miso are made from fermented soybeans and are well tolerated. Published reports are that the fermented soy product, Miso and Tempeh do not interfere with the thyroid function. If you can handle yogurt, use it; if not, try making yogurt from almond milk. You will need to buy a yogurt maker. Sour milk, yogurt, kefir, sour cream and buttermilk are your best choices of protein, other than dietary supplements made from cold processed whey proteins. When all else fails, almond milk or brown rice milk are well tolerated for most persons.

Foods that Heal
Vegetables

All vegetables are recommended in the IED except iceberg head lettuce that has little or no value.

Vegetables most recommended are - Sprouts (wheat grass, red clover, radish and alfalfa), artichokes, asparagus, avocado, bamboo shoots, banana pepper, endive, escarole, parsley, Boston lettuce, dandelion greens, beet greens, beets, bean sprout, cabbage, collard greens, bok choy, broccoli, cauliflower, chinese cabbage, kale, kohlrabi, carrots, celery, eggplant, garlic, onions, jalapeno pepper, lamb's quarters, leek, okra, olives (green and ripe), potatoes, sweet potatoes, rutabagas, turnips, green peas, green beans, pumpkin, radish, red sweet pepper, sea kale, shallot, spinach, squash (all varieties), Swiss chard and turnip greens, ripe olives, green olives and sauerkraut. Note: sauerkraut contains lactic acid, which is beneficial, but does not contain friendly flora. All raw foods contain friendly flora - Cultured cabbage juice is a rich source or friendly flora and lactic acid.

Flaxseed oil

Flax oil - 1 or 2 Tablespoons daily - mix with cottage cheese or yogurt. Other oils - Olive oil or hazelnut oil. These oils may also be blended 50/50 with butter. Note to Hemophiliacs: Flax oil may thin the blood - limit to 1 teaspoon daily.

Seasonings and spices

Paprika, Crushed red pepper, Spike, Braggs Liquid Amino (use in place of Soy sauce), hot peppers, seaweed - nori, kombu etc., apple cider vinegar and thyme are highly recommended. There are several herbal seasoning mixes on the market. Go easy when cooking with black pepper. Use black pepper in moderation. Do not use Lite salt or salt substitutes containing potassium chloride. Potassium chloride suppresses the sex drive and may contribute to hardening of the arteries, according to some reports. It is best to use natural sea salt that contains some naturally occurring trace minerals. Do not go on a salt-free diet, unless you need to lose weight.

Gluten-free grains

Rice - white or brown, corn, rye crisp crackers, Millet, Spelt, Quinoa, Amaranth, Rye or Kamut and any other gluten-free grain.

Fruits

Raw lemons, raw limes, raw grapefruit, raw pineapple and natural unsweetened applesauce.

Use all other fruits in moderation (limit to one serving per day).

Sweetners - use in moderation

Raw, unfiltered unheated honey, maple syrup, sucanat, raw cane sugar, brown sugar, date sugar and blackstrap molasses. Raw unfiltered honey is the only one in this group that will not support thrush or yeast growth.

Water and beverages

Reverse Osmosis, Distilled water, Filtered water, Spring water and Mineral Water are your best choices. Do not use city water without first running it through a charcoal filter. Charcoal filters will remove chlorine but not the sodium fluoride. Sodium fluoride interferes with intestinal enzyme activity and will be an irritant to the intestinal tract. Sodium fluoride can be converted to its natural form, calcium fluoride, by adding a teaspoon of Lime water (calcium hydroxide) to a quart of filtered city water. The metallic taste of sodium fluoride instantly vanishes.

Decaf coffee should be avoided as it lowers HDL cholesterol and may predispose you to hardening of the arteries. Avoid coffee and other high caffeine drinks. Regular tea is a better choice and green tea is a healthy choice that improves HDL levels. Both green tea and regular tea contain some caffeine. If you want to spice it up, use ginger root.

*Warning on Tap water: Chlorinated city water may contain small amounts of Cryptosporidium, a parasite that can cause diarrhea and weight loss. Cities using ozone to disinfect the water will not have this problem. When using chlorinated city water, always take from the hot water side that is likely to have pre-cooked out the pathogens. However, do not use the hot water side of the faucet if it is pretreated in a salt water softener.

Meats – Crock-pot or low-temperature cooking is best

When your body temperature is normal, and you have a real craving for meat, then, boiled meats may be added, like boiled chicken or sliced turkey. Cooking meats in a Crock-pot at a low temperature (175_F) for 6 to 8 hours will give you the tenderest and most easily digestible meats possible. When adding meats or broiled fish, note any discomfort you may feel in the stomach area, or if a feeling of fullness lasts for several hours or your stools the next day are small in diameter, - this is an indication of a constricted intestinal tract, caused by inflammation. All these signs could indicate either a deficiency of hydrochloric acid or allergic and inflammatory reactions to the food. If you notice these, stop eating whatever caused the problem. Consider using hydrochloric acid capsules and digestive enzymes. Always listen to your body. Each of us has some unique biological differences.

Seven gems for better health

The seven foods listed below will help restore normal digestion, a normally functioning liver and significantly increase friendly flora in the colon. The bottom line is that including these 7 foods in your daily diet will improve your digestion, increase your energy level and well-being.

1. Garlic - (build up CD8s and Natural Killer cells)

One person from California, who has been HIV+ for 10 years and is symptom-free, attributes his good health to Kyolic garlic. Garlic is a naturally rich source of zinc and sulfur. It has a 5,000 yr. history as an infection fighter. During the middle ages, it was used along with apple cider vinegar to stop the plague. Legend tells us that during the bubonic plague, four thieves drank a potion of vinegar and garlic and would rob the graves of the dead. They believed the garlic and vinegar mixture protected them from the plague. Garlic has been reported in some studies to be more effective than the anti-fungal drug Nystatin in killing various strains of yeast and fungus. Several studies have shown that garlic inhibits viral replication (1). Dr. Edward Delaha of George Washington University showed that garlic inhibited many acid-fast bacteria, including tuberculosis (1). Dr. Lou reported in his book, "Garlic for Health," that he and his students were testing various drugs for their anti-microbial activity. He stated:

"Upon returning to my laboratory, I prepared diluted garlic extract, introduced it to several of the cultures, and stuck them in the incubator overnight. The next day I was astounded to find that the diluted garlic extract did indeed stop the growth of those cultures, more effectively, in fact, than some of the potent drugs we were testing at the time."

A medical student working with Dr. Lou reported that the HIV virus did not grow well in the presence of garlic in tissue cultures (1). Garlic has been reported in several studies effective against several forms of cancer (1).

In commenting on the use of garlic for AIDS, Dr. Lou writes: "That's a very difficult question; once the disease is fully developed, it is not likely that any single agent or approach will be effective in its treatment. I recall all I have learned about garlic: garlic can inhibit the growth of viruses; garlic enhances the function of phagocytes and natural killer cells; and garlic nullifies some of the toxins that impair the immune system. It thus appears that this natural product has all the good qualities to ensure a healthy host. For this reason, I believe it can be used, to advantage, together with a sound healthful lifestyle, to prevent diseases even as dreadful as AIDS."(1). Dr. Lou cites 108 references to studies on garlic in medical journals.

KHA recommends 3 cloves of raw garlic daily. The garlic should never be eaten straight, but should be sliced and placed on salads, mashed potatoes or on rye crisp. Lab tests show that fresh raw garlic is more potent as an antibiotic than Kyolic or other prepared forms of garlic. Garlic's enhancement of natural killer cells and expansion of CD8s makes it a very important supplement for persons immune-compromised.

A study published in the German Medical Journal "Deutsche Zeitshrift" in Oct, 1989 by T.H. Abdullad, D.V. Kirkpatrick and J. Carter, reports on the results of 7 AIDS patients taking 5 grams of garlic daily as an aged extract, similar to Kyolic garlic. They said that 6 of the 7 patients had normal NK cell activity after 6 weeks and that all had normal NK activity after 12 weeks. Five of the 7 had significant improvements in their T4/T8 ratios, after 12 weeks, with 3 returning to normal reference ranges of 1.0 or higher. They also reported a lessening of diarrhea in one patient with Cryptosporidia, fewer outbreaks of Herpes, Thrush, Candidiasis and Sinus infections.

The authors also wrote: "The antimicrobial spectrum of garlic by in vivo and in vitro studies include many of the opportunistic microbes associated with AIDS, such as Herpes, Cryptocci, Candida, Histoplasma, Mycobacteria, Salmonella, and Entamoeba. In one patient, we observed a platelet count increase from 103,000 to 280,000 mm3 in four months. Recently, a study in China demonstrated the potent antiviral activity of an intravenous preparation of garlic in reducing the morbidity and mortality of the Cytomegalovirus (CMV) in bone marrow transplant patients."

Mark Abbruzzese, M.D. of Washington, recently tested fresh raw garlic in his lab against various pathogens like Tuberculosis and various strains of yeast and found that raw garlic killed them all. The same anti-bacterial effects were not found from over the counter garlic pills.

1. "Garlic for Health," Dr. Benjamin Lou, M.D. Lotus Light Publications, PO Box 2, Wilmot, WI 53192. $3.95 a copy. Add $2.00 for postage.

2. Lemons

Lemon juice stimulates the liver and improves digestion. It helps in the digestion of proteins by stimulating production of hydrochloric acid. It helps dissolve minerals in the food you eat and stimulates saliva flow to assist in digesting carbohydrates. It helps in digesting fats. More than any other substance, lemon juice will improve assimilation of nutrients from food you eat. Taken with meals, it will help raise saliva pH. It will help in weight gain. It also possesses natural anti-viral properties.

3. Olive oil- "Cold Pressed or Extra Virgin" is preferred for most purposes. Olive oil has been shown in recent studies to reduce the incidence of breast cancer. It has been recommended by many holistic health care practitioners to help detoxify the liver. Olive oil should be used with lemon juice on salads. Use Light olive oil for certain bakery (pancakes, cookies etc) – it is debittered and still has 90% monounsaturated fats.

4. Shiitake mushrooms -

Studies in Japan have found that Shiitake mushrooms build up Natural Killer cells. Fresh shiitake mushrooms are sold in many grocery stores and are a better buy than the pills. Use them raw on salads or use them in an egg omelet. Avoid overcooking - warm them slightly for stir-fries.

5. Cayenne -

Cayenne (red pepper) is good to increase body heat, heal ulcers and intestinal inflammation. It stimulates circulation, warms the body, and is beneficial to the liver and digestion. It benefits conditions of congestion, lung problems and helps fight infections.

6. Beets

Beets contain betaine hydrochloride, an aid in protein digestion. Raw beets have natural anti-cancer properties, anti-KS properties and are very beneficial for healing the liver.

7. Squash

Squash, along with beans and corn, are known to Native American Indians as the three sisters. Squash is very high in beta-carotene, which promotes friendly intestinal flora. Squash and other foods high in beta-carotene will help build up T cell counts.

Flax oil/cottage cheese combination
Improving the oxygen carrying power of the blood

Dr. Budwig M.D. of Germany recommends, once a day, a serving of cottage cheese blended with a tablespoon of flax oil. Dr. Budwig M.D. has shown, under microscopic examination, that the combination of flax oil with the sulfur-based protein, cottage cheese, actually changes the color of the hemoglobin from a yellowish green color to a bright red in as little as 3 hours after it is consumed. The red color signifies increased oxygenation of the blood. Dr. Budwig specializes in treating cancer patients with weak immune systems.

Caution: One PWA reported a significant drop in cholesterol levels after using 2 or 3 tablespoons of flax oil daily. Persons with total cholesterol levels below 125 should not use flax oil. Also, Hemophiliacs should not use it either, as it thins the blood.

An important concluding observation

If you eat wholesome foods, you will not need to take 50 to 100 pills each day to supplement your diet. The body needs a smorgasbord of nutrients to function properly and the food you eat is your best medicine. Wholesome foods will provide you with most of the nutrients you will need. The bottom line is to never trust any pill or combination of pills as an effective substitute for a good diet.

22

Symptoms and Remedies
Basic instructions

Allergic reactions: Avoid any food, herb or treatment that is known to induce in you an allergic reaction, without first consulting with a health care professional. When using any new product (herb or any item listed in this book) for the first time, start off with a small amount to test your body's response to the product. If you tolerate it well without allergic reactions (elevated pulse rate, difficulty breathing, feeling cold and clammy, elevated blood pressure etc) or other serious side effects, gradually increase the dosage until you reach the desired or recommended level. If the product is in capsule form, break it open and place 1/4 or 1/2 of the contents under your tongue to test its effects. If you have an adverse reaction or feel uncomfortable, contact your physician.

Notice: To prevent drug inter-reactions, if you are taking any drugs or other doctor-prescribed medications, we recommend taking these drugs either one hour before or one hour after using herbal and nutritional supplements referred to in this chapter. This is to prevent drug interactions in the stomach. When taking any new herb for the first time, start off with a small amount and wait a half-hour to determine how your body is reacting to the new substance. This is important, to avoid serious allergic or metabolic reactions like an elevated pulse rate.

Note: a sudden drop in body temperature or an increase in pulse rate are warning signs to avoid that product and certainly difficulty breathing would require immediate medical attention.

Avoiding herbal side effects

Avoid experimenting with herbal combination on your own, without first getting expert advice. Two observations:

Herbs with strong sedative properties (lobelia, skullcap, lemon balm and valerian) should be only used ALONE and not mixed together).

Avoid herbs like Ma Huang, Kola nut, Yohimbe that can be over stimulating and raise blood pressure. Do not mix any stimulant herbs with sedative herbs. In March, 2001, a reader called to tell me a friend, who used Yohimbe every day to stimulate his sex drive, died of a heart attack earlier this year. I know of one person whose blood pressure went over 250 after taking several Yohimbe capsules. A number of unethical dietary supplement companies, who market Yohimbe through the mail, as a sex stimulant, are telling people Yohimbe is safe. Don't believe it for one second.

As for Ma Huang, the FDA has documentation on numerous deaths caused by weight loss herb. Be careful about buying any herb or herbal combination without knowing the ingredients in it, and don't believe everything you read in newpapers or see on television, nor judge the value of a product because it has a fancy label or is on sale. When prices are very low or the deal sounds too good to be true, it is probably because it is. The ingredients could be rancid, contaminated with other substances like maltodextrin or cheap fillers or may have been purchased at an internet auction site.

In some instances, there has been actual fraud, that is, some cut-rate vitamin companies have sold supplements that have up to 90% less in the pills than what they claim on the label. Any time you deal with a new vendor who sells supplements at prices that are too good to be true, ask for a "Certificate of Analysis." Check with the firm's local Better Business Bureau to see if complaints have been filed and how they were solved.

Do not buy ground olive leaves in pill or capsule form as there are factors other than the active ingredient, "oleuropein," that may be irritating to the intestines. Buy only an olive leaf extract that has 15 to 20% or more oleuropein as determined by HPLC testing or make your own olive leaf tea as described in this book. Do not use olive leaf extract, if you have low blood pressure, as it lowers blood pressure. If you have elevated blood pressure, olive leaf extract and olive oil are good choices. Blackstrap molasses is a good choice for most types of high blood pressure unless you have elevated potassium levels, a condition that is very rare.

Do not use licorice root if you have high blood pressure, as it will raise it further. If your blood pressure is low or normal, use licorice root in small amounts to begin with, to determine how it affects you before increasing the dosage. Licorice root stimulates adrenal function, and when adrenals are exhausted, it is best to use it more often in small amounts.

If you are taking prescribed drugs, check with your physician to see if there are any herbs you should avoid using at the same time. Most of these inter-reaction problems can be avoided, if one hour of time elapses between taking a prescribed medication and an herbal supplement. Vitamin and mineral supplements should usually be taken with meals.

Emergency antidotes to adverse reactions, when immediate medical attention is not possible.

1. Elevated pulse rate (over 100 beats per minute) - take 1 or 2 tablespoons of blackstrap molasses. (If molasses is not available, drink 3 or 4 glasses of pure fruit juice - grape or apple or take 2 tablespoons of honey - the darker in color the better, indicating a higher mineral content). The pulse rate usually drops in 10 to 15 minutes. Note: Elevated pulse rate could be due to an allergic reaction. Keep track of what you eat and its effects on your pulse. Eat a single food at a time, and if the pulse rate increases 10 or more beats per minute, you are most likely allergic to that food. These reactions will occur within 30 minutes of eating the food to which you are allergic.

2. Low body temperature - dropping below 96_F - Take 3 or 4 cayenne (red pepper) capsules or 1 teaspoon of cayenne with a glass of water or eat some hot salsa. Body temperature should increase in 15 to 20 minutes.

3. Tightness in the chest or difficulty breathing - 1. Take cayenne (up to 1 teaspoon or 4 capsules) and 2. Soak a towel in one cup of 3% hydrogen peroxide (works better if warmed up in a pan) and place towel on the chest area for 30 minutes or longer (provides immediate oxygen to the heart, as the H2O2 is broken down in the cells). Relief of symptoms should be noticeable in 10 to 15 minutes. Sublingual DiMethylGlycine (DMG) can also relieve chest pains.

Note: if symptoms follow indigestion related to a meal, also take digestive enzymes - 3 or

4 tablets or capsules with the cayenne. For gas - digestive enzymes plus ginger root, followed by charcoal capsules if needed.

Before, during or immediately after using these procedures, obtain medical assistance.

For emergencies, keep these four items in stock.

1. Cayenne (red pepper)
2. 3% Hydrogen Peroxide (from your drugstore) or preferably 6% food-grade H2O2.
3. Blackstrap molasses.
4. Vegetarian Digestive enzymes (for proteins, fats and carbohydrates). (Ginger root and charcoal capsules)

Other items to stock

Be prepared for future problems by storing some items in advance for future needs. A home made ointment made from fresh garlic and coconut oil is effective against all kinds of fungal, bacterial and skin infections and many kinds of rashes. It is also effective for sinus infections and may be applied to any part of the body directly except the eyes. See end of this chapter for the recipe. It is called GOOT.

Other important items to have on hand are Nutribiotic grapefruit seed extract, lomatium dissectum, wormwood (artemesia annua), colloidal silver, fresh garlic cloves and ginger root. Colloidal silver, which is effective against over 600 kinds of infections, would be a good item to store. It is best to buy this one and use it only when needed. The continuous use of colloidal silver is not recommended.

Herbal teas and extracts

Raw herbs are packaged for sale in capsule form for convenience. Bulk herbs and extracts are also available. The best and most effective herbal teas are made at home, using bulk tea that is steeped in hot water. Steep leaves for 5 minutes and roots and bark for 10 minutes in very hot water. Strain to remove the pulp and chill with one or two ice cubes before drinking. The brewed teas are totally assimilated into the blood stream. Persons who are very ill will respond better to herbal teas and extracts over capsules. Herbal extracts with alcohol may irritate the stomach. The alcohol may be removed by placing a day's portion of the extract in a glass of water heated to 110 degrees F. and let it stand for 30 minutes. Always use a Thermometer.

Symptoms and Remedies

Aching joints and muscles:
Often accompanied by fatigue and are arthritic in nature. Evening Primrose Oil often brings fast relief, as does the whole lemon drink. Rub OxySpray on joints. To make your own equivalent of OxySpray, mix equal parts of 3% hydrogen peroxide and aloe vera juice. Spray and rub this mixture on sore joints twice a day. Warm it up in a pan and massage it

into joints or areas of your body that are sore and aching. If the symptoms are related to arthritis or rheumatism, you may get relief with Glucosamine sulfate and Chondroitin sulfate. Magnesium Chloride (Alta health Products) or MSM works well for many persons with aching muscles and joints. Take 2 tablets or capsules 2 or 3 times daily. Relief of symptoms is quite rapid – usually in a few days.

Tart cherry juice - use about 4 to 6 ounces daily to relieve the symptoms of arthritis, fibromyalgia and aching muscles and joints in as little as two weeks. Cherry juice also reduces uric acid, which causes painful gout. Avoid foods to which you have allergies, and avoid hard cheese made from rennet. Rennet can cause rheumatoid arthritis.

Allergies:

Hay fever and Asthma – Oralmat (Nutricology) Oralmat is an extract of sprouted rye that is used sublingually and has a good track record for treating asthma. .

Food allergies - Intestinal Flora needed L-Plantarum (lowers IgE) and B Longum (increases mucosal IgA). Use with each meal - Vegetarian digestive enzymes with meals - avoid foods that you are allergic to or eat them only once every 5 days - rotation diet. Avoid wheat products. You may also be allergic to corn derived products and some dairy products. Use a Fiber/pectin/probiotic blend.

Common sources of environmental allergies are dust, dogs and cats, house plants, pollen in the air, chemicals emitted from new carpeting or furniture, conditioning agents used to soften clothing in laundries or other chemicals. Everything is suspect, including soaps, deodorants, hair sprays, bug sprays, etc. Try glycerin or oatmeal soap. Use personal and laundry soap labeled "hypoallergenic."

Avoidance of suspected allergens is the best remedy. Installing a good quality filter on your furnace will help, as will an air purifier and/or a Negative Ionizer. As for foods, the only way to know for certain is to obtain an IgG test for 90 food groups. Have your physician call ImmunoSciences Labs at 800-950-4686 to arrange a test. The IED diet will eliminate problem foods for most people, but not for everyone. A physician who specializes in treating allergies may help by giving you shots to gradually build antibodies to the substances you are allergic to. Check with your physician for a specialist.

Alfalfa tablets or capsules. Butyrate supplementation, Red clover tea and or Tumeric (Curcumin) plus low-dose natural cortisone (Cortef) 10 mg daily along with desiccated thyroid (both prescription items). Review chapter on the adrenals and thyroid. Other herbs for relief from allergies are - Burdock, Evening Primrose oil, Pumpkin seed, Flaxseed, Eyebright, Papaya, Parsley, Spinach. Also consider taking Vitamin B6 and manganese. Consider squash, yellow onions and Blue-green algae. Ojibwa Tea. For more information on Ojibwa, call 303-322-7930 or www.ojibwatea.com

Anthrax

Conventional antibiotics are usually prescribed. Additional help for the immune system can come from a transfer factor product now being developed by Chisolm Biological Labs that will be anthrax specific. Ask for a product called Biostress. For more information, call 803-663-9618

Appetite stimulants (to help gain weight)

Herbs to stimulate your appetite: **Gentian, Marijuana, Alfalfa, Angelica,**

Horseradish. I suggest trying Gentian root tea first. If more help is needed, you can experiment with the other herbs to determine which ones are most beneficial for you. **To stimulate your appetite, add a teaspoon of blackstrap molasses and one Tbsp of fresh lemon juice to a cup of hot water. Drink this before meals and take 3 capsules of cayenne.** Avoid taking Megace or high dose steroids that increases your susceptibility to infections. Balance your saliva pH. Other: whole lemon/olive oil drink daily, balance your pH - use limewater (calcium hydroxide) or coral calcium if saliva pH taken between meals is less than 6.4. Some drugs affect the taste buds and may reduce your appetite. .

Athlete's foot:

Caused by fungus overgrowth. The best treatment for athlete's foot is GOOT (Garlic and Coconut Oil Ointment). See end of this chapter for recipe. I personally witnessed a person with the worst case of athlete's foot I have ever seen, completely clear up in 2 weeks using GOOT. In addition, all his Planter's Warts fell off and disappeared.

Wear shoes that breathe (no man-made materials) or go barefoot. Wear cotton socks, no nylon or other synthetic material. Use a moisture-absorbing foot powder to keep feet dry. Diet: Avoid sugar and alcohol and go easy on fruit. There are many other over the counter treatments for athletes foot in most pharmacies.

Cancer: See separate chapter Cancer and on Immune-based therapies

Candidiasis:

(Immunological cause: low NK cell function, low neutrophil function and lack of CD8 Killer T cells) - an excess of Th2 cytokines and a lack of friendly flora in the intestines. **Selenium - plant-based (Phytosel, SelBroc) only** to restore neutrophil function. Use 400 mcg twice daily until candida symptoms are gone. **Beta Glucan** - 100 to 500 mg daily or eat 2 or 3 **raw mushrooms** daily **for sulfated glucan (Shiitake** etc) . .L. Salivarius is also beneficial in treating yeast overgrowth as are Acidophilus, B Longum and L Plantarum.

Thrush, yeast infections, itchy skin, insomnia and fatigue are all conditions associated with overgrowth of Candida Albicans, a common strain of yeast. It is very important to avoid sugar, sweets, alcohol and most kinds of fruits. The yeast feed on these. The IED diet should be strictly followed. Use supplements: to normalize body temperature, Use Oregamax (Northern Spice and Herb Co) - 2 or 3 capsules 3 times daily. Other products that kill yeast infections - Caprylic acid, Oregamax and Venus Fly-trap extract, "Yeast Fighters"(by Twinlabs), raw garlic, coconut oil, Thyme, Oil of Oregano; (Pure Purple Lapacho and White Oak Bark Tea combined 3 times a day). Daily enemas with raw garlic cloves. vinegar and chlorophyll added. Apply GOOT (an emulsion of fresh garlic and coconut oil) directly to infected areas. Nystatin is available on prescription.

Candidiasis: selenium, Beta glucan, Coconut oil, raw garlic, caprystatin, Ojibwa tea, sugar free diet, Perfect Colon Formula or make your own fiber/pectin/probiotic blend and Transfer Factor Plus. Also check out this web site www.candidaprogram.com or call 808-521-5797.

Chest Pains/Circulation/Clogged Arteries:

If the pain starts in the center of the chest and spreads outward, go immediately to the

Emergency section of the nearest hospital. You could be having a heart attack. An emergency procedure to stop the heart attack is to take 1 level teaspoon of red pepper (cayenne) in a glass of water, followed by 2 Tablespoons of Blackstrap molasses or a glass of fruit juice and then 3 or 4 digestive enzyme tablets. Then, spray Oxy-Spray or 3% H2O2 over your chest area and massage it in. Di-Methyl Glycine dissolved under the tongue can also relieve chest pains. A herbal extract called "Night Blooming Cereus" (GAIA Herbs) effectively relieves chest pains. It is also called "Cactus Grandiflorus." Chronic chest pains are usually caused by lack of oxygen and indicate an impaired circulation of blood in the arteries.

Very important. To remove calcium buildup that causes hardening of the arteries, drink reverse osmosis water and take a product called Formula No 1 Original Formula (by Golden Pride www.goldenpride.com). It contains EDTA, the primary ingredient that removes lead and calcium buildup along with magnesium chloride, royal jelly and honey. Dosage: Take 2 teaspoons 4 times a day. After using 3 bottles (27 ounces each), reduce dosage to one tsp twice a day. Don W who needed bypass surgery for arteries 80% blocked when he was 60 years old has used this product for the past 15 years. His arteries have been found by doctors in the past few years to be free of any blockage. Don is now 75 yrs old and remains in good health. Don W 414-529-1787

Other helpful suggestions. 1 Tbsp of lecithin granules twice daily with meals. The most important herb for the heart and circulation is Hawthorne berries. "Hawthorne Supreme" by GAIA Herbs is an extract. Take 1/2 tsp. twice day.

Relaxation: Use controlled visual relaxation or self-hypnosis to induce a deep state of relaxation. Other considerations: Follow a salt-free diet that is very low in saturated fat. Eat hot chili with lots of chili pepper or red pepper added. Eat small meals and only when you are hungry. The amino acid, L-Carnitine, metabolizes fat and lowers Triglyceride levels while raising the level of High Density Lipoproteins (HDL). This amino acid is valuable for the prevention and treatment of heart disease and helps reverse hardening of the arteries. Take 500 mg of L-Carnitine twice a day and 400 i.u of Vitamin E. Use salmon or sardine oil. Avoid all high temperature processed foods cooked with vegetable oil or hydrogenated oils.

Cholesterol level - high or low:

If the total cholesterol count, (for both HDL's and LDL's combined), is over 225, it is too high and should be lowered. To lower your total cholesterol level, go on a diet high in fiber, low in fat - especially saturated fat, and get plenty of exercise and fresh air each day. Use fish oil with DHA/EPA (Max DHA)

If your cholesterol level is below 135, it is too low and it is depressing your immune system. You will need to raise your cholesterol level to get your immune system back on track. The fastest way to do this is to boil two eggs for three minutes, until the whites are cooked, but the yolks are soft; or poach two eggs until the whites are cooked, but the yolk is still liquid. Place them over mashed potatoes or over two rice cakes and make this your breakfast. Do this once a day. This should help raise your cholesterol level and boost your immune system. Also, eat butter. Do not use margarine, as it has dangerous transfatty acids that can damage your arteries. Supplements: Lecithin - 2 capsules twice a day. Use triple strength lecithin (PC-35) and L-Carnitine - 500 mg twice a day.

Cholesterol levels (low HDLs):

HDL stands for "High Density Lipids". HDLs are the good cholesterol, as they dissolve the LDLs and prevent them from settling on the arterial walls. Exercise, plant oils high in monounsaturated fats - includes olive, avocado oil, macadamia nut, hazelnut oil or specially grown Safflower oil that contains 90% monounsaturated fats, Palm oil – naturally solid at room temperature), Green tea, Lecithin, Niacin, L-Carnitine and Omega-3 fatty acids (salmon, sardine oil, cod liver oil) are the best natural substances to raise HDL's. Lecithin is sold in capsule or in granular form. Mega PC 35 (Jarrow Formulas) is a highly purified form of lecithin, with excess soy oils removed. Beverages: Avoid decaffeinated coffee. It lowers HDLs. Drink green tea, instead, which has a beneficial effect on raising HDL levels. Take L-Carnitine, 500 mg twice a day. This will raise your HDLs and lower your Triglycerides (a bad fat), which is usually too high in advanced HIV. Niacin - take 100 mg 2 or 3 times daily. Butter substitute – use "Smart Balance" that contains palm and olive oil. Never use Canola oil, marjarine, any partially hydrogenated fats or vegetable oils high in PUFA's (PolyUnsaturated Fatty Acids). PUFAs with the natural antioxidants removed are rancid and immunosuppressive and increase the bad LDL cholesterol, while lowering the good HDL cholesterol.

Cholesterol Level - Ratios of HDL to LDL

The total cholesterol count is less important than the ratio of HDLs to LDLs. LDLs stand for "Low Density Lipids". If the ratio is 4 or less, you are in good shape and your arteries are not being plugged up with LDLs. To determine the ratio, divide the HDLs into the total cholesterol count. For example, if your total cholesterol count is 200 and your HDL's are 50, your ratio is 4. (200 divided by 50 = 4). You are right on the borderline, but OK. However, if your total cholesterol count was 180 and your HDLs were 30, your ratio is 6 (180 divided by 30 = 6). This means your arteries are being plugged up with cholesterol since you have an insufficient amount of HDLs to dissolve the LDLs. You need to follow a program to raise your HDLs. Get plenty of exercise. Exercise will raise your HDLs. Eat lots of bran and foods high in beta-carotene and fiber. Take 2 tablespoons of ground flaxseed meal daily. Grind it fresh from whole flax seeds. If you follow these procedures, your numbers will start looking better in a short time. EDTA chelation therapy helps remove calcium and heavy metal deposits from the arteries.

Chronic dry cough:

The cause is mucus buildup in the bronchial tubes and surrounding areas. Raw lemon juice, distilled water and grapefruit will help break up mucus. Except for butter, avoid all dairy products - milk, cheese, ice cream and yogurt, as these are very mucus forming. Wheat is the next most mucus forming food and should be avoided. Raw spinach will break up mucus. Horseradish and red pepper are also good mucus busters. Supplements: Fenu-Thyme (by Nature's Way) will help break up mucus and kill Candida Albicans in the blood. Take 3 capsules twice a day. Vitamin C - take 1,000 mgs every 2 hrs. Herbs: Marshmallow Root tea and/or Mullein tea. It helps relax bronchial tubes and expel mucus from the lungs. Oxy-Spray rubbed into upper chest area and placing a magnetic pillow or north pole ceramic magnet over the bronchial area that is irritated and tight. If no infection is present, place the south pole of a magnet over the bronchial tubes and it will improve the flow of air almost instantly.

Chronic Fatigue Syndrome: See separate chapter

Crohn's disease:
Have your physician check for intestinal infections and consider treatment options, if any underlying infection is found. Follow Rapid Recovery Procedures, until your condition has improved, then phase in the Immune Enhancement Diet. Avoid wheat, oats and barley or other products with gluten. Follow suggestions for restoring normal intestinal flora (fiber/pectin/probiotic blend. Use coconut milk - 1/2 cup or more daily.

Colds (head and sinus):
Option 1. Mix one teaspoon of fresh lemon juice with one tablespoon of water or liquid chlorophyll and hold in the palm of your hand in a cupped position. Sniff this up your nostrils. It will burn slightly. In a few seconds, your mouth will fill up with mucus that you should spit out. Keep spitting out the mucus until it stops.

Option 2. Turn a hair dryer on low. Hold it about 12 inches away from your face. Let warm air blow up your nose as you breathe in. If throat is sore, open mouth and let warm air blow against back of throat. The heat destroys the cold virus.

Option 3. Use Zinc lozenges. Take about 50 mgs of zinc daily. Also consider procedures for Chronic Dry Cough. If you take zinc sulfate daily, you should have no need for the zinc lozenges.

Option 4. Golden Seal and Echinacea tea. Alternate with Blue Vervain and Oregon Grape root tea. Drink one cup of tea every hour for severe conditions. Hot chicken-flavored rice soup.

Option 5. FOR STAPH AND STREP INFECTIONS. Mix one tsp of apple cider vinegar, 1 clove of garlic and a small amount of ginger root in 1/2 cup of water. Place in a blender for 60 secs. Gargle this mixture and then swallow it. Repeat hourly, if staph or strep infection is present. Also, for Staph or Strep, drink one cup of Oregon Grape root tea every two hrs until you are relieved of all symptoms. Oregon Grape root tea should be steeped in very hot water for 15 minutes before drinking it.

Option 6. A product called "Nutribiotic Liquid Concentrate" may also be used. It is an antimicrobial liquid, made from grapefruit seeds that have been tested effectively against more than 20 pathogens. Use 10 drops in a glass of water every 2 or 3 hours.

Option 7. Check your urine and saliva pH. If the average of the two is above 6.4, you are too alkaline to effectively fight off this infection and you should consider a short fast of lemon juice or apple cider vinegar, raw honey and distilled water. Also Vitamin C, V8 vegetable juice, Hyssop or Rose Hip tea will lower saliva pH, when it is too alkaline.
Other suggestions: See Pneumonia

Dietary Considerations: Eat chicken rice soup. Something in it is good for colds. Avoid all dairy products and all wheat products. Herbal teas for colds: Yarrow and Mullein - great for lung problems and to promote sweating, Hyssop, Ginger, Garlic, Blue Vervain, Oregon Grape Root (kills strep and staph), Bayberry, Rose Hips, Golden Seal, Lemon-grass and Horehound. Yarrow is especially good to induce sweating. Yarrow is highly recommended when there is no sweating. Once sweating starts, toxins leave through the pores of the skin and the person recovers much quicker.

Guaifenesin 400 mg daily will prevent most sinus infections and can be used 3 times daily to help trat them as well.

Cryptosporidiosis:
Follow diet for diarrhea. One person with AIDS told me he wiped out cryptosporidium in 14 days with the following combination protocol: **Colostrum Specific** - contains immunoglobulins for cryptosporidium (Jarrow Formulas) two capsules four times a day; **Humatin** (prescribed drug) 2 capsules (250 mg) 4 times a day.

Locally, one person stopped Cryptosporidium diarrhea in 3 days using Jarrow Formulas **"Colostrum Specific"** as a monotherapy. Dose was 2 capsules 4 times a day. Duration of treatment should be 3 weeks and until stool specimen tests show the cryptosporidium is gone. Since this was reported, 4 more persons with have told me they completely eradicated the cryptosporidium with Jarrow Formulas product called "Colostrum Specific." They used 2 capsules four times a day for 21 days straight, then stopped, without the return of diarrhea.

Other suggestions:
Coconut oil - use 2 tablespoons cooked with white rice daily 3 times a day. Coconut oil is used in India to treat cryptosporidium in cattle. Garlic: Add 1 tsp. of Psyllium to a glass of water and cut up a fresh garlic clove in 3 or 4 pieces. Place the garlic cloves in your mouth and swallow them immediately with a glass of water with the psyllium added. This will create a timed release effect to bring the garlic cloves into the small intestines to kill the Crypto. Do this 3 times a day. Also, do a retention enema with up to 3 raw garlic cloves, 1/2 tsp. of black walnut and 2 Tbsp of chlorophyll added once a day. Mix in a blender.

Diet: Eat rice, steamed vegetables, and badly burned toast. Drink black and orange Pekoe tea (do not add sugar). Avoid dairy products, sweets and all fruits except lemons. Take 3 herbs (green-black walnut, wormwood and cloves) or drink tea made with cloves.

Check with your physician for the latest drugs to treat crypto. All the treatments listed here may be combined together.

Cytomegalovirus retinitis (CMV or HHV-6A?):
BHT for CMV/HHV-6A Retinitis: An article by Charles Caulfield suggested the use of BHT for CMV. BHT (Butylated Hydroxytuolene) is an anti-oxidant food preservative used to prevent rancidity in fats and oils. It is sold over the counter in health food stores (Twinlabs). Caulfield writes: "Researchers believe that 250 mg. taken daily with a fat containing meal will prevent outbreaks of Herpes. 500 mg. daily during acute outbreaks will shorten the length and decrease the severity of the outbreak. Higher doses may be needed in the case of shingles...It is thought that 2,000 mg of BHT will stop the progression of symptoms of CMV. and that after a period of treatment for acute symptoms, the dosage may be decreased to 1,000 mg per day to prevent reactivation."

Caulfield suggests taking BHT with olive oil to improve assimilation of the BHT. Taking it with the "Whole Lemon Drink" that has olive oil added to it would be good combination. Caulfield also suggests supplementing the diet with the amino acid L-Lysine (1,000 to 2,000 mg daily) and avoid L-Arginine rich foods such as chocolate, barley beer, fresh corn and many kinds of nuts. Avoid all foods (canned soda, pastry, candy bars) containing white sugar, corn syrup, dextrose and all other forms of sugar. These will feed the growth of CMV and Herpes.

Caution: One source I read said that BHT in doses of 2000 mg might elevate liver enzymes in some persons. Monitor liver enzymes, if you take more than 1000 mg daily on a continuous basis.

Update: In two cases, persons with AIDS told me that taking 1000 mg of BHT twice daily in the whole lemon/olive oil drink, plus the use of Ganciclovir, wiped out retinitis in 2 weeks. Note: if you do not use BHT with the whole lemon/olive oil drink, then take it with a high fat meal to improve absorption.

CMV infection frequently occurs in PWAs whose CD8 counts fall below 600 or who have less than 50% of normal NK cell function. CMV is a virus that is thought to cause blindness in HIV seropositives, who have depressed immune systems. It belongs in the Herpes family of viruses. Foscarnet and Ganciclovir are the main drugs currently used for CMV. However, recently, several researchers have now found that HHV-6A is causing retinitis. The jury is out as to which one, or if both viruses, are involved. Both CMV and HHV-6A belong to the herpes family. Several persons have told us that implants of Ganciclovir in the eye have been the most effective without the side effects and immuno-depression of taking it intravenously.

6/8/95 update: Persons with low CD8 counts who develop CMV or HHV-6A retinitis have often been on a heavy protocol of antibiotics, steroids or various drugs for several months preceding the CMV activity. Sugar may feed replication of CMV. Avoid sweets and canned soda, and especially avoid chocolate that increases viral replication.

Lutein: The antioxidant Lutein is found in Kale and Spinach and other dark green leafy vegetables. An article published the Journal of the American Medical Assn, Nov. 8, 1994, on studies in senior citizens, showed that Lutein helps reduce macular degeneration of the retina of the eyes. Lutein has an affinity to deposit in the retina of the eye and prevents oxidative stress and macular degeneration. HHV-6A and CMV can cause oxidative stress in the retina, doing damage that can lead to blindness. Lutein is now available as a dietary supplement. Suggested dosage if CMV/HHV-6A is active is to take two 20 mg capsules three times a day. A local PWA with visual fogginess took 40 mg of Lutein twice daily and 500 mg of BHT twice daily with COD Liver Oil. After two weeks, he reported his vision was normal.

Bilberry is an herb that has proanthocyandins and other powerful antioxidants. Take 500 mg daily. It helps remove eye floaters. It improves clarity and visual acuity. Look for tablets with a coating rather than lose capsules that may absorb oxygen into the capsule, reducing its effectiveness. (Source Naturals or Scandinavian Natural Products have the tablet form).

Ozone: I.V. or autohemotherapy has shown itself to be effective against CMV. Dr. Shallenberger M.D. (ph no 702-782-4164) reports of one case where all CMV activity stopped for 2 and 1/2 months after 10 days of IV ozone. Previous to IV ozone, the patient had used IV Ganciclovir and would start losing his eyesight, if he stopped using it for more than one week. Persons saying the Pieta Prayers have a promise from Jesus to protect their five senses (See the chapter on Prayers, Promises and Miracles). One PWA with a T4 count below 10 told us that he takes 4 BHT capsules (250 mg ea.) every evening to prevent CMV. He has done this for the past 6 months and has had no problems with his eyesight. He also does ozone rectal insufflation 3 times a week.

I should add that no controlled study using ozone or BHT for CMV has been undertaken. Ganciclovir and Foscarnet are effective drugs against CMV, but can have depressing effects of the CD4 levels. A better treatment for CMV is needed. 500 to 1,000 mg of BHT should be taken daily as a CMV preventative in PWA's with CD8 counts below 600. BHT (by Twinlabs) is sold in health food stores. Use Lutein and Bilberry and 3 garlic cloves daily along with BHT for the best results.

A study published in the German medical journal "Deutsche Zeitshrift" in Oct, 1989, by Abdullas, D.V. Kirkpatrick and Carter refers to a Chinese study where an infusion of Garlic extract killed the CMV in immune depressed bone marrow transplant patients. Our recommendations: Eat 3 cloves of fresh raw garlic daily. Between two slices of whole grain bread, slice two cloves of raw garlic and add fresh parsley sprigs.

Since CMV is in the herpes family, some of the following herbs may be effective against CMV and HHV-6A and need to be tested in a controlled study. Herbs effective against herpes type viruses are Black Walnut, Thuja, Oregon Grape root, Lomatium Dissectum, Venus Fly-trap, Slippery elm, Butter nut (bark and leaves. One source listed Butter Nut to help restore lost vision.

Dementia
(May also be good for Alzheimer's):

1. Vitamin B-6. 100 mg taken twice daily by itself. Do not take as part of a B complex formula or it won't work.
2. Oralmat.3 drops 3 times a day or 500 mg Beta Glucan
3. Sugar-free diet.
4. Ginkgo Biloba Extract - 1/2 tsp. 2X.
5. Exposure to Natural Sunlight - 1 to 2 hours daily. Wear no sunglasses - minimum clothes.
6. Ozone therapy to kill off viruses causing inflammation in the brain.
7. Ground Flaxmeal - 1 to 2 Tablespoons daily.
8. Use Blue-Green Algae or Spirulina - 1 rounded tsp. daily and Magnesium Chloride - 600 to 1200 mg daily.
9. Brewer's Yeast - 9 tablets 2 or 3 times a day.
10. EDTA chelation therapy.

(See chapter on antiviral treatments for HHV-6A)

Depression:

Mental depression is usually caused by toxins emitted by fungal infections or other body infections, low endorphin and serotonin levels and a lack of oxygen to the brain. Depression and fatigue go hand in hand. Herbs: St. John's Wort. Ginkgo Biloba, Siberian Ginseng and Green tea made together. B-complex vitamins are good in countering depression. If you are not allergic to brewer's yeast, it is your best source. Otherwise, take sublingual Coenzymated B vitamins (Source Naturals). Follow a candida control diet. Candida Albicans overgrowth is a common cause of toxins and depression. Ozone in the ears: Hold stream of ozone gas about 1/2 inch from each ear for 30 seconds each day. Breathe through your nose instead of your mouth to help get more oxygen to the brain. (See candidiasis). Exercise (light, fun and aerobic) increases endorphin levels and vanishes depression. Try dancing to your favorite music.

To increase serotonin levels, fast one meal each day or one day a week of whole grain bread and water. Do not add butter or fat, or it won't work. Note: During the fast, raw vegetables may be eaten with the whole grain bread, but add no oil or salad dressing that has oil in it. A meal of pure carbohydrates without added fat, oil or meat, fish, nuts or cheese will quickly increase serotonin levels and elevate your mood and spirits.

Diarrhea:

Diet: Black or orange Pekoe Tea (no sugar), cooked brown rice with blackberries or blueberries added and badly burned toast. The best over the counter treatment for diarrhea is Imodium AD. Eat no raw foods, until the diarrhea stops. Eat small meals of cooked foods - steamed vegetables.

The use of charcoal tablets is also an effective way to stop diarrhea. Charcoal acts like a vacuum cleaner, absorbing fluids, toxins and pathogens throughout the G.I. tract. Try 2 or 3 capsules every 4 to 6 hours, until the diarrhea stops. In one experiment, five HIV seropositives with diarrhea were placed on a gluten-free diet. Within a few days, the diarrhea stopped in all five patients. This was reported in HIV and Nutrition (Source - FDA). Grapefruit seed extract - 10 drops in a glass of water with 1 tsp. of psyllium added - take once every 3 hours. *Colon implants of raw garlic clove dipped in olive oil - use before bedtime or take a daily enema with raw garlic cloves and liquid chlorophyll added. Ozone rectal insufflation will stop most types of diarrhea, except for Cryptosporidium. See Cryptosporidiosis and Parasites.

Dry skin:

Dry skin conditions are usually caused by a deficiency in GLA (gamma linolenic acid), due to the body's inability to produce GLA, because of a lack of zinc, magnesium and B vitamins in the diet. B vitamins are produced by bifido-bacteria in the colon. It takes a diet high in fiber to support the growth of friendly flora.

A healthy body should be able to convert EFA's in flax oil or pumpkin seed oil to GLA. However, if taking 1 Tbsp of either of these two oils daily does not alleviate the dry skin condition, I recommend taking Primrose Oil capsules (1300 mg ea) two capsules, three times a day. Cod liver oil is also beneficial for dry skin conditions. Notice: If the dry skin condition is accompanied by white flaking, it may be due to Candida overgrowth. See Candidiasis. Low Glutathione levels also are associated with dry skin and rapidly aging skin.

Epstein barr virus:

EBV is associated with Candida and other fungal overgrowth. Take supplements to normalize body temperature. Monolaurin capsules or granules – 1500 mg 2 or 3 times a day. Take 20 drops of Lomatium Dissectum in water every 4 hrs until symptoms are alleviated. Avoid sugar and alcohol. Clean the colon - Drink 1/2 cup of cultured cabbage juice three times a day. Follow a diet to control Candida. EBV grows with Candida. Consider Ozone or Hydrogen Peroxide therapy. *Colon implants of raw garlic clove dipped in olive oil - use before bedtime or use GOOT. Avoid chocolate. See protocols for herpes and cytomegalovirus.

Eye strain from using a computer

Computers put out radiation that can cause mental confusion and eyestrain. A screen that you can attach to the front of your computer is made by Belkin and is sold in stores that sell computer supplies. The Belkin screen is a Premium Glare Filter and blocks 99% of all ELF and VLF radiation. This is a must for anyone who spends several hours a day in front of a computer, and it is very helpful in reducing computer-related fatigue. Costs about $15.

Fatigue:

Many factors can cause fatigue, including adrenal exhaustion, liver toxicity, acidosis, thyroid dysfunction, viremia or other infections, thrush, candidiasis and insomnia to name a few. Malnutrition and malabsorption are also contributing factors. Follow Rapid Recovery Procedures for fastest results. A very common but overlooked cause of fatigue is yeast and fungal overgrowth. Thrush is an indication of yeast activity. In his book, "The Yeast Syndrome," Dr. Trowbridge reports on over 20 kinds of poisons emitted by various strains of yeast, including Candida Albicans. These toxins (poisons) are frequently a major cause of fatigue and depression. Avoid sugar and alcohol. Eat more raw foods and sprouts.

Specific supplements that give energy and reduce fatigue: Cat's claw, Sun Chlorella, Spirulina, Klammath Falls Blue Green algae (capsules or powder only, not tablets), Siberian Ginseng, Green Tea, dark green leafy vegetables, Blackstrap molasses.

6/8/95 update: Two PWA's have reported that the herb "Cat's Claw" significantly increased their energy levels. Dose take was 2 or 3 capsules daily.

Fever:

First of all, say "Thank You" to your immune system. It is actually working. A fever is an indication that your immune system is functioning. Fevers that don't rise too high have a lot of healing power in them. Don't be too quick to quash a fever. However, don't let it get out of control either. To break a fever, sip on a cup of hot **Yarrow** and **Echinacea** tea combined. This is a powerful infection fighting formula and will stimulate the immune system while breaking the fever. If more is needed, take a cup of Golden Seal leaf tea between your Yarrow/Echinacea teas or take Golden Seal root capsules - about 2 every 4 hours. **Golden Seal** tea is an anti-viral herbal infection fighter. Diet - abstain from solid food while fever lasts. Eat soups, drink vegetable and fruit juices and consider taking "Designer Protein" by Next Nutrition. If the fever lasts more than one day, simply follow "Rapid Recovery Procedures." Freshly squeezed juice is best. However, you may drink orange, grapefruit or Concord grape juice, if a juicer is not available or you have no one to wait on you.

Lobelia is another very powerful herb to fight infections and fevers. It works, when all else fails. To make Lobelia tea, use 1/2 tsp. in a cup of hot water. Strain after 5 minutes. Drink one cup every 4 to 6 hours. Other: bathe in cool water to cool off an overheated body.

Gas (upper):

Recommendation: Take digestive enzymes and ginger root. Grapefruit seed extract - 10 drops in a glass of water. This will kill bacteria causing upper gas. Then take 3 or 4 charcoal capsules. You might consider opening the capsules and mixing them with water. Bacterial infections can sometimes cause upper intestinal gas. Many of these can usually be knocked out with cultured cabbage juice. You can sip on half a cup three times a day for 3 to 5 days, or until all symptoms have vanished.

Food Combining: Upper intestinal gas can also be caused by food allergies or improper food combining. Never eat fruits or desserts right after the main course of any meal. Try eating only one food at a time and see how your body handles it, before eating another food. Consider what you ate at the last meal and see if the same symptoms occur when you eat the same food again. If a food allergy is present, eliminating the offending food will stop the symptoms from reoccurring. Some of the most common foods that cause allergies are milk, eggs, wheat, corn, yeast, soy, citrus fruit, lunchmeat and some sea foods. Chemical additives like monosodium glutamate (MSG) often cause hidden food allergies.

Herbs for Gas: Wild Yam root, Ginger, Papaya, Raw Pineapple, Anise. Do not consume hydrogen peroxide, carbonated water or aloe vera with or just after mealtime; they will dilute hydrochloric acid, which is necessary for protein digestion. Charcoal capsules or Gas-X and other products for gas are sold in drugstores OTC.

Gas (lower - flatulence):

Some flatulence from the lower colon is a sign of a healthy colon. Lower gas is a cause for concern, only if it has a cheese like odor. This would indicate Candida overgrowth. If this is the case, consider colonics or enemas. Flatulence after you eat beans is normal, and odor-free flatulence is normal and indicative of a healthy colon. An unhealthy condition would be stools that sink to the bottom of the toilet and where no gas is present. This means that there is too much E Coli in the colon and that the colon is too alkaline to produce gas. You must take steps to restore normal (floating stools). A diet high in squash, garlic, onions, cultured milk, dark green vegetables and cultured cabbage juice are recommended. Herbs: Wild Yam root, Ginger, Papaya, Raw pineapple, Anise. *Colon implants of raw garlic clove dipped in olive oil - use before bedtime.

Hemoglobin (low levels):

One person successfully increased his Hemoglobin levels by taking 1 Tbsp of liquid Chlorophyll in water 3 times a day. Food sources: dark green vegetables, Spirulina, Chlorella, wheat and barley grass. We have heard of other reports of similar results. Note: A blood transfusion is the fastest way to increase hemoglobin levels.

Hepatitis (B or C)

Thiamine – vitamin B 1 – Persons report less fatigue and more energy in 2 or 3 days. A low cost way to reduce viral load for hepatitis B and C – dose 100 mg taken 3 times a day 8 hours apart. Thiamine as well as alpha lipoic acid helps process iron out of the liver. Iron is used by HBV and HCV to help in viral replication. For more information, go to www.mercola.com/2001/apr/21/thiamine.htm. Additional help: Take 1 Coenzymate B Complex (Source Naturals) sublingually twice daily and eat one raw potato as a source of natural alpha lipoic acid. Dip raw potato chips in olive oil and sprinkle on basil for flavor. Silymarin or Milk thistle is critical to protect the liver from oxidative stress and prevent disease progression Use 400 to 800 mg daily.

Selenium: Two readers report a 90% drop in HCV viral load within 2 months after taking 400 mcg of plant-based selenium 3 times daily. No adverse effects were reported after one year of using 900 to 1000 mcg daily. High selenium mustard greens (Phytosel) or high selenium broccoli or yeast. Castor oil packs over the liver area daily to reduce enzymes and prevent cirrhosis.

Chlorophyll – a potent natural antibiotic and antiviral to cleanse the intestines and purify the liver. Consider 5 grams daily of chlorella, Spirulina or wheat grass How friendly is your flora? Consider Fiber/pectin/probiotic blend. Did you know hepatitis viruses live in the intestines?

Nutricology has a new Chinese herbal formulation (Eurocell) that has some really good data on it for treating Hepatitis C infection. www.nutricology.com.

Hepato C, a Chinese herbal formulation with 15 herbs has reportedly cleared Hepatitis B and C in several cases after 3 months of use. Dose: 2 capsules twice a day. For more info contact Pacific Biologic at 800-869-8783.

Transfer Factor Plus (4-Life Products) or Immax (www.immunefoods.com)- good anecdotal data available for Hep B or C. Take ProBoost Thymic Protein A daily.

Transfer Factor for Hepatitis A, B and C. (Chisolm Biologicals) 1 day – use DS or T grade product. I have reports of viral load declining 80 to 90% after 3 months. No adverse effects reported.

Ozone therapy is very effective against all strains of Hepatitis. Follow the protocol for serious infections. One daily enema with chlorophyll and raw garlic added. Add 2 Tablespoons of liquid chlorophyll to a glass of water and drink 3 times a day. Silymarin - take 200 mg twice a day. Take 2 dandelion root capsules twice a day. If jaundice is present, take "Fringe Tree" herbal extract - 15 drops under the tongue 4 times a day. Drink one cup of lobelia tea before bedtime and use a colon implant of raw garlic. Eat no meat, but lots of raw foods. Have regular medical checkups for status of hepatitis virus. *Colon implants of raw garlic clove dipped in olive oil - use before bedtime.

Ultraviolet light therapy. Dr. Wm Douglass MD at an Ozone convention in Dallas, TX in 1994 told of a case where he removed a pint of blood from a patient with Hepatitis and exposed the blood to full spectrum light with UV for 20 minutes and then reinfused the blood into the patient. After this single treatment, the patient was cured.

Levamisole for hepatitis B – protocol developed by Prof Humberto Saconato and Ewerton Cortez if Rio Grande do Norte, Brazil Tel:55-84-221-6320 saconato@summer.com.br.

Lamivudine (Epivir) aka 3TC and alpha interferon – standard therapies from your physician.

Herpes (genital):

Treatment: BHT, Lomatium dissectum, Red Marine Algae, Olive Leaf Extract, Venus Fly-Trap, Lemon Balm, Ozonated olive oil, BioPro Thymic Protein A and Monolaurin. Choose one or two of these items at a time and continue down the list until you find what works for you.

A chest or head cold usually accompanies cold sores around the lips and herpes in the genital area. Concentrate on getting rid of your cold by following a mucus-free diet. The main mucus forming foods to avoid are those containing lactose and glutens. Candidiasis and yeast infections often accompany herpes, so alcohol and foods high in white sugar must be avoided. Canned soda, pop and fruit drinks are troublemakers. Clean the colon or use enemas. Consider raw garlic suppositories dipped in coconut or olive oil and inserted into colon before bedtime. Even better, do the enemas with raw garlic and chlorophyll added.

For topical application, use Orlamat or ACNO, Lomatium Dissectum (diluted with water), ice cubes - apply directly to lesions, zinc oxide, Super-Lysine Plus - sold in Health food stores or Venus Fly-Trap extract. In one case, ozonated olive oil completely cleared all Herpes lesions in 1 week. Ozone in a Sauna Bag completely eliminated Herpes in another case. For internal Herpes, use Ozone Rectal Insufflation.

After applying liquid treatments, dust generously with a moisture absorbing athlete's foot powder such as Desenex powder or Dr. Scholl's foot powder. Do not touch sores. Wash hands if you do touch them, as you could spread the virus to other parts of your body. It is especially important to keep your hands away from your eyes. For Herpes infection in the eyes, add 3 drops of Lomatium dissectum to 1 tablespoon of sterile water and place in an eyecup over eye for 5 minutes 3 times daily or see your doctor. Avoid touching your eyes after touching the sores and you can prevent this problem. *Colon implants of raw garlic clove dipped in olive oil - use before bedtime.

Relax - reduce stress and take these supplements: Zinc sulfate - 220 mg daily (provides 50 mg elemental zinc) Vitamin B-12 - 1,000 mcg daily, 400 mg of Vitamin E, 2 times a day during outbreaks, reduced to 400 mg daily after healing of sores is completed. To prevent spreading the virus to others, avoid all sexual activity until the sores have dried up and all tingling and itching sensations have disappeared.

I received a letter from one reader who had a chronic Herpes condition for 2 years. He claims that after taking Red Marine Algae for 6 weeks, his condition was 80% improved. He took 2 grams a day (2,000 mg). The strain of Red Marine Algae used by our reader was from the species "Dumontiaceae." Red marine algae is distributed at www.dynamune.com.

Avoid chocolate, nuts and foods high in L-Arginine. The Herpes virus is stimulated by L-Arginine. Avoid all foods containing white flour and white sugar and avoid alcohol.

One person reported that since taking 1 teaspoon of Lemon Balm extract (GAIA Herbs) 3 times a day, he no longer needs Acyclovir. He says the Lemon Balm is more effective than the Acyclovir in preventing herpes outbreaks.

Histamines:

Natural anti-histamines are Pycnogenol (extracted from a species of Pine bark), rinds of lemons, vitamin C, Vitamin B-6 and Quercitin (found in Spirulina and yellow onions).

Human Papilloma Virus (HPV):

Genital warts caused by Human Papilloma Virus (HPV) can be treated with Aldara Cream - available from your physician. Aldara cream is FDA approved and works about 50% of the time. Beta-Mannan, a product developed from aloe vera by Dr. Joe Glickman MD. He reports a 95% cure rate for HPV infection. Two persons who used Beta Mannan told me it got rid of the HPV warts. More info at www.alotek.com or call 406-863-9824. One person used a combination of equal parts of colloidal silver and DMSO, applied topically to get rid of these warts.

Immune systems (other factors that depress it):

Electric blankets or any other strong alternating current field. Living close to a Radio or TV station or other source of alternating electronic waves, Microwave ovens, wearing clothing made from nylon, rayon, polyester and other unnatural materials. Being influenced by negative thinkers, or persons who are chronically depressed. Eating foods with chemical preservatives and drinking city tap water, with either chlorine or fluoride added. Smoking tobacco, drinking alcohol, taking street drugs, lack of deep restful sleep can stress the body. Use organically grown foods, if available.

Indigestion:

Indigestion has many causes, one of which is low body temperature. Eating when you are not hungry, eating too fast and not chewing your food well and mixing too many foods together, can cause stomach distress. Try eating proteins first at each meal. Follow with vegetables. You may eat grains and vegetables together or carbohydrates and vegetables together. Never eat sweets or fruit with vegetables, or you will have a real case of indigestion. Mix as few foods as possible. Never eat fast or when under stress. Chew food slowly and salivate each mouthful.

For more information, read the book by Shelton on Food Combining Made Easy. (Sold in health food stores). Do not consume hydrogen peroxide, carbonated water or aloe vera with, or just after, meals; They will dilute hydrochloric acid, which is necessary for protein digestion. Herbal Digestive aids: Add 1/2 tsp. of Gentian root and 1 tsp. of fresh sliced ginger root to a cup of hot water. Drink with or after meals. Fresh ginger root is sold in grocery stores. Cayenne strongly stimulates digestion. A product sold in health food stores called "Swedish Herbal Bitters" is a time proven digestive aid that has helped millions. Lemon juice with meals is a great aid to digestion. Also, cayenne and other hot peppers. If more is needed, take 1 betaine hydrochloride tablet and Vegetarian Digestive enzymes with each meal.

The Australian Herbalist, Peter de Ruyter, recommends a Spice tea to put the fire (heat) back into the stomach. It is made from Fennel seeds, Dill seeds, Caraway seeds, Anise, Coriander seeds. 1/4 teaspoon of each is added to one cup of boiling water and left to stand in a covered teapot overnight. Strain and bring liquid to a boil. Remove from heat and add one tsp of Slippery Elm. This creates a jelly like product, when it cools. Peter de Ruyter recommends this tea to be eaten by the spoonful for any kind of gastro-intestinal inflammation or ulceration. He warns against using an aluminum teapot, as the herbs can inter-react with the soft aluminum metal. He recommends using stainless steel, porcelain or glass.

Insomnia:

For insomnia, try the following before bedtime: First choice: One **Scullcap** capsule (Nature's Herbs) plus a small glass of **sour cherry** juice. Scullcap is a herb that works like a dream and Cherry juice contains natural melatonin.

Second Choice: Drink a cup of tea made of Thyme and Marjoram. Use 1/2 tsp. of each herb to make the tea. Coral calcium – 1/2 teaspoon powder in the evening, or Calcium lactate - 1 tsp. in water or 5 capsules or eat half a cup of cottage cheese. Other: juice of 1/2 lemon in water and/or 1 betaine HCL and 1 digestive enzyme tablet.

Synthetic Melatonin tablets - take 1 to 3 mg. before bedtime to induce sleep. Available in drug stores and health food stores. Melatonin is a natural hormone produced in our body. A few persons have reported that 3 mg is too much and knocks them out. Liquid melatonin is now available that lets you take a smaller dose. Take a walk for 30 minutes before retiring for the night. Avoid heavy meals at least 3 hours before bedtime.

Other choices: **Essential oils** – sprinkle 3 or 4 drops of lavender, marjoram, neroli or clary sage essential oils on your pillow or vaporizer before retiring at night for a deeper more restful sleep.

Sun tanning outdoors or in a salon indoors – 15 to 20 minutes 2 times each week improves calcium absorption and promotes deeper sleep.

NEW: Listen to music and go to sleep. "Healing Music" by Alan Roubik (Positive Health News, Report No 21). Several persons report this CD really works. They just fall asleep every time they play it. Do not play this CD, while you are driving a car! More info can be found at www.roubikrecords.com/menu.htm or by calling 818-597-9358 Ask for the "Four Seasons" CD that was formerly called "HADO Music – Series I." A new CD released is "Keys to my Heart" and Alan Roubik, the producer said several people have reported using this CD to induce deep sleep.

Jaw TMJ
- stiff jaw or cracking sound under your ears when you swallow:
   Evening Primrose oil - 1000 mg three times a day.

Kaposi Sarcoma:
   See the Chapter on Cancer

Lipodystrophy:
   Elevated triglycerides, cholesterol and fat accumulation in the upper back and tummy area. Lipodystrophy is caused by protease inhibitors used to treat HIV and especially when they are combined with Zerit (D4T) or AZT. Dr Bernard Bihari MD has found that Naltrexone 4.5 mg daily prevents and helps reverse this condition in most persons with HIV.

Lung Infections : See Pneumonia

Lymph nodes (swollen):
   Swollen lymph nodes in AIDS are an indication of active viral activity, due to HHV-6A, or it could be a sign of other problems like leukemia or lymphoma. Twenty out of 24 PWA's who had swollen lymph nodes have reported a complete remission in one week to 10 days using the Whole Lemon/Olive oil drink daily. Surprisingly, a few reported no change. When this happens, saliva pH should be checked. In my own observations with PWA's, a saliva pH of less than 6.0 has been associated with lymphadenopathy. When saliva pH is chronically acid, it calls for an alkaline diet. For more information, see the chapter on "Balance your pH."
   Other lymphatic cleansers are aloe vera juice and spirulina. Oxy-spray may be rubbed directly on the swollen lymph nodes. A vibrator with a built-in heat pad is great to move lymph fluid. Walking, jumping rope or jumping on a trampoline are also excellent ways to clear out the lymph system. A man from Chicago reported that sleeping with a ceramic magnet under his pillow completely reduced a swollen lymph node under his armpit in just two days. When using a magnet, the north-pole should be oriented toward the body. Ozone Therapy - Rectal insufflation and/or Sauna Bag is very effective and will eliminate swollen lymph nodes in 2 to 3 weeks.

Lyme disease:
   Early treatment – use antibiotics as prescribed by our doctor. If no cure after after 60 days of antibiotic treatment, consider a herbal product called **SpiroKete** (Kroeger Herb Co www.kroegerherb.com). Take 2 capsules twice daily for 4 days per week. On the 3 days off each week, use **Venus flytrap extract** – 40 drops 3X . Continue treatment for at least 8 weeks and then get a re-examination from your physician. **Cat's claw** - 2 cups of the tea may be used daily along with the other treatments.

MAC/MAI:

Antibiotics are usually used to treat mycobacteria infections. Raw Garlic kills MAC - use 3 to 5 cloves daily. MAC/MAI usually occurs when your cell mediated immunity is low due to low levels of CD8 Killer T cells, usually below 600 per UL or low CD4's – usually under 100. Prescription drugs are usually needed, if your immune system is severely depressed. See your physician.

Meningitis:

Eucalyptus oil - inhale vapors of 10 drops on pillow or handkerchief every 15 to 30 minutes each hour and rub the essential oil on the chest. 3% H2O2 - one teaspoon in a glass of distilled water taken on an empty stomach hourly, until condition stabilizes or as directed by your physician. Suggestion for physicians: add a few drops of eucalyptus oil to humidifier, when administering oxygen to patients. Orally - 5 drops of Eucalyptus oil in a glass of water every 2 hours.

Microsporidium:

One reader had good results using Albendazole (Zentel) for this condition. The dose was 400 mg twice a day. The reader reported a complete cessation of symptoms in 14 days. If Albendazole does not work, consider treatments used for Cryptosporidium.

Molluscum:

Apply **Oralmat** drops (Source: Nutricology). This skin condition should improve in a few days. Oralmat is imported into the US by Nutricology and is sold in health food stores. Other: **Neem seed oil**, tea tree oil, lavender oil.

Mouth sores:

White Patches - Use coconut oil or apply GOOT directly to sores. Rinse mouth with 3% hydrogen peroxide. For stubborn sores, soak a Q-tip directly in 35% H2O2 and apply against the sore. Sore will usually disintegrate. Place a ceramic magnet, magnetic pad or pillow against the facial area where the sore exists. Use north pole energy. Sores will usually decrease after 1 hr of exposure. Herbs: Oil or Oregano or Lomatium dissectum. Myrrh Gum extract. Also Bee Propolis dissolved in the mouth is very effective. Rinse your mouth and gargle with ozonated water. Also see Candidiasis.

Nausea:

Herbs: Ginger root capsules or tea.

Neuropathy:

Neuropathy is a disorder affecting the nervous system. HIV or diabetes are common causes, as is HHV-6A infection. The most effective treatment for neuropathy is the Whole Lemon/Olive oil drink done daily, along with lecithin supplementation. One tablespoon of lecithin granules should be blended into the whole lemon drink and consumed each day. Other supplements: Magnesium Chloride – 2 tablets 2X, Methyl B-12, Coral calcium - 1000 to 2000 mg daily. One person reported that Vitamin B-6, 100 mg twice daily improved his condition 60% in 2 weeks. Neuropathy can be caused by some prescription drugs. Check on the side effects of the drugs you currently use.

Night sweats:

From Balmain, Australia, Herbalist Peter de Ruyter (B.Sc Ag, Reg. Nurse, Med. Herb. Homeopathy, Cert. Reiki II and Iridology) writes: "Night sweats are extremely easy to stop with common Sage herb (Salvia officinalis). Use 1 Tablespoon of Sage per 3 cups of boiling water. Leave the cover on the teapot and let it stand overnight. The next day, have the person drink 2 or 3 cups of the tea. The night sweats will stop within a few days. Sage tea is very drying and should not be used continuously, but used only when needed. Persons with chronic night sweats should have their physician check for T.B. or syphilis as these infections can also cause night sweats. Sage is a seasoning sold in grocery stores and in health food stores."

Night sweats results from overheating the body. Undigested proteins from your last meal may be a contributing factor. Grains, alcohol and sugar are also contributing factors, as is yeast overgrowth. If you wake up sweating, take 2 digestive enzymes (HCL and Vegetarian Digestive enzyme tablets). Squeeze the juice of 1/2 lemon and take with ice water. Also, you can take a spoonful of apple cider vinegar in water. If you think indigestion is related to the night sweats, get up and take a walk for 1/2 hr to 1 hr. The walk will aid the digestion of your last meal. Before going back to bed, drink a cup of Marjoram and Thyme tea.

You may need colonics or high enemas to remove candida (yeast) and parasites and toxins from your lower bowel. For a colonic, look up a colon therapist in the Yellow Pages under "Colonics", or ask your local health food store if they know of one in your area. Use colon implants of raw garlic before bedtime.

Pancreatitis:

Pancreatitis is an inflammation of the pancreas. It is usually caused by the consumption of alcohol along with drugs like DDI or other toxic drugs. The immediate solution is to stop all alcohol consumption, including herbal extracts with alcohol in them, and all drugs suspected of bringing on this condition. To help reduce inflammation, place the north pole of a magnet over the pancreas area for 1 hour twice a day. Herbs: Juniper Berry tea - 1 cup 3 times a day. Cayenne - with meals - two capsules 3X, Dandelion root Capsules - Two 3X with meals. Castor oil packs daily over the left side of abdomen. Gentian root.

Parasites:

Symptoms of parasites are diarrhea and weight loss. Chlorinated public water supplies and well water are possible sources of contamination. Distilled water or Reverse Osmosis water should be free of all parasites. The most effective treatment is a combination of black walnut, cloves and wormwood tincture. Use 30 to 50 drops 3 times a day with meals. Raw garlic cloves also kill parasites. Eat one clove on rye crisp every four hours. *Colon implants of raw garlic clove dipped in olive oil - use before bedtime. Herbs: Black walnut, raw garlic. Frozen castor oil capsules - take 1 or 2 before bedtime - kills parasites in the colon. Also see the protocol for Cryptosporidium. Imodium A-D can be helpful to stop diarrhea in between.

Platelet count (low):

Use **ProBoost Thymic Protein A** (Longevity Science) - one packet daily under the tongue to increase platelet counts. See Thrombocytopenia.

Pneumonia (PCP):

Symptoms are tightness in the chest, pain in the chest and shortness of breath. Normal drugs prescribed to treat PCP are Bactrim/Septra or Dapsone, all sulfa based drugs. When these drugs cannot be tolerated, because of allergic reactions/rashes, Mepron is the drug of choice, as it is well tolerated by most persons.

SEES-2000: I have talked to several PWA's in the Houston, TX area who swear by the effectiveness of a special herbal preparation called SEES-2000, an herb that has a high sulfur content. SEES-2000 contains the ground roots of the herb - Radil Lomatium Nevadensis, aka "Lomatiuim Dissectum." Of 50 persons I have followed using SEES-2000 on a daily basis, one capsule a day is reported to prevent PCP 98% of the time. When pneumonia is present, one capsule every 4 hours is recommended for 3 to 5 days until symptoms are gone. Four persons have reported rapid recovery from PCP who have taken this herb.

Side effects of SEES-2000. One in 7 persons report getting a rash. If this happens, stop using the SEES-2000, until the rash is completely gone. Then resume taking the SEES-2000. So far, most persons who have followed this procedure and resumed taking the SEES-2000 have not had the rash return. Note: if you get PCP before you start on SEES-2000, take one every 4 hours along with antibiotic therapy. Separate the herb from the antibiotics by one hour, to avoid any unknown drug/herbal inter-reactions. If you should get PCP after using SEES-2000, follow the same procedure.

Desensitizing yourself to Sees-2000: To reduce the chance of getting a rash, start off with Sees-2000 using one capsule once every 3 days (i.e. Mon and Thurs) for the first two weeks. In weeks 3 and 4, take one Sees-2000 every other day. Choose even or odd numbered days. In week five, take one a day. Note: Desensitization to Bactrim, a sulfur based drug, has also enabled people to tolerate this drug, who previously would break out with a rash. I would advise against using both Sees-2000 and Bactrim/Septra together - use one or the other.

Note: In January 1997, a friend in a local hospital (Milwaukee, WI) with PCP was being treated with antibiotics. However, his condition was so bad that the doctors told him he had only a 50% chance of recovery and should get his affairs in order. The next day, while in the hospital, and with his doctor's permission, he started using Sees-2000 - one capsule every 4 hours, plus the antibiotics he was receiving. Within hours, his blood oxygen levels began to increase. He improved so rapidly that he was sent home 3 days later.

Fenugreek-Thyme. It is especially valuable when excess mucus is present. It has a drying effect on the lungs and kills fungal infections in the lungs and head area. Take 2 capsules 3 times a day. It may be used along with SEES-2000. Sold under the brand names "Nature's Herbs" and "Nature's Way." It is found in health food stores.

Another treatment for pneumonia is **oral hydrogen peroxide - food grade**. Take hydrogen peroxide orally as follows: Take 1 teaspoon of 3% H_2O_2 (drugstore variety) in a glass of distilled water every hour, up to one hour before meals or 3 hours after. This can be repeated up to 8 times in one day. Do not take any supplements with iron in them, while using the H_2O_2. Discontinue using the H_2O_2, after the lung infection has cleared.

Herbs: **Pleurisy root tea or Lobelia tea** are the most important of all the herbal teas to drink for pneumonia. You could alternate these teas every 2 hours apart. Herbal teas: Pleurisy Root or Lobelia. Other herbs: marshmallow root and mullein made together. Drink it and/or inhale the steam.

Several options may be used together, until the infection has cleared. Note: If body temperature is below normal, take supplements (cayenne) to increase body heat. If you have a question about what options are compatible, consult your physician.

Manufacturer of Sees-2000 is Sharon and Jane Barlow of Generation II, PO Box 1008, Sandy, Utah 84091 866-688-6757

Pruritus, Folliculitis and Psoriasis:
UVB light has been used to clear these 3 conditions. However, for tanning, use UVA that penetrates deeper into the body and does not promote skin cancer, as does UVB light. The product, ACNO, from Australia, has cleared up a number of skin problems of unknown origin. A homeopathic ointment called Florasone (Boericke & Tafel). This topical cream relieves itching and skin rashes. Available in health food stores.

A low fat diet is very important - use little or no butter, cheese or chocolate and avoid fried foods. Also, take Silymarin - 175 mg 2X, Oregon Grape Root tea - 1 cup daily made with 1 tsp. of the herb steeped in hot water, Lecithin - two 19 grain caps with meals 3X, Cod Liver Oil - 1 Tbsp - 2X, Good oils are Flax oil, Olive oil, marine lipids and Evening Primrose oil.

Red blood cells - low:
Take liquid sublingual B-12 with folic acid (Bricker labs) or Methyl B12. B-12 builds up red blood cells. Vitamin B-6 is also reported to help build up red Blood cells. Check your body temperature. Low body temperature has been linked to low red blood and white blood cell counts. Conventional treatment for anemia is Procrit.

SARS (Sudden Activated Respiratory Syndrome) A new easily transmitted disease that can be fatal. See treatments for Pneumonia.

Scar tissue (from radiation, burns or surgery)
Castor Oil packs: Internal scar tissue in the abdominal area (intestines, uterus etc) can be removed by doing warm castor oil packs over the area 1 hour daily for about 3 months. If scar tissue is in the lungs, throat or bronchial tubes, do castor oil packs over the upper part of chest and throat area daily for 2 to 3 months. For external scar tissue, warm castor oil packs followed by pure topical applications of vitamin E. Fresh aloe vera emulsion: Blend one cup of the white inner part of aloe vera leaves with 1/2 cup of water. Drink this daily, or use it as an enema or douche or apply topically. Aloe leaves may be stored in a refrigerator for up to 3 weeks. Fresh organic aloe leaves can be shipped to you from - Aloe Supply Co., PO Box 93, Belle Glade, FL 33430 (863-467-6200).

Seizures -
Deficiencies of magnesium, potassium and vitamin E may contribute to seizures. Dilantin, a prescription drug, is usually effective in preventing seizures. If an actual seizure occurs, seek emergency medical help. To help prevent a seizure, give any available source of magnesium such as Epsom salts (mg sulfate) and water. Start with 1 Tsp. Epsom salt and water. Follow this with 2 Tablespoons of blackstrap molasses, a rich source of potassium, magnesium and trace minerals. To help prevent seizures, avoid alcohol that depletes magnesium reserves and take a supplement with magnesium daily along with Vitamin E -

400 I.U daily. Consider Blackstrap molasses - 1 or 2 Tbsps daily or Magnesium Chloride tablets – two twice daily.

Shock (anaphylactic)-
A severe allergic reaction to a food or medicine that causes body temperature to fall rapidly, saliva pH to go acid, pupils to dilate and smooth muscles to contract. If you should sense these conditions happening to you, after taking some medication, new herb or food, call Emergency for help (dial 911) and then immediately take 1 tsp. of cayenne with water, kelp or any herb to raise body temperature and 2 tablespoons of blackstrap molasses. You may substitute honey, if molasses is not available. Also, you can take some Dimethylglycine (DMG) under the tongue. These supplements will act to turn off the shock reaction. You may do all of the above. Turn on the heat and get as warm as possible. Get immediate medical attention.

Sinus infection:
Supplements: For long-term relief, take 400 mg **Guaifenesin** and 220 mg of **zinc sulfate** once a day. Other: Take 1 tsp. of fresh lemon juice in 2 Tbsps of water and sniff up your nose. It will burn a little, produce a lot of mucus, but also open up your sinuses and help kill viral infections in that area. Consider getting a humidifier, if the air is too dry. **Avoid all wheat and dairy products containing lactose and casein.** A negative ionizer will also help. Hold ionizer near nose. Breathing ionized air will frequently open plugged sinuses. Stay away from dairy and wheat products. **Sniff Colloidal Silver up your nose.** A Colloidal Silver Nasal Spray by Source Naturals works fine. See Colds. See Pneumonia. **Inhale vapors of Eucalyptus oil.** Note: **Short-term use (5 to 7 days) of oral hydrogen peroxide is very effective against sinus infections.** See chapter on Bio-oxidative Therapies.

Skin - dry, wrinkled, hard; loss of elasticity and smoothness
Use Evening Primrose Oil to overcome dry skin conditions. Vitamin A - 10,000 to 25,000 i.u. daily (Cod Liver Oil capsules – 6 to 12 daily). Kombuchu Tea. Excess free radicals in the blood cause skin to become wrinkled, hard and have a loss of smoothness and elasticity. Pycnogenol is a free radical scavenger and improves skin smoothness and elasticity, helps protect collagen binding, reduces edema and swelling in legs, reduces fragility of capillaries and inhibits histamines. Elderberry extract and bilberry are very high in proanthocyandins, the same substance found in Pycnogenol. Increase your intake of vegetables and fruits high in red, blue or orange pigments. These pigments contain flavinoids that are free radical scavengers. Take supplements to increase Glutathione levels. Increasing Glutathione levels stops breakdown of the skin.

Sore throat:
Place a glass of water in a blender. Add 1 tablespoon of apple cider vinegar and one clove of garlic in half cup of water. Blend until smooth. Gargle half and spit out. Swallow the other half. Repeat this every hour until desired results are obtained. Consider a cup of Blue Vervain and Oregon Grape root tea every two hours. These two may be mixed together. Other Herbal teas: Mullein and Yarrow. Consider gargling with 3% H_2O_2 or ozonated water every few hours. (See Colds).

Sore stomach:
Drink 1/2 cup of cultured cabbage juice three times a day or eat raw cabbage and raw potatoes. Consider - Slippery Elm Tea and Licorice root tea. Other herbs: Golden Seal tea, White oak bark. Magnetic Therapy - North Pole of pad over stomach area for 1 to 2 hours daily. Bland diet - Have yourself tested for any infections in the stomach area.

Thrombocytopenia (low platelet count):
ProBoost Thymic Protein A gives very rapid results for increasing platelet counts (distributed by Klabin or Threshold and available in health food stores). Also, the whole lemon/olive oil drink combined with the Castor Oil packs increased platelet counts in several cases. Two persons who have had ozone autohemotherapy have told me that they started out with very low platelet counts, which climbed rapidly within 3 weeks and returned to their normal reference ranges.
HHV-6 LINKED TO ITP. USE OZONE TO BUILD UP PLATELET COUNTS. An article written by Neenyah Ostrom in The New York Native (Oct 10, 1994) cites an article appearing in The Lancet (Sep. 17, 1994, by K. Kitamura "Idiopathic Thrombocytenic Purpura after Human Herpesvirus 6 infection." It is HHV-6, variant A that is causing widespread damage in both AIDS and CFIDS progression. Ostrom reports that HHV-6 (A) can infect and kill natural killer cells and CD4 cells can infect and damage the brain, spinal cord, lymph nodes, heart, bone marrow, liver, kidney, spleen, tonsils, adrenal glands, pancreas and thyroid.

Toxoplasmosis
See your physician for a prescription antibiotic first. A parasitic protozoan causes this condition. Household cats are common carriers. Usually, anyone with toxoplasmosis infection of the nervous system or brain is under intensive care in a hospital. **One teaspoon of Colloidal Silver twice a day completely reversed toxoplasmosis in one case, where the person had very low T cells.** Also consider Ozone therapy or take **40 drops (1/2 tsp) of 6% H2O2 (food-grade quality)** solution in a glass of water every 4 hrs. Consider retention enemas, with garlic and chlorophyll added, once a day. Take supplements to raise body temperature. **Raw garlic** - 3 cloves daily.

Triglyceride levels too high:
Dr. Bihari, in an article published in POZ magazine, Jan. 1996, linked high tryglyceride levels to high Tumor Necrosis Factor (TNF) levels. The primary cause is HHV-6A. The problem is that your CD8 counts are too low, as are your NK cells, to control the HHV-6. High triglycerides predispose you for a heart attack. Bihari has found that Naltrexone (4.5 mg) daily reduces Triglyceride levels. Olive leaf extract with 20% oleuropein – 2 caps twice daily. Take Max DHA with EPA (Marine lipids, L-Carnitine - 500 mg twice a day. Exercise - walk for 1 hour twice a day. North Pole magnetic therapy will also help reduce triglyceride levels. L-Carnitine lowers triglyceride levels. Exercise burns off triglycerides by stimulating the body to convert L-lysine into L-Carnitine.

Warts (HPV):
Genital or vaginal warts caused by Human Papilloma Virus (HPV) can be treated with **Aldara Cream** - available from your physician. Aldara cream is FDA approved and works

about 50% of the time. **Beta-Mannan**, a product developed from aloe vera by Dr. Joe Glickman MD. He reports a 95% cure rate for HPV infection. More info at www.alotek.com or call 406-863-9824. One person used a combination of equal parts of colloidal silver and DMSO, applied topically to get rid of these warts. Another person here in West Allis applied **"Miraculous Water"** from San Damiano in the vaginal area daily for several months. When her physician examined her several months latger, the PAP nodules were completely gone.

Wasting syndrome: (See chapter on Weight Gain).

West Nile virus

West Nile Virus is spread by bites from infected mosquitoes. Over 200 Americans died from this virus in 2002. A transfer factor product is now being developed by Chisolm Biological Labs that will be antigen specific for stimulating a strong immune response against the West Nile Virus. For more information, call 803-663-9618 Other: **Oral hydrogen peroxide drops** - see the chapter on Bio-oxidative therapies.

White blood cells - low

Use **ProBoost Thymic Protein A. Daily castor oil packs** over liver area. Supplements to increase Glutathione levels (ImmunePro, Designer Protein, Alpha Lipoic acid). Beta-carotene - 50 mg 3X; Cod Liver Oil – 6 capsules twice daily; sun tan up to 1 hour daily or up to 30 minutes in a **Tanning salon** using UVA light therapy.

An Acupuncturist told me of another Chinese herbal product for increasing white blood cell counts. It is called **"Marrow-Plus."** It is manufactured by Institute for Traditional Medicine (ITM), 2017 SE Hawthorne, Portland, OR 97214. Ph No 503-233-4907. Take 3 capsules 3 times daily until WBC counts are 7000 UL or higher, then use only as needed to keep WBC's in a normal reference range. ITM only sells through health care professionals. Prescription drugs: Neopogen increases WBCs rapidly.

Zits (red pimples):

If zits are weeping like open sores, suntan or go to a Tanning Salon. Do up to 1/2 hour daily with UVA light, until the zits are gone. UV light kills topical infections. If the zits are an allergic response, consider a homeopathic equivalent to cortisone is called Florasone (Boericke & Tafel). Consider 1% hydrocortisone cream – use up to 1/2 teaspoon daily.

Other: bathe them in 3% H2O2, and then place aloe vera gel over them. As multiple infections disappear from your intestinal tract, blood stream and lymphatic system, the zits will also disappear. Ozone in a Sauna Bag is very effective for all skin problems or apply ozonated olive oil over topical infections or irritations.

A formula that will produce miracles - GOOT
Garlic oil ointment
Anti-infective/Anti-fungal/Anti-parasites

Warm 3 tablespoons of Coconut oil over stove until melted and add 3 tablespoons of olive oil. Remove from heat and add 1 tablespoon of fresh chopped garlic. Blend at slow speed, then at high speed for 2 minutes. Use a blender or coffee grinder. Pour mixture through a screen to remove chunks of garlic that the blender may have missed. Pour into a wide mouth jar and label it "GOOT." Place in a refrigerator.

GOOT turns into a thick soft paste after 1 hour. GOOT, rubbed into the skin, transfers raw garlic oil directly into the blood stream. Apply on the feet of children or infants to fight infections. Rub on chest for chest colds, pneumonia or rub into nostrils for sinus infections. Apply directly to sores inside the mouth. Rub on Athlete's foot and genital area for jock itch. Insert GOOT into vagina or rectum for yeast or other related infections. Apply on rashes any place. Place on cotton swab for ear infections. GOOT kills Candida, parasites, bad bacteria and virus by direct application. In addition, it treats systemic infections by absorption through the skin into the blood supply and travels throughout the body. After two weeks, make a new batch of GOOT.

23

CANCER

Signs & symptoms of Cancer
From the American Cancer Society's website www.cancer.org

A symptom is an indication of disease, illness, injury, or that something is not right in the body. Symptoms are felt or noticed by a patient, but not easily observed by anyone else. For example chills, weakness, achiness, shortness of breath, and a cough are symptoms that might indicate pneumonia.

A sign is also an indication of illness, injury, or that something is not right in the body. But, signs are defined as observations made by a physician, nurse or other health care professional. Fever, rapid breathing rate, abnormal breathing sounds heard through a stethoscope are signs that may indicate pneumonia.

The presence of one symptom or sign may not provide enough information to suggest a cause. For example a rash in a child could be a symptom of a number of things including poison ivy, a generalized infection like rubella, an infection limited to the skin, or a food allergy. But, if the rash is associated with a high fever, chills, achiness and a sore throat, then all of the symptoms together provide a better picture of the illness. In many cases, a patient's signs and symptoms do not provide enough clues to determine the cause of an illness, and medical tests such as x-rays, blood tests, or a biopsy may be needed.

How does cancer produce symptoms?

Cancer is a group of diseases that may cause virtually any sign or symptom. As cancer progresses, it goes through many stages, producing symptoms as it goes. The symptom produced will depend on the size of the cancer, the location of the cancer, and the surrounding organs or structures. If a cancer metastasizes (spreads), then symptoms will be very different, again depending on size, location, and surrounding structures. As a cancer grows, it begins to exert pressure on nearby organs, blood vessels and nerves. This pressure creates some of the signs and symptoms of cancer. If the cancer is in a critical area, such as certain parts of the brain, even the smallest tumor can produce early symptoms.

Sometimes cancers form in locations where symptoms may not be produced until the cancer has grown quite large. For example, some pancreatic cancers do not produce symptoms until they begin to grow around nearby nerves, causing a backache. Unfortunately by the time a pancreatic cancer causes back pain, it has usually reached an advanced stage. A cancer may cause generalized symptoms such as fever, fatigue, weight loss, etc. The cancer cells may release substances that alter metabolism. Or, the cancer may cause the immune system to react in ways that produce these symptoms.

Sometimes, cancer cells release substances into the bloodstream that cause symptoms not generally thought to result from cancers. For example, some cancers of the pancreas can release substances that affect blood clotting and cause blood clots to develop in veins of the legs. Some lung cancers produce hormone-like substances that affect blood calcium levels, affecting nerves and muscles and causing weakness and dizziness.

Why is it important to recognize symptoms?

The treatment of cancer is most successful when the cancer is detected as early as possible. It is possible to detect some cancers before symptoms occur. The American Cancer Society, and other organizations, encourage the early detection of certain cancers before symptoms occur by recommending a cancer-related checkup and specific early detection tests for people who do not have any symptoms. For additional information on early detection tests, see the American Cancer Society document on Cancer Detection Guidelines.

However, these recommended early detection tests do not diminish the importance of reporting any symptoms to your doctor. Sometimes symptoms are ignored because the person is either frightened by their implications and refuses to seek medical help or does not recognize the symptom as being significant. It is very easy for individuals to think that a backache or fatigue is a "part of life" or that a breast mass is probably a cyst that will go away by itself. Whenever a symptom occurs, it should not be discounted or overlooked. This is especially true if the symptoms have been going on for a period of time, such as weeks.

General cancer symptoms

It is important to know what some of the general (nonspecific) signs and symptoms of cancer are. They include unexplained weight loss, fever, fatigue, pain, and changes in the skin.

Unexplained weight loss: Most people with cancer will experience weight loss at some time with their disease. An unexplained weight loss of about 10 pounds may be the first sign of cancer, particularly cancers of the pancreas, stomach, esophagus, or lung.

Fever: Fever is very common with cancer. Almost all patients with cancer will experience fever at some time, particularly if the cancer or its treatment affects the immune system and reduces resistance to infection. Less often, fever may be an early sign of cancer, such as with Hodgkin's disease.

Fatigue: Fatigue may be a significant symptom as the cancer progresses. It may occur early, especially if the cancer is causing a chronic loss of blood as in some colon cancer or stomach cancers.

Pain may be an early sign with some cancers, such as bone cancers or testicular cancer. Most often, pain is a symptom of advanced disease. Skin clues: In addition to cancers of the skin, some internal cancers can produce visible skin signs such as darkening of the skin, or hyperpigmentation; reddening, or erythema; itching; and excessive hair growth.

Cancer's seven warning signs - specific cancer symptoms

In addition to the above general symptoms, the American Cancer Society has established the following seven common symptoms that could lead to a diagnosis of cancer.

1. A change in bowel habits or bladder function. Chronic constipation, diarrhea, or a change in the size of the stool may indicate colon cancer. Pain with urination, blood in the urine, or change in bladder function could be related to bladder or prostate cancer. Any changes in bladder or bowel function should be reported to your doctor.

2. Sores that do not heal. Skin cancers may bleed and resemble sores that do not heal. A persistent sore in the mouth could be an oral cancer and should be dealt with promptly, especially for patients who smoke, chew tobacco, or frequently drink alcohol. Sores on the penis or vagina should not be overlooked.

3. Unusual bleeding or discharge. Unusual bleeding can occur in early or advanced cancer. Blood in the sputum is a sign of lung cancer. Blood in the stool could be a sign of colon or rectal cancer. Cancer of the lining of the uterus (endometrial cancer) or cervix can cause vaginal bleeding. Blood in the urine is a sign of possible bladder or kidney cancer. A bloody discharge from the nipple may be a sign of breast cancer.

4. Thickening or lump in breast or other parts of the body. Many cancers can be felt through the skin, particularly in the breast, testicle, lymph nodes (glands), and the soft tissues of the body. A lump or thickening may be an early or late sign of cancer. Any lump or thickening should be reported to your doctor. You may be feeling a lump that is an early cancer that could be treated successfully.

5. Indigestion or difficulty swallowing. These symptoms may indicate cancer of the esophagus, stomach, or pharynx (throat).

6. Recent change in a wart or mole. A change in color, loss of definite borders, or an increase in size should be reported to your doctor without delay. The skin lesion may be a melanoma that, if diagnosed early, can be treated successfully.

7. A nagging cough or hoarseness. A persistent cough that does not go away is a sign of lung cancer. Hoarseness can be a sign of cancer of the larynx (voice box) or thyroid. These are often late signs of cancer.

End of excerpts from the American Cancer Society's website

Metabolic and immune factors linked to cancer predisposition

1. **Elevated interleukin 6 levels**. Adrenals are exhausted - chronic fatigue. - Free cortisol levels are low while bound cortisone and estrogen levels are elevated. Liver is toxic and sluggish. When muscle mass is wasting away, tumor necrosis factor (TNF) is elevated.

2. **pH profile of a cancer patient** or early stage– first urine pH reading in the morning is very alkaline (7.0 or h higher) and saliva pH is very acid- less than 5.8. A typical pH profile would be a urine pH of 7.5 and a saliva pH of 5.5. As recovery from cancer is underway, the pH profile reverses itself and the first urine pH reading becomes acid – less than 6.0 while the saliva pH moves closer to a normal 6.4.

3. **Stool profile – small diameter – always sinks to bottom of toilet bowl** – will not float on water. Person will develop multiple food allergies and intolerances. Low bifido bacteria count and low butyrate levels in stools.

4. **Urine characteristics**: Clear or cloudy with strong odor of ammonia – not yellow unless B vitamin are taken daily.

5. **Cravings** – sweets (refined sugar, corn syrup) and foods high in fat – usually the wrong kind (i.e. vegetable oils like soybean or canola etc all bad choices).

6. **Sleep – interrupted – not restful.**
7. **Stomach and intestines** – appetite and digestion poor – sore spots may exist in tummy area.
8. **Mineral deficiencies of calcium, magnesium and selenium** as measured in blood serum. Tendency to develop osteoporosis. Also, as cancer likes to hoard iron, look for low iron levels. Note: iron supplements feed the growth of cancer.
9. **Hypothyroid - body temperature – low** or below normal.
10. **Hormones – estrogen dominant – high level of bound or total Cortisone and low levels of Free Cortisol. Adrenals exhausted.**
11. Skin test for **Delayed Cutaneous Hypersensitivity** (DCH) Result is no response or a condition called **Anergy**.
12. **Natural Killer cell Function test** – less than 50. When cancer is present, NK function is less than 20.

Review sections of this book that address these 12 preceding factors linked to cancer and what remedies, if any, are available. Additionally, smoking cigarettes and exposure to chemical and industrial pollutants and electromagnetic pollution, including cell phones, will increase the cancer risk.

Precautions

1. Avoid most synthetic vitamins, especially vitamin C. Do not use vitamin C supplements with Chemotherapy or the chemotherapy will fail. Chemotherapy is based on oxidative responses to kill cancer cells. Other oxidative therapies include ozone, hydrogen peroxide, a type of wormwood called artemesia annua (artemisim) and Venus flytrap extract. The use of vitamin C and other synthetic antioxidants must be avoided or all these therapies will be neutralized and will fail. The antioxidants in wholesome foods are not a problem. Exceptions to this advice is B-12, niacin and co-enzymated B complex (sublingual) by Source Naturals.
2. Avoid all man-made iron supplements. Cancer cells sequester iron and use iron to assist in their metabolism and growth. Iron supplements feed the growth of cancer cells. All iron must come directly from plant or animal sources.
3. Avoid all man-made amino acid chelates, complexes or proteinates.

Plant/animal based vitamins and minerals to use

Natural vitamins found in whole foods will always cost a little more than their cheap synthetic counterparts. Be aware that there are many manufacturers of dietary supplements that compete to have the lowest-priced vitamins and supplements on the market. The lower the price means there is less quality in the marketed product and the greater probability that the dietary supplement will have little or no health benefits. While they cost more, in my experience I have found natural vitamins are 1000% or more effective than their synthetic counterparts. Synthetic vitamins may also produce side effects at high doses whereas plant or animal derived vitamins do not. However, not all synthesized vitamins are necessarily bad. Coenzymated B vitamins and Methyl B12 are possible exceptions. Some antioxidants like lutein are derived from plants and have significant health benefits for the consumer.

However, most of the Vitamin C sold in pill form today while called " natural" is actually synthetic and is not extracted from any plant source but synthesized. Studies have found DNA damage and oxidative stress from synthetic vitamin C used at a dose of no more than 500 mg daily. No study has found these adverse effects from natural plant based vitamin C (e.g. oranges, camu, rose hips, acerola etc). The safety of natural vitamins may be due in part to the accompanying co-factors found in whole foods that affect their function in the body; co-factors that are missing in their cheaper synthetic counterparts.

a. Vitamin A and D – Cod liver oil capsules or desiccated liver tablets for vitamin A, D and B complex.

b. B complex – other sources - desiccated liver tablets or brewers yeast tablets, Royal jelly, Chlorella or Spirulina from the ocean only or wheat, kamut or rye grass juices, parsley or other dark green vegetables, bananas, whole rye bread or other gluten free whole grains. Note: If you need to use high potency synthetic B vitamins, consider "Coenzymate B Complex" by Source Naturals or Methyl B12.

c. Vitamin C and bioflavinoids – whole rose hips powder, extract or tea. Acerola cherries, Camu. – one teaspoon daily. If you need to use a high potentcy synthetic vitamin C, use the one synthesized from beets from Nutricology. It is preferable to the synthetic vitamin C synthesized from corn that is the most common form on the market.

d. Vitamin E – from wheat germ oil or use wheat germ oil or natural mixed tocopherols.

e. Vitamin K – parsley and dark green vegetables. – 1/2 cup daily.

f. Calcium and magnesium – Calcium Lactate (6 caps daily) or 1 teaspoon of coral calcium powder daily plus 2 or 3 magnesium oxide, mg citrate or mg chloride tablets twice daily (Alta Herb Co) or magnesium sulfate (Epsom salts) – 1/2 tsp daily. If anemia exists and iron is needed, use only liver, brewers yeast, spinach and/or blackstrap molasses. If you use iron pills, it will cause the cancer to grow rapidly.

g. Selenium – Use Phytosel – 800 mcg daily or 400 mcg selenium plus 4 Brazil Nuts for a total of 800 mcg daily of selenium..

h. D'glucarate – 1600 to 2000 mg daily if in pill form. However, in my opinion, the preferred choice is to eat 1 cup of broccoli daily plus 6 apples or oranges or the juice of 6 fresh apples or oranges to give you a total of about 2300 mg of glucaric acid. Glucaric acid blocks cancer growth in 3 different ways (1).

Lack of glucaric acid and increased beta-glucuronidase has been found in breast, ovarian, lung, colon, liver, bladder and prostate cancer. Glucaric acid is found in some fruits and vegetables and Calcium D'Glucarate is available as a dietary supplement. Persons under a toxic overload should try to consume 1500 to 2000 mg daily of glucaric acid. Because it is processed quickly out of the body, it is best to consume a food with glucaric acid once every 3 or 4 hours throughout the day. Apples that are tart like Granny Smith or Winesap are highly recommended. Eat one apple every 3 hours or 3/4 cup of raw applesauce or 1/2 cup of fresh pressed apple juice (not canned or pasteurized) every 3 hours throughout the day. If you prefer a dietary supplement, take D'Glucarate – 2 capsules every 4 hours or 8 total each day.

Apples and broccoli are the preferred choice for glucaric acid, as the acid in oranges or lemons may not agree with some people. Note: Grapefruit should be avoided, as it interferes with the P450 liver detox enzymes. Tart cherries or cherry juice have about 200 mg glucaric acid per cup and 4 to 8 ounces of cherry juice before bedtime will also help with sleep, as cherries contain natural melatonin.

1. D-Glucarate – A Nutrient Against Cancer – Thomas Slaga, A Keats Health Guide, (found in health food stores).

Other supplements that are very important: Naltrexone - 4 mg daily late evenings and low-dose hydrocortisone - 20 to 30 mg once daily in the AM. While Naltrexone improves NK function, low-dose hydrocortisone lowers IL-6 and TNF.

Natural Killer cell function test

Natural killer cells are a type of white blood cell that have an innate knowledge of what is self from non-self. Functional NK cells attack and destroy what is non-self - cancer cells along with various other foreign viruses and antigens. An NK function test actually measures the ability of this white blood cell to lyse or kill cancer cells in a laboratory. The effect of killing cancer cells is measured in "lytic" units. This is not the same as a count of the number of NK cells in your blood. You could have a large number of NK cells that are non-functional or useless.

Ask your physician for a Natural Killer Cell Function test. If the number of lytic units is below 35, you do not have good immunity against cancer. See the chapter on Immune-based therapies for more information on NK function tests and protocols to increase NK function. Take a Fiber/Pectin/Probiotic blend. Every cancer patient I have talked to, who has active cancer, has intestinal dysbiosis and stools that sink to the bottom of the toilet bowl. Also, the first pH reading in the morning is acid saliva and alkaline urine. See earlier chapters in this book on how to reverse and normalize pH, as well as restore normal bowel flora. The result will be noticeable floating stools.

Conventional, complementary or immuno-therapies?

Conventional therapies for cancer are surgery, chemotherapy, hormonal regulation and radiation. Complementary therapies are those designed to be used with conventional therapies, while alternative therapies are used in place of chemotherapy, radiation and surgery. Generally, immunotherapies, also called immune-based therapies, can be used with conventional therapies or alone or in combination with other alternative therapies. Tamoxifen is a drug that obstructs estrogen binding in the breast area to prevent the return of breast cancer. Tamoxifen would be considered a hormone-based treatment. Herbs that have similar properties to Tamoxifen and have phytoestrogens that block excess estrogen binding to cells include red clover, tumeric, thyme, yucca and hops with special emphasis on red clover, which is widely reported to be used as an anticancer treatment from several different cultures and areas of the planet. The same can be said for tumeric.

Immune-based therapies for cancer

See separate chapter on **Immune based therapies**. Immune modulators usually activate natural killer cells and/or CD8 killer T cells and include low-dose hydrocortisone, Naltrexone, IP6, aged garlic extract (Kyolic), transfer factor, fresh aloe vera leaf juice, shiitake and maitake mushrooms and others. Natural Killer (NK) cells, that are functional, hunt down and kill (lyse) cancer cells anywhere in the body.

Finding help at Cancer Treatment Centers of America

If you are a person who wants to keep all options open and are considering using both conventional and complementary therapies at the same time, you may want to contact the Cancer Treatment Centers of America. They offer all of the conventional treatments in combination with diet modification, detoxification and acupuncture. On the internet you can reach them at www.cancercenter.com. Their phone number is 800-577-1255

Gerson cancer treatment and "The Gerson Primer"

For alternative therapies for cancer that are effective, it is my opinion that the Gerson Institute sets the gold standard. Briefly, the treatment consists of a number of freshly prepared juices, especially apple combined with carrot, and then green juices, initially given at specific times during the day. Yogurt with flax oil and several supplements are also given daily including thyroid (1 grain), potassium iodide, pancreatic enzymes, niacin, desiccated liver, B-12, colostrum, royal jelly and much more, including castor oil packs. All the supplements are listed along with the diet plan in The Gerson Primer. The two books will tell you how to treat cancer, but you will need a helping hand to move from concept to reality. A person with cancer will need a full time assistant, family member or friend, to help prepare the meals and juices and will need to consult with a local physician, trained in the Gerson method.

From 1928 to 1958, Charlotte Gerson's father, Max Gerson MD, pioneered and developed the original Gerson method of treating cancer and published it in a book called, "A Cancer Therapy – results of 50 cases." What is so remarkable about the Gerson cancer treatment is that an impressive number of terminal cancer patients recovered, and some went on to live another 40 years cancer-free. The Gerson method, if used, should be assisted by a physician trained at the Gerson Institute. Taking shortcuts and leaving out parts of a protocol will undermine the effectiveness of the treatment. The best decision - and often this will depend on available fund - is to go directly to the Gerson Institute in Mexico for a 2 or 3 week stay for treatment. Short of that, both books, "A Cancer Therapy" by Max Gerson and "The Gerson Primer" should be purchased for the person who is unable to travel. Both books should be considered required reading. "The Gerson Primer" also contains a section on lab data and interpreting lab results. To order "The Gerson Primer" and "A Cancer Therapy," call 619-685-5353, or write to Gerson Institute, 1572 2nd ave, San Diego, CA 92101 or visit their website at **www.gerson.org**.

Note: The use of high doses of plant based selenium (1000 to 1600 mcg daily) along with 400 i.u of vitamin E, Ip6, Butyrate, Aged Kyolic garlic, aloe vera, Maitake or shiitake mushrooms, Transfer Factor plus (4-Life Products) and Naltrexone can be included with the Gerson protocol.

To order supplies for the Gerson protocol (desiccated liver, thyroid, potassium iodide, pancreatin etc) listed in "The Gerson Primer," or to arrange a visit to the Gerson clinic in Mexico, call 011-5266-4680-1103 from the US. Note: Call either the phone number in Mexico or the US number for help in finding a local physician trained in the Gerson method of treating cancer.

Additional treatments that may be used in conjunction with the Gerson method include high doses of plant-based selenium (1000 mcg or more daily), Aged garlic extract – 5 grams daily (Kyolic formula 100), IP6 – 4 to 6 grams daily, Maitake or shiitake mushrooms – 5 grams daily, magnesium chloride 6 tablets daily from Alta Herb Co and; oxidative therapies that include (ozone, hydrogen peroxide, a type of wormwood called artemesia annua (artemisim) and Venus fly trap extract). Artemisim is available through Allergy research (Nutricology). It is important not to use any man-made vitamin C with any of the oxidative therapies or they will fail, and supplements with iron will cause the cancer to grow. Safe sources of vitamin C and iron must be 100% natural and plant based or animal based – for iron – liver (desiccated liver), molasses, spinach and for vitamin C – oranges and rose hips powder, extract or tea.

Editor's Note: In my opinion, if the patient's estimated survival time is (1) less than 60 days (end stage); the patient is in (2) constant pain or (3) has lost more than 20% of their normal body weight, then the Gerson treatment (an entirely nutritional approach and a much more intensive treatment program than offered by conventional Oncologists or the Cancer Treatment Centers of America) offers the best chance for recovery. Any person with cancer, who has one or more of the 3 preceding conditions, should, if at all possible, make arrangements to go directly to the Gerson Institute in Mexico for treatment.

Persons who have one or more of the 3 conditions listed her,e and attempt self-treatment, usually make treatment decisions that are too little and too late. An example would be a cancer patient with wasting syndrome, who is on pain killers daily and decides to use Sutherlandia alone to reverse their wasting condition. The patient does not incorporate the Gerson diet, supplements and juices, but instead dines on pizza, pasta, pastries, soda, and avoids raw vegetables, and fresh vegetable juices and continues to use the pain killers, instead of coffee enemas, to get rid of the pain. This patient's prospects for recovery are slim.

As a secondary, but better choice, than self-treatment alone, anyone who is not able to go directly to the Gerson clinic for treatment, should contact the Cancer Treatment Centers and then, in consultation with their doctor, also use information from the two Gerson books to incorporate as much of their dietary and detox protocols as possible into their daily treatment program. Additional treatment options can also be found in John Boiks book on Natural Compounds in Cancer Therapy.

"Natural Compounds in Cancer Therapy" by John Boik

Natural Compounds in Cancer Therapy is a scholarly, balanced review of the actions and potential clinical use of over three dozen carefully selected natural compounds. Nearly 4,000 references are included. It provides a comprehensive and systematic examination of the actions, pharmacology, toxicology, and potential clinical use of natural compounds as anticancer agents. This is the sequel to the author's first book, Cancer and Natural Medicine, which received excellent reviews in medical and lay journals worldwide.

Persons who will benefit from this book include cancer patients as well as students and professionals in oncology, nursing, cellular and molecular biology, pharmacology, toxicology, veterinary medicine, herbal medicine, health sciences, and natural products chemistry.

Topics covered: Comprehensive examination of the effects of natural compounds on the biological processes involved in cancer progression, including effects on cell proliferation, angiogenesis, invasion, metastasis, and the immune system. Also contains a detailed review of dose, pharmacology, toxicology, and other issues of clinical and scientific importance. Natural compounds discussed include, for example, vitamin A, selenium, plant flavinoids, mushroom extracts, garlic, and ginseng. See www.ompress.com for the Table of Contents and additional information.

John Boik received his Masters Degree in Acupuncture and Oriental Medicine from the Oregon College of Oriental Medicine in Portland and his Bachelors degree in civil engineering from the University of Colorado in Boulder. He is currently enrolled in a Ph.D. program at the University of Texas Health Sciences Center, Houston, where he studies the anticancer effects of natural substances. He serves on the scientific advisory board for the natural products firm, Hauser Inc., and on the editorial review board for the journal, "Alternative Medicine Review."

"This authoritative and thorough review of the use of natural products [in cancer treatment] is one of the best in the field of herbal medicine. ...This valuable resource is highly recommended for physicians and their patients, researchers, pharmacists, nurses, educators, and laypersons seeking reliable information about complementary cancer therapies."

"A jewel...clear, crisp, concise and useful. The scope is incredible. Not simply a regurgitation of the literature, but a thoughtful and well-balanced interpretation and analysis of the data."

"Natural Compounds in Cancer Therapy," by John Boik provides invaluable information with scientific research and documentation on complementary therapies that can be used in conjunction with the Gerson Therapy or conventional treatment approaches. The book can be obtained at local book stores or by calling 800-610-0768 or 763-389-0768; Fax: 612-395-5239 Web: www.ompress.com   Oregon Medical Press 520 pages 8.5" x 11 ISBN:0-9648280-1-4

"Cancer Therapy" by Ralph Moss, PhD.

For researching possible additional treatments to use in conjunction with the Gerson treatment, Ralph Moss's book, "Cancer Therapy," is another valuable aid with short articles on more than 80 alternative cancer treatments, including the well-known Gerson treatment. However, with over 36 possible treatments listed for breast cancer alone, it can quickly lead to information overload. Also, the specific details on how to use each treatment are usually not provided and require further research, so information that can be implemented quickly in a practical application is not immediately available. This book is a valuable tool for the researcher or individual who wants to see the full scope of available treatment options, along with significant references to contact resources.

Ralph Moss has created a summary guide for 80 cancer treatments used in treating 19 types of cancer. However, I have found some serous flaws in his summary charts, so many that I would skip this section of his book, and certainly not buy into the sections on using Megace or synthetic vitamin C. The potential for DNA damage from using large doses of synthetic vitamin C is real and is supported by credible research. Only vitamin C found naturally in oranges, rose hips and Acerola cherries and other food sources should ever be used. There is no research that has linked natural vitamin C to DNA damage. Unfortunately, rose hips and acerola cherries often have synthetic vitamin C added to "standardize" the vitamin C content. If you see a rose hip or acerola cherry product that is standardized to contain 5% or 25% vitamin C, then you know it has been spiked with the synthetic C. Look for bulk rose hip powder or acerola cherry powder with nothing added. Add one tablespoon once or twice daily to a shake, applesauce or yogurt as a source of completely natural vitamin C. In spite of my critical comments here, the book is a valuable resource for the researcher.

"Cancer Therapy" by Ralph Moss PhD is available from Equinox Press, Brooklyn, NY phone 718-636-4433 or your local health food store or bookstore ISBN 1-881025-063.

Other optional treatment specifics - fresh aloe vera drink – contains beta-mannan, a powerful cell detoxifier/healer

A critical part of the healing process is detoxification. Water itself is a great healer and fresh aloe vera juice is a miraculous detoxifier. You can make your own whole leaf aloe vera juice at home with fresh aloe leaves. Wash leaves and remove the spines on the edge. The spines contain a laxative. To make one cup of whole aloe juice, cut up one cup of aloe leaves. You can leave the green skin on the leaf for the benefits of the bitter factions. Place chunks of aloe in a blender. Add one cup of distilled water. Blend at a slow speed for 10 seconds and then strain through a screen type strainer or cheesecloth. Drink 1 or 2 cups daily. You may make larger batches and store in a refrigerator for up to 5 days. Aloe leaves may be stored in a refrigerator for up to 3 weeks. Source of fresh aloe leaves that can be shipped to your house: Aloe Supply Co., PO Box 93, Belle Glade, FL 33430 (863-467-6200). Using fresh aloe vera leaves is a very cost effective way of healing the gut and detoxifying the lymph system, a better choice than buying processed aloe vera products and costs less than $1.00 a day. Aloe vera juice is especially valuable for healing the intestines and removing scar tissue.

Prostate Cancer - PC-Hope replaces PC-Specs – lowers PSA

The main symptoms associated with prostate cancer, and often with other prostate problems before cancer, can be detected, as follows: *
Urinary hesitancy (delayed or slowed start of urinary stream)
Urinary dribbling, especially immediately after urinating
Urinary retention
Pain with urination
Pain with ejaculation *
Lower back pain *
Pain with bowel movement
Additional symptoms that may be associated with disease of the prostate: *Urination, excessive at night *Incontinence *Bone pain or tenderness *Hematuria (Blood in the urine) *Abdominal pain *   Anemia *Weight loss *Lethargy

The prostate helps control urination and helps sexual activity. It plays a passive role in the process of urination by controlling the rate urine flows out of the bladder and into the urethra, with the muscles in the prostate that surround the urethra. The prostate has an active role in sexual activity byÊ making a whitish glandular secretion that collects within the prostate and is fed into the urethra during ejaculation. This glandular secretion helps the motility of the sperm in the urethra and makes up about a third of the seminal fluid, thus giving seminal fluid its whitish appearance. A strong (mostly) vegetarian diet, low fat diet or one that mimics the traditional Japanese diet may lower risk.

Early identification (as opposed to prevention) is now possible by yearly screening of men over 40 or 50 years old through digital rectal examination (DRE) and PSA (prostate specific antigen) blood test. P S A (Prostate Specific Antigen) The PSA test is performed to detect the presence of PSA in the blood. A high PSA test is indicative of the presence of Prostate Cancer. PSA is a glycoprotein (a protein with a sugar attached) found in prostatic epithelial cells. It is detected at low levels in the blood of adult men. The PSA level is greatly increased in most men with prostatic cancer, but can also be increased somewhat in other disorders of the prostate.

PC-Specs is a Chinese herbal formulation with an excellent track record for treating prostate cancer and lowering PSA levels, often 90% or more in a short time period. However, because of marketing claims and that PC-Specs did not go through the FDA approval process, they were forced to change the name to PC-Hope and stop making the claims. From our information, PC-Hope is essentially the same product as PC-specs. Some of the things we are hearing about PC Hope include: "PC Hope works!" PC-Hope is available at nutrition 2000 and other sites found on the internet.Ê For more information or to contact Nutrition 2000, call (800)-587-7077 or e-mail Frank at frank@nutrition2000.com. Nutrition 2000 Salina, OK 74365.

Other suggestions for preventing and help in treating Prostate cancer – zinc supplementation and or pumpkin seeds – raw 2 or 3 tablespoons daily –a rich natural source of zinc and Saw Palmetto extract or capsules and a fresh raw parsley sprig eaten daily – about 1/2 cup. However, in considering these other suggestions, PC-Hope should be your primary treatment.

Breast Cancer

Conventional treatments include radiation, chemotherapy and surgery. Research on breast cancer patients has shown that they have up to a 75% reduction in Natural Killer cells. Glucaric acid levels are low and estrogen receptors are high. **Researchers have found that breast cancer return can be substantially reduced with high doses of vitamin A, selenium and magnesium chloride**. (1,2).

Imunological: Test for **Interleukin-6 levels** (IL-6) and **Natural Killer** (NK) cell function and monitor **Estrogen** and free urinary **Cortisol** levels.

Alternative treatment specifics: **Black Cohosh** capsules 2 three times daily **See chapters on "Osteoporosis" and on "Immune based therapies." Naltrexone, Low-dose hydrocortisone, low dose Amrour Thyroid, Miraculous Water** applied topically.

Some persons have reported mixing 6% hydrogen peroxide solution with pure aloe vera juice and applied it topically on lumps in the breast and other areas topically. They report the lumps have reduced in size or gone away completely. One person said he injected pure ozone gas into the center of a cancerous lump in his wife's breast, and the lump disintegrated and was gone in about 2 weeks. Anyone who gets rid of a cancerous tumor by any oxidative therapy or surgery alone, and does not use immune-based therapies to restore Natural Killer cell function and normal thyroid, adrenal and liver functions, will likely have a return of the tumors at some future point in time.

1. Ramesha A, et al. Jpn J Cancer Res. 1990;81:1239-46
2. Blondell JM. Anticarcinogenic effect of magnesium. Med hypotheses, 1980;6:863-71

Kaposi Sarcoma

Symptoms of KS are red to purplish, flat or raised blotches, bumps, or spots, usually painless, occurring on or under the skin, inside the mouth, nose, eyelids, or rectum, that don't go away. Initially, they may look like bruises, but usually are harder than the skin around them. Usually, these blotches are preceded by yellowing of the skin and are indicative of active KS lesions.

Before AIDS, Kaposi Sarcoma (KS) was a rare disease in Africa associated with malnutrition, particularly protein calorie malnutrition. Yellowing around KS lesions is a sign of new KS activity. The purple color of the lesions indicates an acid blood condition that is high in carbon dioxide and low in oxygen. Bright red lesions are less threatening as they indicate increased oxygen content. Brown lesions that are flat are basically dead lesions. In KS, as in cancer, cuts and wounds heal slowly.

A KS patient from New Mexico told me in Dec. 1995, that every time he ate pork, he had a flare-up in his KS lesions. HHV-6A has many factors in common with African Swine Fever Virus and Cytomegalovirus. ASFV virus infects pigs systemically. In humans, eating pork may trigger growth of HHV-6A and cause new KS lesions to form. Apparently, this virus likes pork. The activity of HHV-6 could trigger certain cytokines, like Interleukin 6, and hormones like estrogen, that together would act like growth stimulators to the blood vessels. KS patients should strictly avoid ham, bacon, pork, sausage and lunchmeat containing pork.

Potassium is a key mineral to stimulate wound healing, when used in conjunction with amino acids. Rutin is very effective in strengthening capillary walls and should help prevent formation of new KS lesions. Good sources of rutin are - the herbs Rose Hips and Rue, black currants and the rinds of citrus fruits - lemons, oranges and grapefruit, that are also high in bio-flavinoids.

TNF and triglyceride levels are often elevated in PWA's. Dr. Bihari has found that high triglyceride levels are linked to high TNF levels. High triglyceride levels are associated with active HHV-6A. Marine lipids, DHA/EPA lower triglycerides and may be helpful. Max DHA (Jarrow Formulas) or Salmon Oil would be good choices. Low levels of HDL's, the good cholesterol, may be a contributing factor. The liver produces cholesterol and a liver in a toxic state may not be able to produce the quantity needed for normal metabolism. A suggestion that may help lower triglyceride and TNF levels is the Whole Lemon drink with extra virgin olive oil added, which removes toxins from the liver. Note: L-Carnitine lowers triglyceride and TNF levels like the drug - Trental. Trental reportedly reduces K.S. lesions.

The next question is: what effect will L-carnitine have on K.S. lesions? Suggestion: Use 1,000 mg of L-carnitine 3 to 6 times a day.

KS remissions credit Maitake mushrooms. (August, 2001)

I'm writing first to say thank you for such a helpful and inspirational website. I've used the whole lemon/olive oil drink on and off for several years now, with great success, normal liver function being one, despite the heaviest drug regime.

Previous to 1999, I suffered from KS cancer pretty much all over my body. On the advice of a friend who had total remission of his KS from Maitake tablets (7 taken 3 times a day). I took the plunge and started the Maitake*, with a CD4 count of 17 and after 3 months on the tablets, my KS stopped and faded. No one was more surprised than me. I say this because I have NO faith in any type of medicine/remedy/herbs etc. My feeling is that this stuff has to prove itself to me. This same friend lent me your manual on How to Reverse Immune Dysfunction.

    Simon simon@guni.net or simoncaleb@btinternet.com

*Note: Simon used regular Grifon Maitake capsules (about 2000 mg 3 times daily) and not the Maitake D fraction. This is the second case reported where 6000 mg of Maitake mushroom powder daily resulted in a complete remission of the KS lesions after 8 to 12 weeks.

Other protocols for kaposi's sarcoma

Very important - highly effective
1. Norvir (3 caps 3 times a day for adults) plus 2 other drugs like Zerit, Viread or Viramune and Epivir.
2. Hydrocortisone cream applied directly on the lesions daily.
3. Fiber/Pectin/Probiotic blend.
4. DNCB topical weekly applications - apply directly on the KS lesions.

 Note: Several persons using Norvir have reported complete remissions of KS, as well as lymphoma and without using any chemotherapy.

Alternating chemotherapy and immune-based therapies

If chemotherapy is used for KS, Lymphoma or any other form of cancer, it is imperative that the protocol to build the NK cells and the dietary recommendations also be used jointly. Otherwise, the KS, lymphoma or another cancer may quickly return. If they return aggressively enough, they can kill you. Chemotherapy usually works best when someone has a fairly intact immune system. **However, a pulsed therapy should be very effective. By this I mean 2 or 3 weeks of chemotherapy followed by 6 to 8 weeks of the protocols listed in this book.** Once the NK cells are increased to over 200 cells/UL, more chemotherapy should not be needed. Remember, Dr. Bihari has used Naltrexone, which triples NK counts, successfully to treat 3 cases of cancer of the pancreas. This treatment worked, because the restored NK activity eliminated the cancer naturally.

24

Prayers, Promises and Miracles

by Conrad LeBeau

A profound spiritual event occurred to me on June 13, 1956. I was living with my parents and brothers in a farmhouse in the Upper Peninsula of Michigan. I was 13 years old. It was about 8 pm in the evening. My parents and brothers had gone to bed. A thunderstorm that evening had passed over and was fading into the distance. Sometime earlier, a sliver had gotten into the upper eyelid of my left eye that caused severe pain and prevented me from going to sleep. With no one to help me remove the sliver, I began to pray. As a person with Catholic upbringing, I began to say the "Hail Mary." I sat in the living room and quietly prayed and sometimes dozed off to sleep, only to be awakened by the sharp stabbing pain in my left eye.

The praying went on, until I looked at a clock and realized that I had been praying for 2 hours. It was 10 p.m. Thinking that no one up there was hearing me, and being desperate for help, I stood up and said: "Mother of Jesus, help me!" Hardly had the words left my lips, when I felt a pair of fingers touch my left eyelid and the sliver pass through it into the thin air. At that moment, I was energized and wide-awake. For an instant, I was startled, speechless and felt as transparent as a glass of water. I felt the presence of the Virgin Mary standing in front of me, although I couldn't actually see her. I knew she had touched my eyelid and removed the sliver. I sensed that off to my left was an Angel who accompanied her. I said "Thank You" several times and finally went to sleep. For a long time, I told no one about the events of that summer evening.

I decided to share with you this experience I had in 1956, because it was so personal and so profound. In my lifetime, I have had prayers answered hundreds of times. However, none to date have equaled this unique experience of June 13, 1956. The event gave me great faith in the existence of God, Jesus and the Virgin Mary. I also learned that, with prayer, persistence is the key to having a prayer answered. It is even more important than belief that it will be answered.

In the past 2,000 years since the birth of Christ, Jesus and the Virgin Mary have appeared literally hundreds of times, if not thousands, to give messages to the world. The latest ongoing apparitions are in Medjugorje, Yugoslavia, where the Virgin Mary has been appearing daily to 6 children, since 1981. In her earlier visits, she asked for many prayers to prevent the civil war that later broke out in that nation. An uneasy truce between the three warring sides went into effect in Nov 1995. I have read that the Virgin Mary has promised that God would, at some unknown date in the future, leave a permanent sign in Medjugorje (www.medj.org or www.gospa.com) that the whole world would see. The bloody civil war has left over 200,000 people dead. When the Serbs fired mortar shells at the church built in honor of Our Lady of Medjugorje, the shells did not explode. One that did, twisted a cross several hundred feet away. Shortly after this, the Serbs became very ill and retreated.

Today, with the overthrow of Slobodan Milosovec, and the United Nations keeping the peace, the terrible atrocities and war in the Balkans is finally over. Unfortunately, in its place, war clouds now hang over the Middle East, while in Rome the Pope appeals for prayer and fasting to avert war. Millions march across the globe for peace.

The prayers and promises given to St Bridget
"I shall preserve and guard his 5 senses"

In August, 1993, a friend who had been to Medjugorje on a spiritual retreat, sent me a prayer book called "Pieta" that he had purchased there. The book is filled with many prayers and each set contains some unique promises given by Jesus to those who say these prayers daily. One prayer that especially interested me was a set of 15 prayers given to a Saint from Sweden in the 13th Century named Bridget. Of the 21 promises given to those who say these prayers daily, there is one special promise - No 13: "I shall preserve and guard his 5 senses." When I read this, I immediately thought of persons with Retinitis, who fear losing their eyesight or who have already lost their eyesight, due to this affliction. Assuming these prayers are for real, I thought, then anyone saying them can have their eyesight restored.

I said the prayers once in November 1993. Before I prayed, I asked God to show me a sign, if these prayers were for real. It took about 25 minutes, as the set includes not only the 15 prayers to St. Bridget, but also 15 "Our Fathers" and 15 "Hail Marys." When I was finished, I noticed the scent of fresh flowers in my room. In my apartment, there are no flowers and since I lived alone at that time, I knew no one had placed any deodorants there to create the scent. I knew the scent of the flowers was placed there by God to let me know that he will honor the promises he made to those who say these prayers.

In Dec., 1993, I read the 21 promises given to St. Bridget and found one that said: "He will obtain all he asks for from God and the Virgin Mary." However, to receive the blessings of the 21 promises requires saying the complete set of prayers daily for one year. What would happen, if someone said the prayers for one year and asked God to bring forth a cure for Cancer and AIDS? To prevent the outbreak of a Third World War? In the past year I found that my busy schedule prevented me from saying the complete set of prayers each day, so I would often say half of the set one day and the other half the next.

What is unknown about prayer is how long one has to pray to see results. Of the prayers given to St. Bridget, I only said them 4 times in 1993, once in November and three times in December. On both occasions, I am convinced God answered my prayers. The question we need to ask ourselves now is, "what do we want God to do for us when we say these prayers?" Are you a Hemophiliac, who wants his normal clotting factors restored to his blood? Are your underweight and want to gain weight? Do you want to be cured of cancer, Lyme disease or AIDS? Should we be so specific, or just ask God to bless our health? As a matter of faith, I am convinced that anyone who recites these prayers daily will experience a personal miracle in his or her life.

Another prayer in the "Pieta" book is a 1900 year-old prayer to St. Joseph, the Foster Father of Jesus. It has rarely been known to fail, if you say it once a day for 9 consecutive days. It takes about 40 seconds to say this prayer. In early August, I tried saying this prayer for a friend who had been unjustly imprisoned for failure to pay a civil forfeiture. His wife said the fine was so large that he would be in prison for 18 years, if he were unable to pay it. I told her I would ask St. Joseph to help. So I said the prayer daily. After 9 days, nothing happened, so I said it for another 9 days and still nothing happened. I then figured it was one of those rare times it would not be answered. Then I forgot about it, and 3 weeks later, I stopped by to visit Chris, his wife. As I approached the door, I could see Chris putting on her jacket, and she had a smile on her face. She said: I'm going to get Glenn - .he has just been released from prison." It was then I remembered the prayer to St. Joseph, and I said: "Thank you, St. Joseph." Chris smiled. She remembered what I had said earlier about saying this prayer.

It is significant that I learned of his release at the moment it was happening. It was St. Joseph's way of saying "I did not forget." Copies of the "Pieta" Prayer book are available from Keep Hope Alive.

"Miraculous Water" from San Damiano, Italy

Several years ago, I wrote about a healing water brought to the US from a well in San Damiano, located in north-central Italy. The well was dug at a location designated by the Virgin Mary, who first appeared to Mama Rosa Quattrini on September 29, 1961, the feast day of St Michael. In her first appearance, the Virgin Mary touched Mama Rosa and cured her instantly of an affliction - abdominal wounds that would not heal. Following this, Rosa Quattrini met with Padre Pio, who told her to return to San Damiano and await a great mission. A series of weekly visions began in October 16, 1964, with messages from Mary to the world that ended in 1981. Her first message to Rosa was:

"My little one, I come from far away. Announce to the world that all must pray, for Jesus can no longer carry the Cross.

I want all to be saved, the good and the bad. I am the Mother of Love, the Mother of all; you are all my children. That is why I want you all to be saved. That is why I have come: to bring the world to prayer because the chastisements are near.

"I will return each Friday and I will give you messages and you must make them known to the world."

Rosa replied: "But how will they believe me? I am only a poor ignorant peasant. I have no authority. They'll throw me in prison!"

The Madonna replied: "Do not fear, because now I will leave you a sign. You will see it, this tree will blossom."

On October 16th, 1964, Mary left a sign of her presence - the pear tree over which she appeared that was full of ripe fruit, then broke out in blossoms later that day. Photographs of the pear tree full of pears and blossoms at the same time were widely published in newspapers throughout Europe.

In 1966, in one of the apparitions, the Madonna directed a well to be dug at a specified location in a Rose garden in San Damiano. It was where a golden beam of light was seen that touched the ground during the apparition. Of the well, the Madonna said:

"Drink this water and have confidence in it. Many will be cured of physical diseases. Many will become holy. Bring the water to the sick and dying. Go often to visit the souls who are mourning. Do not fear, I am with you ...this is the hour when the well will give light. Come, draw the water and take it into your homes and you will receive infinite graces."

The San Damiano Center in Natick. MA

I spoke with Lisa Custodio, whose mother became a friend of the seer, Rosa Quattrini. Lisa's mother, Claire, brought the water and the Virgin's messages from San Damiano to the United States for 35 years until her death on August 10th, 2001. Today, Lisa continues the work of her late mother.

In February 2002, I returned a phone call to Lisa and she told me that many cancer patients had been cured using this water, and some AIDS patients said that they had been helped by the water. She could not, however, give me testimonial letters, without their permission. She said that since the mid 1960's, when she first accompanied her mother to San Damiano, there have been thousands of cures, too many to count. For me, miracles happen every day. Recently she stated she had mailed 5 cardboard boxes full of testimonial letters from persons who used the water to the Vatican. Lisa said she receives more than 200 phone calls a week from persons with incurable diseases and in need of the water.

According to Lisa, the Virgin Mary told Mama Rosa that the water is to be used throughout the whole world and given to the sick and the dying. The Virgin stated that as more water is drawn, more would flow from this well to serve the needs of all mankind. The site where this water is drawn is located in the middle of a tomato patch in north central Italy, in an area where St. Francis of Assisi lived centuries ago.

According to instructions in a book written about the water and the apparitions, only a couple of drops are needed, when used with prayer. Lisa told me of a lady from New York whose daughter had several small brain tumors and was receiving radiation treatments. The lady was in church, and another parishioner saw her crying on a Sunday morning in January 2002. She approached the women in tears and asked her what was wrong. When the lady told her that her daughter had brain cancer, the parishioner said "I think I have something that will help you," and she gave the lady a small bottle of San Damiano water.

According to Lisa, the lady told her that she said a few prayers that accompanied the water and poured some on her daughter's forehead that same Sunday evening. Immediately, the daughter screamed to stop, saying that it was burning her head. Within a few moments, this sensation stopped.

The following morning the lady took her daughter to the hospital for her 7th radiation treatment and the Oncologist ordered new X-rays. When he looked at the x-rays, he said he had been brought the wrong x-rays that belonged to someone else. The nurse told him they were the right x-rays. The doctor then stated that he could not find any tumors on the x-ray. The lady then told the doctor about the water she had used from San Damiano, and the doctor said that this was possibly a miracle, since it is not explainable by modern science.

Lisa told me of another case about a lady whose husband had colon cancer and he had been bleeding daily for 2 months. She received a bottle of the water the day before her husband was scheduled for surgery for a colostomy. She gave him the bottle and he drank a capful and said the prayers. Immediately, the bleeding stopped.

The following morning he went in for the surgery as scheduled. The doctor took x-rays to examine him before the surgery. When the doctor read the x-rays, he could find no trace of the cancer; it had simply vanished overnight. The operation was cancelled.

For more info, write to JMJ San Damiano CTR, PO Box 94, Natick, MA 01760

Miraculous healing water - Jack Fristoe's Experience

CA: 8/13/02: Jack called to tell me about his experiences with the Miraculous Water that had arrived Aug 9th. He used two capfuls daily with the accompanying prayers,. He placed some of the water on the tumor on his right leg that was painful and the size of a silver dollar. "In 4 days, it has shrunk to a half-dollar size and the pain is now mostly gone." Before Aug 9th, he stated he would wake up several times each night to urinate. Now, he sleeps through the night without waking up.

August 23rd: Jack called to tell me that the tumor on his leg has now shrunk to the size of a quarter. He said his overall health continues to improve. August 30th update: Jack called to tell me the tumor is down to the size of a dime. He said: "The water is miraculous .I feel more energy than I have had in a long time…. my colon health has improved too."

In her visitations to the poor uneducated peasant, Rosa Quattrini, in the 1960's, the Virgin Mary said that the Eternal Father has made the water available for everyone for all generations. A golden ray of light was seen to pierce the ground and marked the spot where the well was to be dug. The water is available to help persons of all denominations, of any race, ethnic group or religion, including atheists, non-believers and the worst of sinners.

Jack Fristoe belongs to a non-denominational church. He is 73 years old. He told me that, when he first used the water, it caused a detox effect and gave him diarrhea for a few days. He said he uses only about 3 drops a day along with the 2 sets of prayers in the instructions. By late September, Jack said the tumor had shrunk to the size of a dime and no longer bothered him. Jack said he had used the water sometimes without saying the prayers, but that the water was slower in providing pain relief. He said the water provided faster results when the prayers are used with it.

In October 2002, Susan A of Virginia phoned and told me that for 3 days she had a severe pain in the back of her neck that would not go away. She had a bottle of the water I had sent her, but had not used it. Finally, she was desperate, and took 3 drops under her tongue and then knelt on the floor to pray. When she stood up the pain was gone. She said she was speechless and the pain has not returned.

In November, 2002, a local resident in West Allis, WI, Paul Mandela, whose wife had breast surgery a year earlier for breast cancer, had the reoccurrence of lumps in her chest area that had been recently diagnosed as "atypical," or not normal cells. Concerned that the lumps were cancerous, the doctor recommended immediate surgery. For 3 weeks prior to the operation, Paul's wife sprinkled one drop of the Miraculous Water on each side of her chest and took a few drops under her tongue. She said the 4 prayers once each day. When the operation was completed three weeks later, the doctor had the lumps removed and examined in a lab. In December, 2002, the doctor told Paul the lumps removed in surgery had tested normal and that he could not explain why they had changed in the previous 3 weeks.

Locally, David G, who suffers from depression and severe headaches, said that after using the Miraculous Water with the prayers, that both the headache and the depression left instantly.

Once this past fall, I had developed ringing in both ears that was quite severe. I placed a few drops of Miraculous Water in each ear and said the 4 prayers. The ringing instantly stopped and has not returned.

We have located the Internet site for the San Damiano apparitions, where the well is located. The site is called City of the Roses, the name of a future spiritual and physical healing center that is to be built. It is http://www.cittadellerose.it/. If you are going to Italy, this site has a series of maps that give the exact location of San Damiano di Piacenza. On the home page, click the arrow to the right of the word "home" at the bottom of the page, to bring up the 4 maps. If you are planning a trip there, please contact me. I would appreciate hearing from you.

In August, 2002, I called the City of the Roses in San Damiano, Italy, to see if anyone there would ship some water to us. I also had written to them a week earlier. A member of the clergy answered the phone and spoke Italian. I talked to him in English, and neither of us could understand a word of what the other was saying.

A few days later, a reader in England, who speaks both English and Italian, called the City of the Roses center for me. She found out that they do not ship water out to anyone, because, if they did this for one person, they would have to do it for everyone. The water is free at the well and can be drawn any day of the week. They are concerned that someone might tamper with the water while it is enroute. You would think that someone in the area would draw the water and offer to ship it out for a fee. A search on Google finds no such place exists, at least not on the Internet.

Update: August 2004: Persistence and prayer pays off. After 2 years and countless hours of searching, *and I mean countless hours*, I have finally located a contact in San Damiano, Italy, where a member of a local religous order, who resides a short distance from where the well is located, has shipped us Miraculous Water. This is truely a great gift from God above. Unfortunately, the Miraculous Water remains known to but a few and is so underappreciated. One day this will change and the world will beat a path to San Damiano.

Lourdes Water

Boston MA. The Marist Fathers distribute a monthly newsletter called *"Echoes from Lourdes."* The newsletter reports on the experiences of persons whose association with Lourdes has changed their life beginning with the very first written account by St Bernadette who was visited by the Virgin Mary several times beginning on February 11th, 1858. The Marist Fathers distribute Lourdes Water to their readers and publish reports of their experiences using the water. Here are a few of what is half a dozen or more letters received monthly and published in *Echoes from Lourdes* (Volume 50, No 2 and No 7)

KY. *"My eye doctor was watching me for glaucoma in my eyes for a year and a half. I started using Lourdes Water in each eye every night at bed time six months ago, and now the pressure is down in both eyes and there is no sign of glaucoma. The doctor says my eyes look great. I am so grateful to Jesus and His Mother for this healing!"* AC.

NJ " *"I just want to say thank you to Our Lady of Lourdes and her intercession for me to the Sacred Heart of Jesus. I had a small cyst on my eye lid that grew and became itchy, so my eye doctor worked on it and said I would need minor surgery. He gave me antibiotics and asked my to come back in a month for the surgery. I went home and started applying Lourdes Water on my eye lid everyday. Within one week, the cyst fell off! The doctor said most of the time something is left there but it looks so good that I do not need surgery. I am very grateful to the lady of Lourdes and her intercession...."* C.W.

July 2004., a resident of California writes:

"This is a gift for a special favor received. I have been using Our Lady's Lourdes Water since 1958 when I had cancer, and thank Our Lord and Our Blessed Mother for so many blessings and thank you so much for the Lourdes Center." M.D.

The monthly newsletter that I have been receiving contains many reports from readers of cancer remission and help from the water and from prayers for all kinds of health-related problems, even in situations where hope for recovery was almost nil. For a sample copy of the newsletter, write to Lourdes Center, Marist Fathers, 698 Beacon St, Boston MA 02215.

At Keep Hope Alive, we now have available the healing waters from the Grotto at Lourdes, France, as well as from the Rose Garden in San Damiano, Italy.

APPENDIX

NutraSweet blamed for vision loss, brain damage and insomnia. One death reported.

April 16, 1995: "I had used Equal NutraSweet with Aspartame for 4 years with no idea that it's poisonous, as I assumed that FDA approval means it's perfectly safe to use. I used about 12 paks of Equal in hot coffee each day.

"The first symptoms were depression and vertigo, but I didn't connect them with Equal. My legs cramped constantly and pained at night, and I had insomnia, terrible nightmares and memory loss. My vision deteriorated, until I expected to go blind, but my eye doctor couldn't explain why. My life became a nightmare. I turned to prayer.

It worked! I received a "Nutrasweet is a Neurotoxin" flyer, listing all my symptoms, so I abandoned aspartame in any form. My vision returned, the cramps disappeared and vertigo vanished. It was a miracle because I thought I was dying."

Often the "Experts" are publicity mills, funded by the pirates that make the stuff. It's like asking the Mafia about the crime rate. Both the American Dietetics and American Diabetic Associations get big bucks from NutraSweet. Such organizations propagandize physicians on how safe it is, so doctors are often unaware of the danger."

Gloria Collins, 234B Dunwoody Crossing, Dunwoody, GA 30338.

Chicago Sun Times, 10/17/86: Dr. H.J. Roberts of West Palm Bch, Fl, said that methyl alcohol is a component of Aspartame and is responsible for vision damage. Under certain storage conditions, the sweetener breaks down in part and methyl alcohol is a byproduct. Of 360 patients he has diagnosed as having aspartame-related problems, Roberts said, "about one-fourth had decreased vision or blindness, nearly half had severe headaches and substantial numbers had epileptic seizures, confusion, memory loss and depression." Roberts added that methyl alcohol, in heavy users of Aspartame, is the same as in drinkers of moonshine in Prohibition days: They go blind."

Betty Martini reports that symptoms of Aspartame poisoning mimics Multiple Sclerosis and that "many patients have had their diseases reversed, even blindness, after discontinuing aspartame."

An extensive newsletter, documenting from several sources over 24 symptoms linked to the use of Aspartame, is available from MISSION POSSIBLE, PO Box 28098, Atlanta, GA 30358.

The newsletter reports the death of Joyce Wilson of Stockbridge, GA from Aspartame poisoning. Aspartame is manufactured by Monsanto Corporation, the same corporation that sells the hormone, BGH, to farmers to increase milk production. Betty Martini reports that Monsanto funds the American Diabetic Assn., which endorses the use of Equal/Nutrasweet/Aspartame for their members. Mission Possible recommends the use of the herb "Stevia," as a sugar-free natural sweetener. It is sold in health food stores. No adverse effects have been reported.

Dangerous herbal combination - Ma Huang and Kola Nut

Mrs. Ricardo Wilson, whose husband is a medical doctor in Los Angeles, told Keep Hope Alive that a neighbor friend developed heart damage after using a "pep" pill containing a combination of Ma Huang and Kola Nut. His heart was fine before he used the herbal formula, she told me. Recently the FDA has been doing a critical study of adverse reactions to Ma Huang, an herbal supplement sold in some health food stores. Mrs. Wilson can be reached at 213-876-6820.

Yohimbe causes dangerous high blood pressure

Yohimbe, an herb used to help men get penile erections, may elevate blood pressure to levels so dangerous as to precipitate a fatal heart attack. One source, which asked to remain anonymous, told Keep Hope Alive, that Yohimbe had caused heart attacks in 10 people, 3 few of which were fatal. Aside from this report, which I could not confirm, I talked to a local person I know, who took up to 6 Yohimbe tablets in one day and developed severe chest pains. His blood pressure was so high he should have been admitted to the Emergency room. Fortunately, he stopped taking Yohimbe after I warned him the herb was dangerous enough to kill him if he continued to use it.

A much safer love potion is wheat germ oil, vitamin E and Ginseng.

Patient dies from shock after "live cell" therapy

San Diego, CA: Jay reported that his former lover died from anaphylactic shock four hours after receiving injections of "live cell" therapy at a clinic in Mexico. Live cell therapy usually comes from live animal embryonic or fetal tissues. The clinic in Mexico had no antidote to turn off the life threatening allergic reaction known as "anaphylactic shock." There is always a danger involved in injection of foreign proteins directly into the blood.

Monthly magazines and publications

1. National CFIDS Foundation, 103 Aletha Rd, Needham, MA 02492. Write for sample newsletter Include $3.00 for sample copy. 781-449-3535.
2. SEARCHLIGHT, a publication of Search Alliance. Subscription - $25.00 annually. Free sample copy. Search Alliance, 7461 Beverly Blvd, Suite 304, Los Angeles, CA 90036
3. GMHC Newsletter is a monthly publication. It focuses on experimental AIDS therapies. Provides technical information valuable to medical professionals. Subscriptions are $20 per year. Write: GMHC, Dept of Medical Information, 129 West 20th St., NY, NY 10011. Additional contacts, resources and links can be found on our website at keephopealive.org.

Manufacturers and Sources of supplements

Sources of products are listed throughout the book, usually at the end of the article about the subject discussed. However, phone numbers, websites and addresses and suppliers continue to change over time. If you obtained this book after 2004, you may want to write for an updated list of manufacturers of products mentioned in this book. Write to Keep Hope Alive, PO Box 270041, West Allis, WI 53227 with your request.

Request Form

___Send me _____ copies of Immune Restoration Handbook 2nd Edition at $19.95 ea. Six or more copies are $11.97 ea. Add $2.00 per order for Parcel Post or $4.00 per order for Priority mail.

___Place me on your mailing list to receive future issues of the Journal of Immunity.

___Enclosed is a donation. ____I am financially indigent. Send me a free subscription.

___Send a free sample copy of your latest newsletter.

___Send _____ copies of the latest issue of Journal of Immunity for free distribution to clients or persons in a local support group.

___Send me a list of local Physicians who have purchased this book that I may contact.

___Send an updated list of manufacturers of products mentioned in this book.

___Send me a copy of the Pieta Prayer book. ___English or___ Spanish edition.

Send ___ bottles of the Miraculous Water with built-in dropper dispenser (2 ozs ea) or send ___ bottles of Lourdes Water (2 ozs ea). Suggested donation is $4 per bottle for either Lourdes or Miraculous Water. Add $3 per order for postage.

___Total enclosed is a donation for _____ (check/MO/credit card)

Credit Card No (MC/Visa/Dis/Amx)_____

Exp_____

Name_____

_____

Address_____Suite/Apt _____

City_____State_____Zip_____

Ph. No. _____

Send to - Keep Hope Alive, PO Box 270041, West Allis, WI 53227

Keep Hope Alive interactive: Stay informed of the latest developments and research by visiting our website at www.keephopealive.org.
Ten years of research online – Search Box, Message Board, articles and links. Enjoy!
Phone 414-545-6539 (to leave a message)   Fax - 414-329-0653

Note: if you are financially indigent, you may write for instructions on how to obtain a free copy of the Immune Restoration Handbook or have a copy donated to your local library.

Thank you for your support.

Index

A

Abha Light Foundation.........................129
Acrylamides and Cancer......................127
Adrenal and Thyroid Tests................80
Adrenal exhaustion.........................60, 65
AIDS Research Alliance........................44
Albion selium adverse effects................30
Allergies..125,
Allergies..238
Aloe vera leaf drink...........................127
Alternative treatments for HIV..............149
Alzheimers..................................246
American Cancer Society....................262
Anergy..3
Anthrax......................................239
Antigen presentation.......................9
Antioxidants.....................................103
APPENDIX......................................282
Appetite stimulants......................239
Armour Thyroid..................................82
Artemesia anua................................144
Aspartame......................................282
Athlete's foot..............................239

B

B Vitamins.......................................213
Bernard Bihari, MD...........................154
Beta 1, 3 Glucan..............................168
Beta 2 micro-globulin..........................51
Beta Carotene...........................172, 213
Beta-glucuronidase............................101
Beta-Mannan...................................271
BHT...101
Bio-oxidative Therapies.....................197
Bitter melon Enemas.........................135
Black Cohosh inhibits HIV and Cancer..194
Bob Becks machine...........................147
Body temperature (low)........................51
Bone Mineral Density.........................193
Breast Cancer..................................273
Butyrate deficiency and intestines........122

C

Calcium..217
Cancell...147
Cancer and IL-6............................264
Cancer symptoms.........................263
Cancer Therapy by John Boik..............270
Cancer Treatment Centers of America...268
Cancer's Seven Warning Signs........264
Candidiasis.................................240
Candidiasis and HHV-6........................42
Candidiasis, Cure for............................31

Carnivora..144
Castor oil capsules............................116
Castor oil packs................................113
Cayenne...149
CD8 CTL's......................................152
Cell-mediated immunity.........................2
CFIDS CD4/CD8 ratios......................177
Chemotherapy..................................275
Chest Pains.................................240
Chocolate and herpes..........................38
Cholesterol level..........................241
Chronic dry cough:........................242
Chronic Fatigue Syndrome..................174
Circulating immune complexes.............128
Clogged Arteries..........................240
CMV..244
Coconut oil......................................139
Cod Liver Oil....................................213
Coffee retention enemas....................107
Colds (head and sinus):.................242
Colloidal Silver.................................142
Colostrum Specific.......................243
Complementary therapies...................129
Conrad LeBeau.................................275
Copper...218
Cortisol deficiency...............................60
Cortisol precursors (natural).................73
Cortisol reduces IL-6...........................62
Cortisol treats Cancer..........................71
Crohn's disease:...........................242
Cryptosporidiosis.........................243
Cultured cabbage juice......................126
Curcumin..138
Cytomegalovirus..........................244

D

DCH skin reaction...............................48
Death from "live cell" therapy.............284
Dementia...................................246
Depression.................................246
DHEA.......................................64, 172
Diagnostic Tests.................................48
Diarrhea....................................246
Didi Ananda Rucira............................131
DiNitroChloroBenzene........................164
DNCB...164
Donald Carrow.................................169
Dr Brownstein...............................86
Dr. McGarey....................................115
Dr. Patricia Salvato's Regimen for CFS...181
Dry skin.....................................247

E

Echoes from Lourdes 281
EDGAR CAYCE 115
EDTA chelation 108
Elderberry 103
Emergency Procedures 237
Epstein barr virus: 247
Essiac Tea 133
Estradiol 94
Estrogen 70, 93
Eye strain 247

F

Fatigue 247
Fatigue-inducing cytokines 60
Fever 248
Fiber/pectin/probiotic blend 13
Fibromyalgia 174
Fish Oil 72
Food Allergy test 222
Foods that Heal 231
foreign antigen 9
Fred Walters 191
Free radical scavengers 100
Free radicals 98
Friendly flora 109

G

Gallo, Robert 38
Garlic 111
Garlic increases NK function 135
Gas (lower - flatulence) 249
Gas (upper) 248
Gerson cancer treatment 268
Glucaric acid 101
Glutathione 152
GOOT 111
GOOT recipe 261
Grapefruit seed extract 145
Grass-fed beef 96
Great Smoky Diagnostics 125
Green Coffee Beans 138
Guaifenesin for Fibromyalgia 183
Guaifenesin for sinus infections .. 243

H

H2O2 accidental ingestion 209
HAART and beyond 192
Heavy metals 108
Hemoglobin 249
Hepatitis 152, 249
Hepatitis C 15
Herbal cocktail for HIV 137
Herpes 250

HHV-6 37
HHV-6 and HIV 37
HHV-6A and CFIDS 40
HHV-6A, treatments for 180
Histamines 251
HIV Drug book 193
HIV in the Gut 45
Holy Basil 195
HPA Axis 61
HPV 260
Hulda Clark 143
Human Papilloma Virus 251
Humoral immunity 2
Hydrogen Peroxide 207
HYDROZONE AND GLYCOZONE 205
Hyssop 138

I

IBOM 204
IgA blocks HIV 44
IgA for Mucosal Immunity 5
IgE linked to allergies 5
Immune enhancement diet 222
Immune factors and Cancer 264
immune profiles 119
Immune-based therapies 151
Immune-based therapies for cancer 268
ImmunePro 211
Indigestion 251
Insomnia 252
Interleuken-6 48
Interleukin-6 Test 71
Inteulukin-6 61
Iodine 218
Iodine deficiency 85
IP6 163
Iron 218

J

Jaw TMJ 253
Journal of Immunity 284

K

Kaposi Sarcoma 273
Kombucha tea 112

L

Leaky gut 122
Leaky gut syndrome 4, 124
Lemon/olive oil drink 105
L-Glutathione 8
Licorice 195
Limewater 59
Lipodystrophy 253

Longevity Science..................................172
Lourdes Water......................................281
Low Body Temperature.........................85
Hydrocortisone for Wasting Syndrome....210
L-Selenomethionine................................25
Lyme disease......................................253
Lymph nodes (swollen)......................253

M

Ma Huang and Kola Nut......................283
MAC/MAI..254
Magnesium...219
Magnetic fields.....................................147
Magnets...147
Maitake mushrooms...........................274
Major Autohemotherapy.......................205
Mama Rosa Quattrini............................278
Manganese...219
Manganese inhibits HIV........................133
Mary Enig Ph.D.....................................139
Medjugorje...276
Melatonin...83
Meningitis...254
Mercury, lead...91
Methionine-enkephalin.........................160
Metyrapone..76
Microsporidium..................................254
Miraculous Water.................................277
Mitochondria.......................................87
Molluscum...254
Monolaurin...140
Morphine / Codeine..............................161
Mouth sores.......................................254
Mucosal immunity....................................4

N

Naltrexone..154
Naltrexone treats pancreatic cancer.......159
Naltrexone triples NK cells...................159
Natural Hormones................................83
Natural Killer (NK) cells........................152
Natural Killer Cell Function Test.............48
Natural Killer cells..................................11
Nausea...254
Neem for HIV..129
Neuropathy..254
Night sweats.....................................255
NNRTs..187
Norvir...187
Nucleosides...187

O

Ojibwa te....................................89, 133
Oleuropein...141
Olive leaf...141

Osteoporosis.......................................193
Osteoporosis and HIV Meds.................195
Ozonated Olive oil................................143
Ozone..99, 198
Ozone insufflation................................203
Ozone stops CMV and hepatitis...........199

P

Pancreatitis..255
PCP..256
Pectin...112
pH..53
pH and cancer..55
pH tendencies..55
Pharmaceutical drugs for HIV/AIDS......185
Phytoestrogens......................................93
Phytosel - natural selenium..................26
Pieta Prayer book.................................285
Plant sterols...73
Platelet count (low)............................255
Plechners Protocol.................................77
Plechner's theories................................70
Pneumonia...256
Pork and HHV-6.....................................37
Prayers, Promises and Miracles...........275
Proboost..172
Project Inform......................................193
Prostate Cancer - PC-Hope..................272
Protease Inhibitors...............................186
Prunella vulgaris..................................137
Pruritus, Folliculitis and Psoriasis......257
PSA..272
Pycnogenol..100

R

Ralph Moss, PhD..................................271
Red blood cells - low.........................257
Red Clover...194
Red Sage Root.....................................138
Rife technology....................................146
Royal Jelly...73

S

S.O.D...99
Saliva pH...58
Salt - adverse effects...............................6
San Damiano Center in Natick. MA.......278
San Damiano, Italy...............................277
SARS...257
Sauna bag - for Ozone therapy............204
Scar tissue (from radiation, burns).....257
SEES-2000...256

U

Urine therapy / enema...........................73